Integrated Cardiopulmonary Pharmacology

INTEGRATED CARDIOPULMONARY PHARMACOLOGY

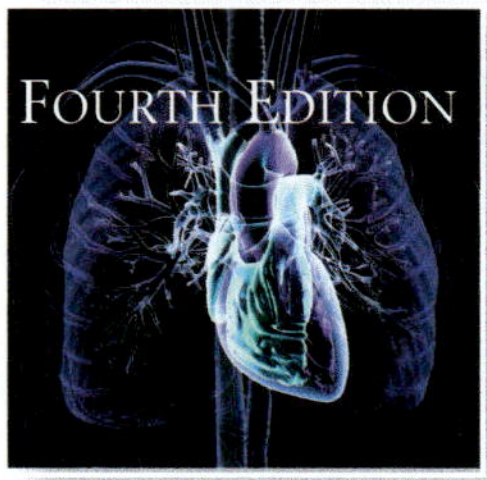

BRUCE J. COLBERT, MS, RRT
Director of Allied Health
Associate Professor
University of Pittsburgh at Johnstown

LUIS S. GONZALEZ III, PharmD, BCPS
Director, Pharmacy Practice Residency Program
Manager, Clinical Pharmacy Services
Conemaugh Memorial Medical Center
Johnstown, PA

BVT Publishing
Better textbooks, better prices
www.BVTPublishing.com

Publisher and Director of Business Development: Richard Schofield
Business Development and Ancillary Manager: Shannon Conley
Higher Education Editor: Nate Shankles
Graphic Designer/Typesetter: Esther Scannell
Typesetting Manager: Rhonda Minnema
Managing Editor: Anne Schofield
Pre-production Manager: Suzanne Schmidt
Production and Fulfillment Manager: Janai Bryand
Proofreader: Tara Joffe
Permissions Coordinator: Logan McDonald

Photo Credits: On the front cover and repeated throughout the book, Getty Images (Hank Grebe)

Some ancillaries, including electronic and print components, may not be available to customers outside the United States.

Loose-Leaf ISBN: 978-1-62751-617-4

Soft Cover ISBN: 978-1-62751-618-1

TEXTBOOK[Plus] (Loose-Leaf Bundle) ISBN: 978-1-62751-619-8

Dedications

In memory of my parents, Robert and Josephine Colbert, who taught me the importance of family and education, and to my loving wife, Patty, and two great children, Joshua and Jeremy, who continue to teach me its importance.

—Bruce J. Colbert

In memory of my father, Luis Gonzalez Jr., who taught me the value of hard work, and to my mother, my wife Stephanie, Stephen, Christopher, and Luke for their love and support.

—Luis Gonzalez III

About the Authors

Bruce Colbert is Clinical Associate Professor and Director of the Allied Health Department of the University of Pittsburgh at Johnstown. He has authored ten books, developed an interactive worktext and DVD program on student success, and given over 300 invited lectures and workshops at both the regional and national level. Many of his workshops are with educational programs on improving teaching effectiveness by utilizing active teaching and learning techniques to make the medical sciences relevant to today's students. Bruce is most proud of his volunteer work with wounded veterans, helping them to successfully transition into the workplace.

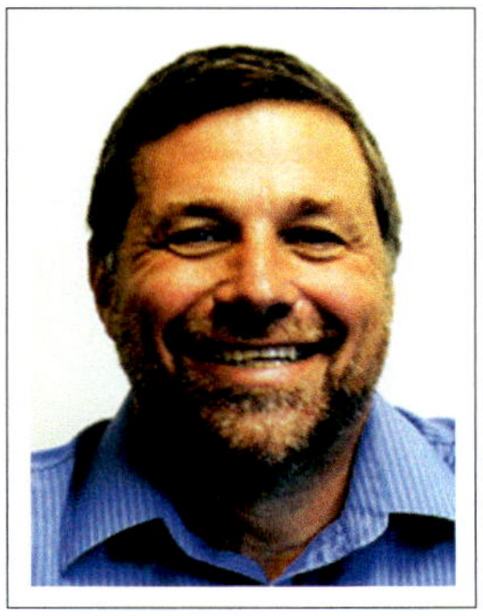

Dr. Luis S. Gonzalez III is an Associate Program Director in the Department of Internal Medicine Residency Program at Conemaugh Memorial Medical Center, where he also serves as the Clinical Coordinator for Pharmacy Services and directs a Pharmacy Residency Program. He is a Clinical Associate Professor for the Schools of Pharmacy at the University of Pittsburgh, Duquesne University, and Ohio Northern University. He has authored numerous peer-reviewed publications and has presented at regional and national conferences. Dr. Gonzalez was one of the original founders of the Johnstown Free Medical Clinic.

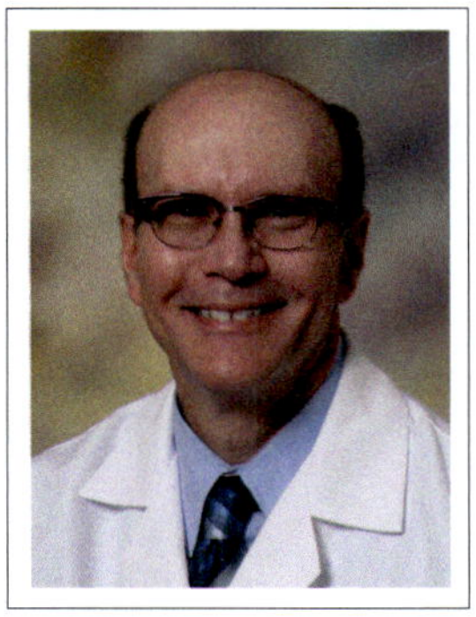

Contents

Foreword

Pharmacology is often perceived as one of the more difficult subjects in a medical curriculum. There are several possible explanations for this. First there are the difficult concepts and terms that are inherent to this subject. Second there is the massive amount of information that must be covered, which is often presented in a dry and highly technical manner. Finally this is a constantly evolving field of new breakthroughs, drugs, and delivery devices. We took all of these factors into account as we developed and pilot-tested this innovative project. So what makes this book unique and able to address these concerns?

First and foremost this truly is an *integrated* project—this is not just a buzzword thrown into the title. The authors and publisher took very seriously the integrated aspect of this project and sought the interdisciplinary perspective offered by both pharmacists and respiratory therapists. The end result is a book that fully integrates both anatomy and physiology concepts and pathophysiology concepts in relationship to pharmacology and heavily integrates clinical practice and application in all the related therapeutic drug classifications. Moreover, it is integrated in the way the book is set up. Part One covers overall pharmacological principles, dosage calculations, the autonomic nervous system, and medication aerosol therapy to lay the groundwork for the specific drug categories found in Part Two (bronchodilators, mucokinetics, surfactants, anti-inflammatory, anti-asthmatics, anti-infective, cardiac, neuromuscular, and therapeutic gases). Part Three then integrates and "puts it all together" to show the integrated approach to the management of COPD, asthma, infectious respiratory disease, and advanced cardiac life support. All of this integrated material was then incorporated into the text in a style that does not distance the student from the material; the authors took very seriously the concept of writing and strove to encourage learning and relating the material, rather than massive memorization.

Finally there are some things we did not take so seriously. While we were serious about the contents, relevancy, and accuracy of the material, we also had fun writing, researching, and collaborating on this project. We utilized splashes of humor in this textbook, with the underlying idea that what is learned with humor is not readily forgotten. In addition we used a conversational writing style, rich with analogies, to make the learning experience comfortable and relatable. In other words we wrote it for the students and not to impress our colleagues.

ACKNOWLEDGMENTS

The fourth edition of this text has an interesting backstory. After publishing the first three editions, Pearson Publications discontinued their line of respiratory textbooks. As authors, we were gratified by the success of the first three editions and were eager to find a new publisher for the fourth edition. We were very fortunate to find BVT Publishing, whose philosophy of publishing high-quality yet affordable textbooks geared toward the students matched our own.

Pearson deserves a great deal of credit and thanks for their professional help in making this transition a smooth one. We would also like to thank the BVT Publishing team, including Nate Shankles and Richard Schofield, for their professionalism and enthusiastic support of this textbook; our copy editor Anne Schofield; and Shannon Conley and her production team, who helped pull everything together to create this fourth edition. The authors also wish to thank Esther Scannell for her creative design work and Tara Joffe for her thorough proofreading. Bruce Colbert wants to personally thank the University of Pittsburgh at Johnstown's Respiratory Care classes, which continue to give input into the concept of this project and keep the vision student friendly.

Preface

New to This Edition

Working with BVT has given us the exciting challenge of redesigning the book to make it even more user friendly. We were also able to enhance the text with BVTLab®, which further supports instructors and students alike. All materials have been updated with a special focus on the latest available approved drugs in all therapeutic classifications. These updates include the following:

- Updated asthma and COPD information with the latest assessment and treatment guidelines
- Updated therapeutic drug categories
- New tables that concisely present drug categories, dosages, and special considerations
- A new book design and new illustrations and photos enhancing presentation and facilitating visual learning

But it is also very important to note what we did not change: We strove to maintain the same user-friendly writing style that has been well received in the first three editions and to keep the rich use of analogies that has helped students to truly learn the material—rather than requiring them to rely on massive short-term memorization.

Pedagogical Features

Our goal is to continue to produce a truly introductory and interactive pharmacology text that students can connect with and use to learn pharmacology. Several features have been incorporated into the textbook to help accomplish that goal; they include the following:

Learning Hints and Controversies

These special features in each chapter ensure understanding of difficult concepts and stimulate further thought.

Clinical Pearls

Clinical pearls are also interspersed throughout the chapters to connect the knowledge and show the relevancy of learning the material. In addition numerous clinical applications are presented to provide a real-world connection.

Patient and Family Education

Each chapter has a special box that discusses important education issues for both the patient and family.

Life Span Considerations

These boxes discuss issues that may affect the pediatric and geriatric populations pertaining to the concept or drug category being reviewed.

Key Terms

Key terms are boldfaced and included in the glossary. Symbols, units, and abbreviations of medical terms are defined in the chapter opener for easy reference.

Review Questions

Periodic "Time for Review" problems within each chapter help to ensure concept understanding before a student moves on to the next topic. Comprehensive questions—which build from multiple-choice and matching questions to higher-level critical thinking and case-study questions—are also included at the end of the chapter.

BVT*Lab*®

BVT*Lab* provides two areas of support for instructors and students. The Student Study Center includes resources such as eBooks, study guides, practice quizzes, flashcards, chapter summaries, multimedia content and so on, and the Online Classroom incorporates grade book, discussion forums and delivery of online assignments, quizzes, and exams.

Supplements and Resources

Instructor's Supplements

A complete teaching package is available for instructors who adopt this book. This package includes an online lab, instructor's manual, test bank, course management software, and PowerPoint® slides.

BVT*Lab*	An online lab is available for this textbook at www.BVTLab.com, as described in the BVT*Lab* section below.
Instructor's Manual	The instructor's manual helps first-time instructors develop the course and offers seasoned instructors a new perspective on the material. Each section of the instructor's manual coincides with a chapter in the textbook. The user-friendly format starts with chapter summaries, learning objectives, key terms, and detailed outlines for each chapter. Then the manual presents sample answers to chapter review questions and case studies, lecture suggestions, and classroom activities. Lastly, additional resources—books, articles, websites—are listed to help instructors review the materials covered in each chapter.
Test Bank	An extensive test bank is available to instructors in both hard copy and electronic formats. Each chapter has 50 multiple choice, 25 true or false, 10 short answer, and 5 essay questions. Each question is ranked by difficulty and style and referenced to the appropriate section of the text to make test creation quick and easy.
Course Management Software	BVT's course management software, Respondus, allows for the creation of tests and quizzes that can be downloaded directly into a wide variety of course management environments such as Blackboard, WebCT, Desire2Learn, ANGEL, E-Learning, eCollege, Canvas, Moodle, and others.
PowerPoint Slides	A set of PowerPoint® slides is available for each chapter and contains slides for the chapter overview, learning objectives, chapter outline, key topics, and summary and conclusion.

Student Resources

Student resources are available for this textbook at www.BVTLab.com. These resources are geared toward students needing additional assistance, as well as those seeking complete mastery of the content. The following resources are available:

Practice Questions	Students can work through hundreds of practice questions online. Questions are multiple choice, true/false, or short answer in format and are graded instantly for immediate feedback.
Flashcards	BVT*Lab* includes sets of flashcards that reinforce the key terms and concepts from each chapter.
Chapter Summaries	A convenient and concise chapter summary is available as a study aid.
PowerPoint Slides	All instructor PowerPoints are available for convenient lecture preparation and for students to view online for a study recap.

support@bvtpublishing.com
Subject Line: Lab Account Request

...structors and their students. It includes ... and chat room, a homework grading ... and exams, and a host of student study ...

	...uitive interface that allows instructors to ...d grade books, and to replicate them from ...r to semester.
	...udents register for the grade book, which ...ds all homework, quizzes, and tests.
	... threads to a class forum and then monitor ...
...esources	...xtbook are available in BVT*Lab* in digital form.
eBook	Students who have purchased a product that includes an eBook can download the eBook from a link in the lab. A web-based eBook is also available within the lab for easy reference during online classes, homework, and study sessions.

Customization

BVT's Custom Publishing Division can help you modify this book's content to satisfy your specific instructional needs. The following are examples of customization:

- Rearrangement of chapters to follow the order of your syllabus
- Deletion of chapters not covered in your course
- Addition of paragraphs, sections, or chapters you or your colleagues have written for this course
- Editing of the existing content, down to the word level
- Customization of the accompanying student resources and online lab
- Addition of handouts, lecture notes, syllabus, etc.
- Incorporation of student worksheets into the textbook

All of these customizations will be professionally typeset to produce a seamless textbook of the highest quality, with an updated table of contents and index to reflect the customized content.

Third Edition Reviewers

Laura H. Beveridge, MEd, RRT
Medical College of Georgia
Augusta, Georgia

Megan C. Dixon, BS, RRT, AE-C
Ferris State University
Big Rapids, Michigan

Virginia Forster, RRT
Community College of Baltimore County
Baltimore, Maryland

Idichandi Idicula, MS, RRT, CPFT
El Centro College
Dallas, Texas

Tammy Kurszewski, MEd, RRT
Midwestern State University
Wichita Falls, Texas

Harley R. Metcalfe, BS, RRT
Johnson County Community College
Overland Park, Kansas

Brian Parker, MPH, RRT-NPS, RPFT, AE-C
Baptist College of Health Sciences
Memphis, Tennessee

Marty D. Partida, MHSM, RRT-NPS
Tyler Junior College
Tyler, Texas

Christopher Rowse, MS, RRT-NPS, RPFT, RPSGT
Northern Essex Community College
Lawrence, Massachusetts

Dustin Spencer, PharmD, BCPS
Clarian Health & Affiliated Universities
Indianapolis, Indiana

George A. Steer, PhD, RRT
Jefferson College of Health Sciences
Roanoke, Virginia

Robert Tralongo, MBA, RT, RRT-NPS, CPFT, AE-C
Molloy College
Rockville Centre, New York

Rita Waller, BS, BSN, MSN
Augusta Technical College
Augusta, Georgia

James R. Woods, MS, RRT, RPFT
Florida State College at Jacksonville
Jacksonville, Florida

Previous Edition Reviewers

Kathleen M. Boyle, MEd, NS, RRT-NPS
Southeast Arkansas College
Pine Bluff, Arkansas

Phyllis W. Brunner, BS, RRT, CPFT
Tyler Junior College
Tyler, Texas

Lynn Walter Capraun, MS, RRT
Valencia Community College
Orlando, Florida

Lana Conrad, BS, RRT
Concorde Career College
Kansas City, Missouri

Charles S. Cornfield, MS, RRT
Gannon University
Erie, Pennsylvania

Joseph S. DiPietro, PhD, RRT
Southwest Virginia Community College
Richlands, Virginia

Crystal L. Dunlevy, EdD
Cincinnati State Technical and
Community College
Cincinnati, Ohio

Christine G. Fitzgerald, MHS, RRT
Quinnipiac University
Hamden, Connecticut

Mary Agnes Garrison, MS, RRT
Daytona Beach Community College
Daytona Beach, Florida

Douglas G. Gibson, BA, RRT
McLennan Community College
Waco, Texas

Robert G. McGee, MS, RRT
Walters State Community College
Greeneville, Tennessee

Ann Medford, MA, RRT-NPS
Midwestern State University
Wichita Falls, Texas

Tammy A. Miller, CPFT, RRT, MEd
Southwest Georgia Technical College
Thomasville, Georgia

Leigh Otto, BS, RRT
Pickens Technical Center
Aurora, Colorado

Richard A. Patze, MEd, RRT
Pima Community College
Tucson, Arizona

Charles Vincent Preuss, PhD, RPh
Ferris State University
Big Rapids, Michigan

Joy Reed, RN, MSN
Indiana Wesleyan University
Marion, Indiana

Thomas Schaltenbrand, MBA, RRT
Kaskasia College
Belleville, Illinois

Bruce Spruell, AAS-RRT
Shelton State Community College
Tuscaloosa, Alabama

Stephen E. Swope, BA, RRT
Idaho State University
Pocatello, Idaho

Stephen F. Wehrman, RRT, RPFT, AE-C
University of Hawaii
Honolulu, Hawai

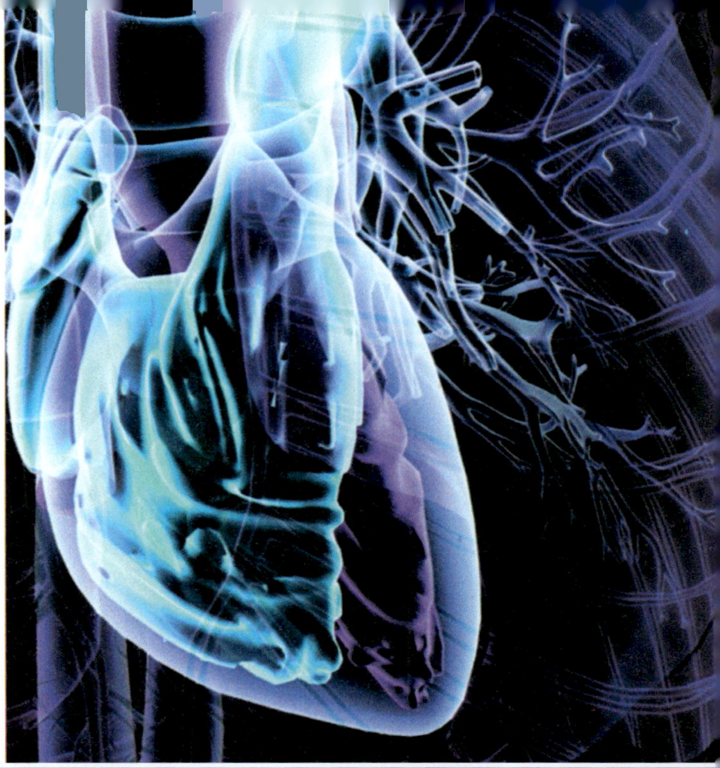

PART 1

The Basics

Chapter 1

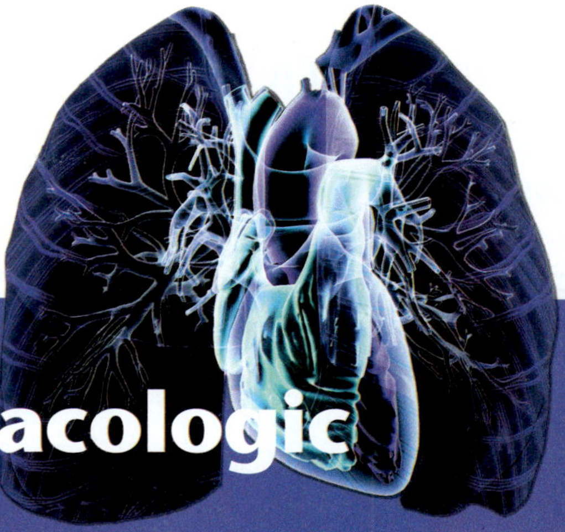

General Pharmacologic Principles

OBJECTIVES

Upon completion of this chapter you will be able to

- Define key terms related to pharmacologic principles.
- Utilize drug reference sources of information.
- Discuss advantages and disadvantages of different routes of administration.
- Describe the processes of drug absorption, distribution, metabolism, and elimination.
- Explain differences in pharmacokinetics, pharmacodynamics, and adverse effects of drugs in pediatric, geriatric, pregnant, and breastfeeding patients.
- Discuss factors that may alter a patient's response to a drug.
- Discuss principles of drug poisonings, adverse drug reactions, and interactions.
- Discuss responsibilities in drug administration.
- Relate the importance of pharmacogenomics to future drug therapy.

KEY TERMS

additive
adverse drug reaction
agonist
antagonist
bioavailability
dependence
desensitization
disease management
efficacy
emetics
enteral route
first-pass effect
formulary
half-life
loading dose
maintenance dose
parenteral route
pharmacodynamics
pharmacogenomics
pharmacokinetics
pharmacology
pharmacotherapy
potentiation
protein binding
racemic
receptor
selectivity
steady state
sublingual
synergism
teratogenic
therapeutic range
therapeutics
tolerance
toxicology
transdermal

ABBREVIATIONS

ACE	angiotensin-converting enzyme
ADR	adverse drug reaction
AHFS	*American Hospital Formulary Service*
CNS	central nervous system
COPD	chronic obstructive pulmonary disease
CPOE	computerized physician order entry
DNA	deoxyribonucleic acid
DPI	dry-powder inhaler
FDA	Food and Drug Administration
GI	gastrointestinal
HIV	human immunodeficiency virus
IM	intramuscular
IV	intravenous
JCAHO	Joint Commission on Accreditation of Healthcare Organizations
MDI	metered-dose inhaler
NG	nasogastric
NIH	National Institutes of Health
NPO	nothing by mouth
OTC	over the counter
PDR	*Physicians' Desk Reference*
PEG	percutaneous endoscopic gastrostomy
PO	by mouth (Latin *per os*)
PR	by rectum
SC	subcutaneous
SL	sublingual
SVN	small-volume nebulizer
$T_{1/2}$	half-life
USAN	United States Adopted Name Council
USP	United States Pharmacopeia
VD	volume of distribution

For the health-care professional, medication administration carries with it many responsibilities. With the vast array of drugs currently used in the practice of medicine, and new ones constantly being tested and developed, it is an impossible task to know every detail about every drug. However, if one is well-grounded in basic pharmacologic principles, one will know where to look and be able to understand the medical language that describes drugs and their interactions within the human organism.

This chapter discusses fundamental principles of pharmacology and strives to provide you with a healthy respect for drugs and knowledge that you can apply daily in pharmacotherapy decision making. After reading this chapter, you will understand the language of pharmacology and the important concepts for safe and effective drug administration.

1.1 BASIC TERMS

Drugs are among the most important aspects of clinical medicine. **Pharmacology**, the study of drugs and their action on the body, is a discipline that hinges on basic and clinical science. Pharmacology has a very long history. Ancient civilizations used plants containing ephedrine to treat breathing disorders, Native Americans used wild mint to treat stomach disorders—the list could go on. There has also been a darker side, when drugs were manufactured for nonmedical reasons. Examples include the infamous opium dens of the past and, in modern times, dangerous designer drugs that have killed many people.

Whereas pharmacology is a broad term that describes the study of drugs in general, **therapeutics** is defined as the study of drugs used to cure, treat, or prevent disease. Often the terms *pharmacology* and *therapeutics* are combined into the term **pharmacotherapy**. Another recent term that relates to these concepts is **disease management**. Disease management refers to the collective management of all aspects of the patient's disease, not just the use of pharmacotherapy. Pharmacotherapy, however, is usually one of the main components of disease management.

Drugs with similar characteristics are grouped together as a pharmacologic classification or class. One can predict how drugs in a class will act. For example drugs in the xanthine class can stimulate the central nervous system (CNS) and have a diuretic effect (i.e., they increase urine output), among other things. Caffeine, found in coffee, and the prescribed drug theophylline are both in this class and have similar effects, which you are probably aware of if you have ever drank large amounts of coffee. Caffeine usually produces diuresis with doses greater than 250 milligrams/day (mg/day). This text focuses on understanding pharmacologic classes and avoids emphasizing massive memorization of the characteristics of individual drugs. This is important because new drugs are approved every day, and the need for knowledge of pharmacology and therapeutics grows constantly.

Drugs can also be classified by their therapeutic category, such as bronchodilators. A therapeutic category can have several different pharmacological classes, and Chapters 5 through 11 are organized by therapeutic categories. For example, the class of xanthines will be discussed in the chapter on bronchodilators, along with other classes of drugs (beta-adrenergics and anticholinergics) that are also used as bronchodilators.

BVT Lab

Flashcards are available for this chapter at www.BVTLab.com.

1.2 DRUG DEVELOPMENT

Drugs are derived from a variety of sources, including plants, animals, minerals, chemicals, and recombinant deoxyribonucleic acid (DNA). Chemicals can be made into drugs synthetically or can be genetically bioengineered. Most drugs today are synthetic, but it is predicted that in the future many will be bioengineered.

The Food and Drug Administration (FDA) is the federal agency that regulates drug testing and approves new drugs for the market. Much to the discontent of animal activists, drugs are first tested on animals. Then each drug must pass three phases of human testing prior to approval. The phases proceed through testing in healthy volunteers (frequently "starving" students of the health-care professions), to testing in people with the disease against which the drug is expected to work, and then to large multicenter trials across the country. Phase IV studies, also called postmarketing studies, are studies performed after the drug is already on the market. They are becoming more frequent and are used to look for rare or serious adverse effects that might not have been fully detected prior to drug approval. The FDA must constantly balance the need to get a medically useful drug to the market quickly against the realization that the safety of the consumer is at stake. A good example of this is the testing and approval of new drugs for the treatment of the human immunodeficiency virus (HIV).

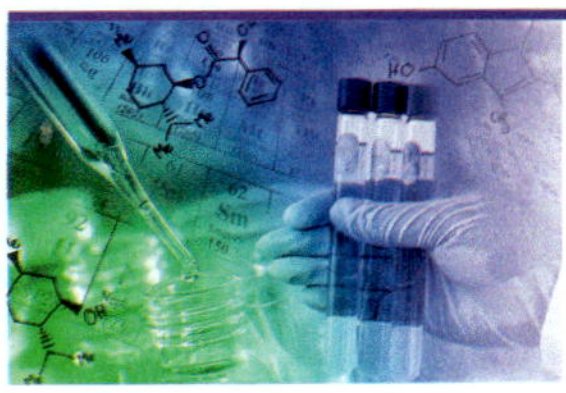

Controversy

The cost to the pharmaceutical industry of developing a new drug is estimated to be between $1.3 billion and $1.7 billion, although this figure has generated quite a bit of debate since this study was funded by pharmaceutical manufacturers. The relationship between drugs and high health-care costs is a topic of frequent public and political debate. High pharmaceutical costs lead some patients to make questionable cost-saving decisions, such as buying drugs from overseas vendors using the Internet or simply not taking their prescribed medicines.

time for review

Describe the process a new drug must undergo for approval. Several ethical, moral, and legal issues are implied in the preceding section on drug development. Can you expand upon them? Can you think of others?

1.3 HERBAL SUPPLEMENTS (NEUTRACEUTICALS)

The use of supplements, also called herbals, is growing in popularity. Frequently patients self-medicate with herbals, and health-care professionals are not even aware of it unless they ask. The FDA treats herbals as dietary supplements, and standards for supplements are different than those for drugs. The long and short of it is that, for herbal products, the manufacturer does not have to prove a product's safety and effectiveness before it is marketed. A manufacturer is allowed to say that a supplement helps a nutrient deficiency, supports health, or is tied to a particular body function (e.g., immunity) if there is research supporting this claim. A claim must be followed by the words "This statement has not been evaluated by the FDA. This product is not intended to diagnose, treat, cure, or prevent any disease." You can visit the National Institutes of Health (NIH) National Center for Complementary and Alternative Medicine for more information.

Patient & Family Education

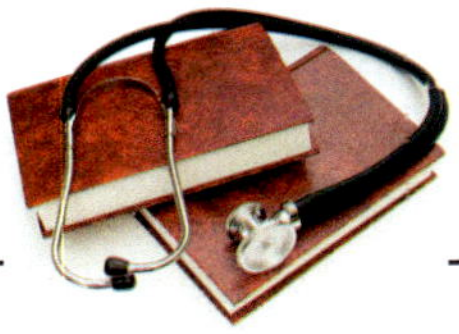

Herbal Interactions

Herbs, vitamins, minerals, and certain other products taken by mouth and not regulated as drugs by the FDA are called "dietary supplements." Manufacturers and distributors do not need FDA approval to sell their dietary supplements. It is a good idea to encourage patients to check with their doctor or pharmacist prior to taking dietary supplements to make sure the supplements won't interfere with their other medical problems or medications.

One good example of why it is important to check with a health professional prior to taking dietary supplements can be illustrated by St. John's wort. This product is a dietary supplement that has been used by people with depression. But combining St. John's wort with certain HIV drugs significantly reduces their effectiveness and may also reduce the effectiveness of prescription drugs for heart disease, seizures, certain cancers, oral contraceptives, and depression.

1.4 DRUG INFORMATION SOURCES

All health-care professionals must recognize the limitations of their knowledge and know where to find information about drugs. Depending on your workplace, a variety of drug references should be accessible to you. Good drug references and sources, in the authors' opinion, include the *American Hospital Formulary Service* (AHFS); *Drug Information,* by the American Society of Health System Pharmacists; and *Drug Facts and Comparisons,* by the Wolters Kluwer Company. *Drug Facts and Comparisons* has useful tables comparing drugs within a class. AHFS provides more information than drug package inserts. For example it lists unapproved medical indications. The PDR, or *Physicians' Desk Reference,* is useful if you are looking for product information required by the FDA, such as drug name, clinical pharmacology, indications, contraindications, drug interactions, adverse drug reactions, dosage, and administration.

Clinical pearl

The United States Pharmacopeia (USP) is the official organization that is responsible for establishing drug standards for the United States. (www.usp.org/aboutusp)

Smartphone versions of the above references as well as several others are also available to health-care practitioners. LexiDrugs, ePocrates, and mobile-MICROMEDEX are several popular electronic drug references. These products vary considerably in terms of the type of drug information provided and cost.

As technology changes and new drugs are developed, you have a responsibility to update your knowledge. No one would deny that this is a formidable task. All you need to do is look at the size of the old PDRs compared with today's. The drug information you learn in school is frequently replaced with new concepts once you are out in practice. This requires that you devise a method of updating your knowledge through self-directed learning and continuing education.

CONTROVERSY

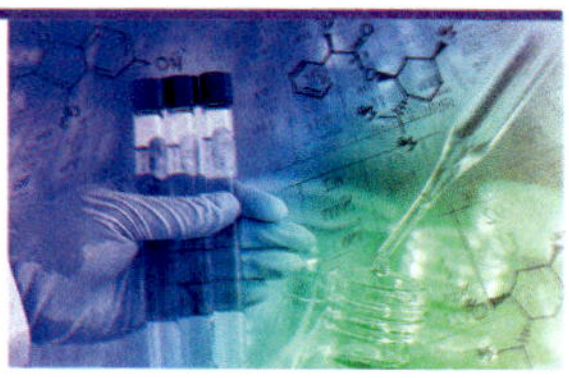

Prescribing patterns and treatments can change daily in response to new research published in medical journals, especially for drug therapy. What would you do if the prescriber were not incorporating the latest research findings into patient treatment?

1.5 INTERPRETING DRUG INFORMATION

Finding a good, valid source of drug information is the first step. Understanding and interpreting the information presented is the next step before one can apply this knowledge in drug administration and evaluation. Some of the typical information presented will include the drug name(s), the clinical pharmacology of how it works, indications and usage, contraindications, drug interactions, adverse reactions, and dosage and administration. We will discuss each of these categories by elaborating upon the specific sections contained in a drug package insert.

1.5a Drug Names

One of the most complicated factors for students encountering a drug for the first time is that it has not one name but at least two—and frequently more. Drugs have chemical names that describe the structure. An example is [4S-(4α,4aα,5aα,6α,12aα,)]-4-(di-methylamino)-1,4,4a,5,5a,6,11,12a-octahydro-3,6,10,12,12a-penthydroxy-6-methyl-1,11-dioxo-2-naphthacenecarboxamide. Imagine asking for that at your local pharmacy! The chemical name is important as a point of reference to manufacture the drug, but it has little practical use for the practitioner or consumer. Minor chemical changes in a drug can greatly change pharmacologic activity. This lesson has been learned the hard way by drug abusers in home labs creating designer drugs that turn out to have dangerous side effects.

Learning Hint

Trade names are traditionally capitalized and may carry a registered trademark symbol—®.

Drugs are also assigned generic names by the United States Adopted Name (USAN) Council. The generic name for the previously given chemical name is tetracycline hydrochloride. Generic names are not owned by any particular pharmaceutical company and therefore are considered the nonproprietary name.

Once a drug is approved, a particular pharmaceutical company can produce and market it under its brand or trade name. The company that originally discovered the drug owns the trade name, which is derived with the help of creative marketing people. The trade name often relates to some aspect of either the generic name or the drug itself. For example, Sudafed is the trade name for the generic drug pseudoephedrine. Some other examples of innovative names are Theo-24 and Elixophyllin. Seeing "24" in the name, you can guess the dosage frequency—once a day, or once every 24 hours. From "Elixo" you can hypothesize that the drug is a liquid (a play on the word *elixir*; elixirs contain alcohol, which aids in dissolving the medicine). Names frequently give clues to drug indications—for example Flovent, for increasing air flow and ventilation. See Figure 1-1 for a portion of a drug package insert related to drug names for the bronchodilator Proventil® HFA.

Learning Hint

Many drugs in a class have generic names that end in the same syllable (e.g., beta-blockers: propranolol, metoprolol, atenolol). Traditionally, generic names are written in all lowercase letters.

Clinical pearl

Drugs may have more than one name. This is because after the patent on the registered trademark expires, a generic drug product containing the same drug and dosage form can be developed by different drug companies. This is why we have both generic and brand names for many drugs.

FIGURE 1-1 Portion of Drug Package Insert Related to Drug Names

Trade Name → **PROVENTIL® HFA**

Generic Name → **(albuterol sulfate)**

Inhalation Aerosol

FOR ORAL INHALATION ONLY

Prescribing Information

Chemical Name → DESCRIPTION The active component of PROVENTIL© HFA (albuterol sulfate) Inhalation Aerosol is albuterol sulfate, USP racemic α^1 [(*tert*-Butylamino)methyl]-4-hydroxy-*m*-xylene-α,α′-diol sulfate (2:1)(salt), a relatively selective beta$_2$-adrenergic bronchodilator having the following chemical structure:

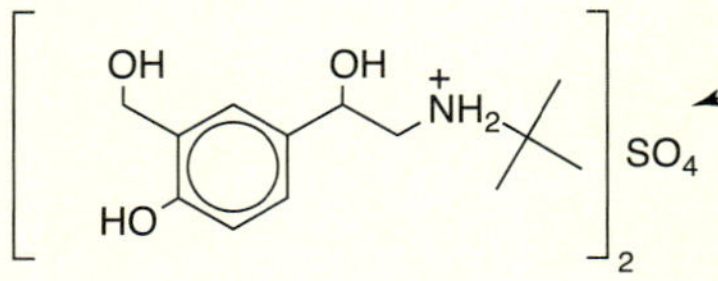

Chemical Structure

Albuterol sulfate is the official generic name in the United States. The World Health Organization's recommended name for the drug is salbutamol sulfate. The molecular weight of albuterol sulfate is 576.7, and the empirical formula is $(C_{13}H_{21}NO_3)_2 \cdot H_2SO_4$. Albuterol sulfate is a white to off-white crystalline solid. It is soluble in water and slightly soluble in ethanol. PROVENTIL HFA Inhalation Aerosol is a pressurized metered-dose aerosol unit for oral Inhalation. It contains a microcrystalline suspension of albuterol sulfate in propellant HFA-134a (1,1,1,2-tetrafluoroethane), ethanol, and oleic acid.

Source: Reprinted with permission from Merck Archives; Merck, Sharp & Dohme Corp., 2015.

1.5b Clinical Pharmacology

In the clinical pharmacology section of the drug insert information, you can learn about the mechanism of action of the drug and its specific classification. More on these topics will be covered in the upcoming pharmacokinetics section and in each specific chapter covering the various categories of drugs. See Figure 1-2 for the clinical pharmacology section of the drug package insert for Proventil® HFA.

FIGURE 1-2 Portion of Drug Package Insert Related to Clinical Pharmacology for the Drug Proventil® HFA

CLINICAL PHARMACOLOGY

Mechanism of Action *In vitro* studies and *in vivo* pharmacologic studies have demonstrated that albuterol has a preferential effect on $beta_2$–adrenergic receptors compared with isoproterenol. While it is recognized that $beta_2$–adrenergic receptors are the predominant receptors on bronchial smooth muscle, data indicate that there is a population of $beta_2$–receptors in the human heart existing in a concentration between 10% and 50% of cardiac beta-adrenergic receptors. The precise function of these receptors has not been established (see **WARNINGS, Cardiovascular Effects** section).

Activation of $beta_2$–adrenergic receptors on airway smooth muscle leads to the activation of adenylcyclase and to an increase in the intracellular concentration of cyclic-3', 5'-adenosine monophosphate (cyclic AMP). This increase of cyclic AMP leads to the activation of protein kinase A, which inhibits the phosphorylation of myosin and lowers intracellular ionic calcium concentrations, resulting in relaxation. Albuterol relaxes the smooth muscles of all airways, from the trachea to the terminal bronchioles. Albuterol acts as a functional antagonist to relax the airway irrespective of the spasmogen involved, thus protecting against all bronchoconstrictor challenges. Increased cyclic AMP concentrations are also associated with the inhibition of release of mediators from mast cells in the airway.

Albuterol has been shown in most clinical trials to have more effect on the respiratory tract, in the form of bronchial smooth muscle relaxation, than isoproterenol at comparable doses while producing fewer cardiovascular effects. Controlled clinical studies and other clinical experience have shown that inhaled albuterol, like other beta-adrenergic agonist drugs, can produce a significant cardiovascular effect in some patients, as measured by pulse rate, blood pressure, symptoms, and/or electrocardiographic changes.

Preclinical Intravenous studies in rats with albuterol sulfate have demonstrated that albuterol crosses the blood-brain barrier and reaches brain concentrations amounting to approximately 5% of the plasma concentrations. In structures outside the blood-brain barrier (pineal and pituitary glands), albuterol concentrations were found to be 100 times those in the whole brain.

Source: Reprinted with permission from Merck Archives; Merck, Sharp & Dohme Corp., 2015.

1.5c Indications and Usage

The indications and usage section will inform you of the FDA-approved clinical indication(s)—that is, why you would consider using this particular medication. However one should note that sometimes drugs are prescribed for uses not listed as an indication in the drug package insert. This is termed *off-label* use. See Figure 1-3 for the indications and usage section of the drug package insert for Proventil® HFA.

FIGURE 1-3 Portion of Drug Package Insert Related to Indications and Usage for the Drug Proventil® HFA

INDICATIONS AND USAGE

PROVENTIL® HFA Inhalation Aerosol is indicated in adults and children 4 years of age and older for the treatment or prevention of bronchospasm with reversible obstructive airway disease and for the prevention of exercise-induced bronchospasm.

Source: Reprinted with permission from Merck Archives; Merck, Sharp & Dohme Corp., 2015.

1.5d Contraindications

The contraindications section contains warnings as to particular patients or situations in which you should not use this medication. This section may also list precautions to follow when administering this drug or situations that may warrant closer patient monitoring. See Figure 1-4 for the contraindications section of the drug package insert for Proventil® HFA.

FIGURE 1-4 Portion of Drug Package Insert Related to Contraindications for the Drug Proventil® HFA

CONTRAINDICATIONS

PROVENTIL® HFA Inhalation Aerosol is contraindicated in patients with a history of hypersensitivity to albuterol or any other PROVENTIL HFA components.

WARNINGS

1. Paradoxical Bronchospasm: Inhaled albuterol sulfate can produce paradoxical bronchospasm that may be life threatening. If paradoxical bronchospasm occurs, PROVENTIL® HFA Inhalation Aerosol should be discontinued immediately and alternative therapy instituted. It should be recognized that paradoxical bronchospasm, when associated with inhaled formulations, frequently occurs with the first use of a new canister.
2. Deterioration of Asthma: Asthma may deteriorate acutely over a period of hours or chronically over several days or longer. If the patient needs more doses of PROVENTIL HFA Inhalation Aerosol than usual, this may be a marker of destabilization of asthma and requires re-evaluation of the patient and treatment regimen, giving special consideration to the possible need for anti-inflammatory treatment, eg, corticosteroids.
3. Use of Anti-Inflammatory Agents: The use of beta-adrenergic agonist bronchodilators alone may not be adequate to control asthma in many patients. Early consideration should be given to adding anti-inflammatory agents, eg, corticosteroids, to the therapeutic regimen.
4. Cardiovascular Effects: PROVENTIL HFA Inhalation Aerosol, like other beta-adrenergic agonists, can produce clinically significant cardiovascular effects in some patients as measured by pulse rate, blood pressure, and/or symptoms. Although such effects are uncommon after administration of PROVENTIL HFA Inhalation Aerosol at recommended doses, if they occur, the drug may need to be discontinued. In addition, beta-agonists have been reported to produce ECG changes, such as flattening of the T wave, prolongation of the QT_c interval, and ST segment depression. The clinical significance of these findings is unknown. Therefore, PROVENTIL HFA Inhalation Aerosol, like all sympathomimetic amines, should be used with caution in patients with cardiovascular disorders, especially coronary insufficiency, cardiac arrhythmias, and hypertension.
5. Do Not Exceed Recommended Dose: Fatalities have been reported in association with excessive use of inhaled sympathomimetic drugs in patients with asthma. The exact cause of death is unknown, but cardiac arrest following an unexpected development of a severe acute asthmatic crisis and subsequent hypoxia is suspected.
6. Immediate Hypersensitivity Reactions: Immediate hypersensitivity reactions may occur after administration of albuterol sulfate, as demonstrated by rare cases of urticaria, angioedema, rash, bronchospasm, anaphylaxis, and oropharyngeal edema.

Source: Reprinted with permission from Merck Archives; Merck, Sharp & Dohme Corp., 2015.

time for review

What is the difference between a generic name and a brand name? What is the difference between an indication and a contraindication?

1.5e Drug Interactions

Often a patient is receiving more than just a single drug, and there is a potential for two or more drugs to interact. Drug interactions can result in unwanted or dangerous side effects by either reducing or increasing the action of one or more of the drugs involved. This usually happens by either increasing or decreasing a drug's absorption or elimination from the body. For example psyllium and digoxin, when given concurrently, will bind together within the stomach and cause a reduction in the amount of digoxin absorbed into the circulation. Therefore, the digoxin may not work as well as expected. Cimetidine is known for inhibiting the liver enzymes that metabolize some drugs. Patients may show increased effects of other drugs they may be taking because now these drugs may not be broken down or metabolized as readily. Phenytoin may increase the metabolism by the liver of certain medications, which would result in a decreased effect of the affected medications. Consulting up-to-date drug interaction information is important both to see if an interaction is possible and then to try and determine its significance.

Drug interactions usually carry a negative connotation among health professionals, but they are not always bad. Sometimes drug interactions can be beneficial. Ritonavir is a medicine used in combination with other HIV medicines only to boost the effect of the concurrently taken drug. This results in fewer pills and a reduction in the number of times per day a patient would need to take his or her HIV medicines. This hopefully also boosts compliance with the prescribed regimen, which is critical since there currently is no cure for HIV-infected individuals.

There are terms related to therapeutic drug interactions. When two drugs are given together and the result of those two can be summed up by the equation $1 + 1 = 2$, the interaction is **additive**. Additive means that the sum of the effects of two drugs given together is equal to each of them given separately but at the same time. This can be beneficial when, for example, you are treating a patient with high blood pressure and you want to avoid the side effects that may occur with high doses of one drug. You can instead give lower doses of two drugs and rely on the additive hypotensive effects being equal to the single drug at a higher dose.

In some cases, giving two drugs together can result in a greater effect than would be expected by giving them together. When two drugs are given together and interact to equal $1 + 1 = 3$, then **synergism** is occurring. Though it is mathematically incorrect, this expression describes the summation of the drug activity exceeding the sum of the two individual drugs. This can be very beneficial in the case of treatment of an infection with a combination of antibiotics. For example, when used together, the antimicrobials rifampin and nafcillin are effective in treating staphylococci; but when patients have joint-replacement infections (e.g., knee or hip), if we were to use one of these drugs alone, it would be ineffective in curing the infection.

If you really want to drive mathematicians crazy, **potentiation** can be described numerically as $1 + 0 = 3$. This means that one of the drugs or substances, while having no direct effect, nevertheless increases the response of the other drug, which normally has a lesser effect. Grapefruit juice, when consumed by patients taking felodipine (medicine for high blood pressure), may lead to a dangerous drop in blood pressure. Grapefruit juice inhibits the metabolism of felodipine in the intestine resulting in a 50%–250% increase in the plasma concentration of felodipine. You can see how this could be confused with synergism, yet it is not synonymous. See Figure 1-5, which shows the drug interactions section of the drug package insert for Proventil® HFA.

Clinical Pearl

Sometimes a drug will have a completely unpredicted or "off-the-wall" effect. This is termed an *idiosyncratic* reaction.

Clinical pearl

The fact that these common drugs are considered "red flag" drugs does not mean that they should not be administered. It simply means that more attention should be paid to the potential for their interaction with other drugs the patient may have been prescribed.

FIGURE 1-5 Portion of Drug Package Insert Related to Drug Interactions for the Drug Proventil® HFA

Drug Interactions

1. Beta-Blockers: Beta-adrenergic-receptor blocking agents not only block the pulmonary effect of beta-agonists, such as PROVENTIL® HFA Inhalation Aerosol, but may produce severe bronchospasm in asthmatic patients. Therefore, patients with asthma should not normally be treated with beta-blockers. However, under certain circumstances, eg, as prophylaxis after myocardial infarction, there may be no acceptable alternatives to the use of beta-adrenergic blocking agents in patients with asthma. In this setting, cardioselective beta-blockers should be considered, although they should be administered with caution.

2. Diuretics: The ECG changes and/or hypokalemia which may result from the administration of nonpotassium-sparing diuretics (such as loop or thiazide diuretics) can be acutely worsened by beta-agonists, especially when the recommended dose of the beta-agonist is exceeded. Although the clinical significance of these effects is not known, caution is advised in the coadministration of beta-agonists with nonpotassium-sparing diuretics.

3. Albuterol-Digoxin: Mean decreases of 16% and 22% in serum digoxin levels were demonstrated after single-dose intravenous and oral administration of albuterol, respectively, to normal volunteers who had received digoxin for 10 days. The clinical significance of these findings for patients with obstructive airway disease who are receiving albuterol and digoxin on a chronic basis is unclear, nevertheless, it would be prudent to carefully evaluate the serum digoxin levels in patients who are currently receiving digoxin and albuterol.

4. Monoamine Oxidase Inhibitors or Tricyclic Antidepressants: PROVENTIL® HFA Inhalation Aerosol should be administered with extreme caution to patients being treated with monoamine oxidase inhibitors or tricyclic antidepressants, or within 2 weeks of discontinuation of such agents, because the action of albuterol on the cardiovascular system may be potentiated.

Source: Reprinted with permission from Merck Archives; Merck, Sharp & Dohme Corp., 2015.

Some drugs are at higher risk of causing drug interactions, and some patients are at higher risk of experiencing drug interactions. Certain drugs are known to be at high risk of causing drug interactions and are even considered to be "red flag" drugs. See Table 1-1, which lists some major red flag drugs.

TABLE 1-1 "Red Flag" Drugs

Drug Name
warfarin
cimetidine
aspirin
phenytoin
theophylline

Clinical pearl

With the recent push to get drugs approved faster and on the market sooner, serious ADRs may not be detected until postmarketing surveillance. Enrolling enough patients in research studies to detect all ADRs before FDA approval is not feasible, so rare ADRs may not be detected until there is widespread use of a drug in a large population.

1.5f Adverse Drug Reactions

Not only can drugs interact with each other, but they may also have unintended interactions within the human body. Contrary to the Hippocratic Oath—which says, "First, do no harm"—at least 5% of reported hospitalizations are the result of an **adverse drug reaction** (ADR). When patients experience unintended side effects from medication, they are having ADRs. Such reactions also occur in patients who are already in the hospital, which can then result in an increased length of stay. Adverse drug reactions can range from a side effect that is mild and goes away with repeated use or discontinuation to a more severe or life-threatening reaction.

One can easily confuse the terms *ADR* and *drug allergy* and mistakenly use the terms synonymously. ADRs include many things, such as tremors, bronchospasms, headaches, changes in laboratory results of renal function, photosensitivity, and so on. An allergy or hypersensitivity is only one example of an ADR, and not all ADRs are allergies. Drug allergies induce a hypersensitivity reaction. This reaction can vary in severity and can be thought of as a continuum. Allergies can be acute and life-threatening—as, for example, in anaphylactic shock—or can be found on the milder end of the continuum, for example, as a dermatologic rash such as hives. See Figure 1-6 for the ADR section of the drug insert for Proventil® HFA.

FIGURE 1-6 Portion of Drug Package Insert Related to Adverse Reactions for the Drug Proventil® HFA

ADVERSE REACTIONS

Adverse reaction information concerning PROVENTIL® HFA Inhalation Aerosol is derived from a 12-week, double-blind, double-dummy study which compared PROVENTIL HFA Inhalation Aerosol, a CFC 11/12 propelled albuterol inhaler, and an HFA-134a placebo inhaler in 565 asthmatic patients. The following table lists the incidence of all adverse events (whether considered by the investigator drug related or unrelated to drug) from this study which occurred at a rate of 3% or greater in the PROVENTIL HFA Inhalation Aerosol treatment group and more frequently in the PROVENTIL HFA Inhalation Aerosol treatment group than in the placebo group. Overall, the incidence and nature of the adverse reactions reported for PROVENTIL HFA Inhalation Aerosol and a CFC 11/12 propelled albuterol inhaler were comparable.

Adverse Experience Incidences (% of patients) in a Large 12-week Clinical Trial*

Body System/Adverse Event (Preferred Term)		PROVENTIL® HFA Inhalation Aerosol (N = 193)	CFC 11/12 Propelled Albuterol Inhaler (N = 186)	HFA-134a Placebo Inhaler (N = 186)
Application Site Disorders	Inhalation Site Sensation	6	9	2
	Inhalation Taste Sensation	4	3	3
Body as a Whole	Allergic Reaction/Symptoms	6	4	<1
	Back Pain	4	2	3
	Fever	6	2	5
Central and Peripheral Nervous System	Tremor	7	8	2
Gastrointestinal System	Nausea	10	9	5
	Vomiting	7	2	3
Heart Rate and Rhythm Disorder	Tachycardia	7	2	<1
Psychiatric Disorders	Nervousness	7	9	3
Respiratory System Disorders	Respiratory Disorder (unspecified)	6	4	5
	Rhinitis	16	22	14
	Upper Resp Tract Infection	21	20	18
Urinary System Disorder	Urinary Tract Infection	3	4	2

*This table includes all adverse events (whether considered by the investigator drug related or unrelated to drug) which occurred at an incidence rate of at least 3.0% in the PROVENTIL HFA Inhalation Aerosol group and more frequently in the PROVENTIL HFA Inhalation Aerosol group than in the HFA-134a placebo inhaler group.

Source: Reprinted with permission from Merck Archives; Merck, Sharp & Dohme Corp., 2015.

Knowledge of ADRs in select populations, such as pregnant women, would be especially useful. However, enrolling pregnant patients in research is not always ethical. Consequently information on how drugs may adversely affect the fetus is not always known or reported. Absorption, one of the concepts of pharmacokinetics to be discussed later in this chapter, needs to be considered when discussing pregnancy and ADRs. When you think of drug absorption for women of childbearing age, it is safest to assume that any drug given to a pregnant woman may also be given to the baby and may be crossing the fetal-placental barrier. The same applies to lactating women, with drugs passing from breast milk to the baby.

A drug that has the potential to damage a fetus in utero when administered to a pregnant woman is called **teratogenic**. The teratogenicity of drugs is classified based on risk and the limited data available. For example, drugs that have shown evidence of fetal risk that outweighs any possible benefit are considered "category X" and are

BVT Lab

Visit www.BVTLab.com to explore the student resources available for this chapter.

absolutely contraindicated. For other drugs, including some for asthma and other chronic diseases such as epilepsy, the risks to the baby caused by the mother not having her disease controlled with a drug can outweigh the risks of drug exposure for the baby. Decisions about drug use in pregnant women need to be made mutually by the patient and the health-care provider.

time for review

What is the difference between an allergy and an ADR?

Some of the most serious ADRs with cardiopulmonary implications are reactions such as acute pulmonary edema, bronchial asthma, pulmonary fibrosis, or respiratory muscle impairment affecting the patient's ability to ventilate. Some of these reactions may occur due to a direct cytotoxic effect on alveolar endothelial cells and can severely impair the vital process of gas exchange. More than 150 drugs have been shown to produce pulmonary ADRs, and Table 1-2 lists some examples of drug-induced pulmonary adverse reactions.

TABLE 1-2 Drug-Induced Pulmonary ADRs

ADR	Drug
Pulmonary edema	methadone IV fluids epinephrine hydrochlorothiazide salicylates
Pulmonary fibrosis	amiodarone busulfan nitrofurantoin
Respiratory muscle impairment	alcohol corticosteroids sedatives penicillamine
Bronchospasm	ACE inhibitors beta-blockers nonsteroidal anti-inflammatory drugs (NSAIDs)

There are also other possible pulmonary complications. Angiotensin-converting enzyme (ACE) inhibitors for the heart, as discussed further in Chapter 9, cause a cough in up to 15% of patients treated. Plain aspirin, which you can buy over the counter (OTC) without a prescription, can cause bronchospasms in up to 20% of patients with asthma. Even topical beta-blocker eye drops can be absorbed enough to aggravate chronic obstructive pulmonary disease (COPD).

1.5g Dosage and Administration

The dosage and administration section of the drug package insert describes the standard dose for the medication. In addition, it should elaborate on how the medication is supplied and whether any special treatment or care should be given to preserve its effectiveness. This section describes the route of administration of the drug. The route of administration is such an important topic that it will be discussed separately in the upcoming section. Please see Figure 1-7 for the dosage and administration section of the drug package insert for Proventil® HFA.

FIGURE 1-7 Portion of Drug Package Insert Related to Dosage and Administration for the Drug Proventil® HFA

DOSAGE AND ADMINISTRATION

For treatment of acute episodes of bronchospasm or prevention of asthmatic symptoms, the usual dosage for adults and children 4 years of age and older is two inhalations repeated every 4 to 6 hours. More frequent administration or a larger number of inhalations is not recommended. In some patients, one inhalation every 4 hours may be sufficient. Each actuation of PROVENTIL® HFA Inhalation Aerosol delivers 108 mcg of albuterol sulfate (equivalent to 90 mcg of albuterol base) from the mouthpiece. It is recommended to prime the inhaler before using for the first time and in cases where the inhaler has not been used for more than 2 weeks by releasing four "test sprays" into the air, away from the face.

Exercise Induced Bronchospasm Prevention The usual dosage for adults and children 4 years of age and older is two inhalations 15 to 30 minutes before exercise.

Source: Reprinted with permission from Merck Archives; Merck, Sharp & Dohme Corp., 2015.

1.6 ROUTES OF ADMINISTRATION

One of the first mysteries of pharmacology is the simple and common question of why some drugs are given orally and others are given by a shot or even by other means. Routes of administration of drugs are selected according to the rate of onset of drug activity desired and physiochemical factors that affect drug absorption. For example, some drugs given by mouth undergo what is called a **first-pass effect**. After being absorbed, drugs with a first-pass effect do not go directly into the systemic circulation but instead go through the liver. In the liver the drug undergoes a metabolic change. The liver enzymes inactivate some of the drug before it reaches the blood circulation (see Figure 1-8). For this reason, the dosage of an orally administered drug may need to be higher than when it is administered by a route that bypasses the liver, such as the intravenous route. Drugs given via the **parenteral route** (by injection) can avoid the first-pass effect, which explains why doses of the same drug vary depending on the route of administration—for example, oral propranolol 40 mg versus 1 mg of the drug intravenously (IV). These two routes, with very different dosages, will produce about the same response.

FIGURE 1-8 The First-Pass Effect

Drugs administered orally are first absorbed through the small intestine and then enter the liver where they begin to be metabolized (broken down) before reaching the bloodstream.

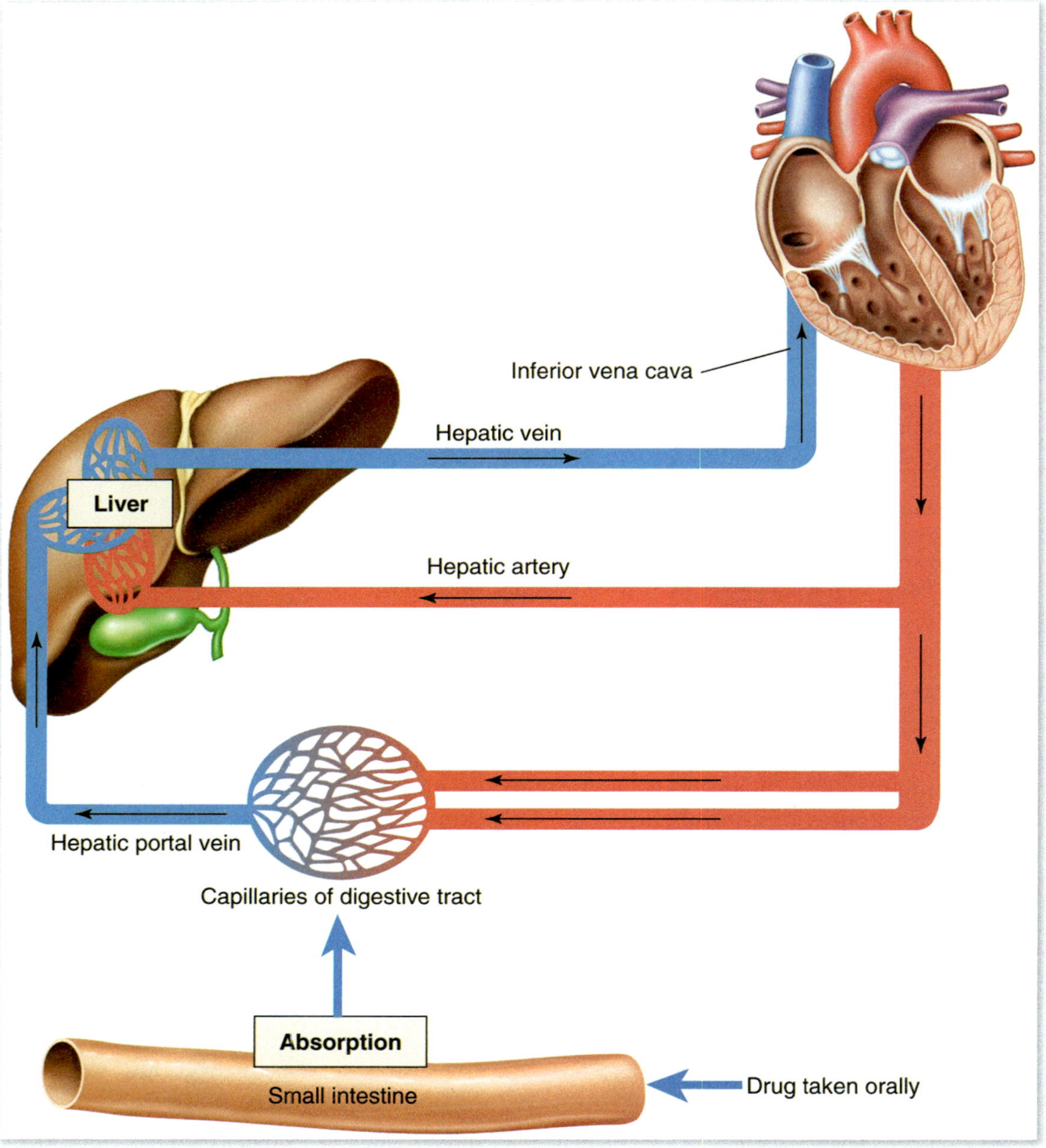

The route of drug administration is also selected based on how compliant the patient is in taking prescribed medication regularly. For example, *depot formulations* of drugs given intramuscularly for noncompliant schizophrenic patients every 2 weeks can keep their disease controlled, whereas they may not take their prescribed oral medications consistently. Depot formulations are drugs that are slowly released once administered, so they only need to be given every week or so, depending on the drug. Some depot drugs are formulated in oil, which allows for slow release into the bloodstream. Depot birth control is an alternative for women who do not wish to get pregnant but who may be less compliant about using other forms of birth control.

1.6a Enteral Routes

Enteral routes of drug absorption are via the gastrointestinal tract for systemic purposes and include the oral (PO), sublingual (SL), nasogastric (NG) tube, percutaneous endoscopic gastrostomy (PEG) tube, and rectal (per rectum or PR) routes. The NG tube is inserted through the nose and esophagus and rests within the stomach. The PEG tube is inserted directly into the stomach. The oral route is usually considered the most common and convenient route. **Sublingual** drugs are absorbed quickly owing to the rich vasculature under the tongue, which explains why this route is chosen for nitroglycerin for quick relief of cardiac chest pain. Rectal drug administration can be very effective for patients ordered "nothing by mouth" (NPO) or those who are vomiting or unable to swallow oral medications. Patients who are receiving enteral nutrition via a gastric tube are frequently given drugs through that tube as well, as long as drug stability and compatibility in mixing with foods and liquids are taken into consideration.

Learning Hint

PO is Latin for *per os*, which means "through the mouth."

1.6b Parenteral Routes

Parenteral routes include the injectable routes. They may be through central lines, intra-arterial, intravenous (IV), intramuscular (IM), or subcutaneous routes (SC). Drugs given parenterally go right into the bloodstream and absorption is rapid, so this route is desirable for emergency situations when an immediate response is needed. Drugs that are insoluble and cannot be dissolved cannot be given intravenously. Some drugs cannot be administered together intravenously because of physical incompatibilities. There are thick reference books dedicated to describing which drugs are compatible with each other in solution.

The rate for IM drug absorption depends on the formulation used. Clear or water-based solutions have a rapid effect. Suspensions that are cloudy or oil-based have a slower rate of absorption. Parenteral administration carries with it the risk of infection, pain, or local irritation.

Learning Hint

The term *parenteral* is derived from the Greek *para*, "apart from," plus *enteron*, "intestine," and technically means any route outside of the oral and intestinal tract. Clinically, it refers to the injectable routes.

1.6c Other Routes

Topical drugs are administered onto the skin or mucous membranes. Examples include nitroglycerin ointment and skin creams. *Inhalation* drug delivery is a form of topical delivery to the lungs that may avoid systemic side effects. *Inhalation* drug therapy or medicated aerosol therapy delivers micron-sized aerosol particles through the bronchial tree to the lungs, providing for rapid absorption. Local administration of a drug to the lungs is advantageous because of their large surface area and location close to the pulmonary circulation. It is also so important in cardiopulmonary pharmacotherapy that it warrants a whole chapter (Chapter 4).

Transdermal delivery of a drug occurs through a skin patch that allows the drug to be released slowly; this provides for sustained blood levels throughout the day without the patient having to remember to take medications (see Figure 1-9). Considering people's busy lives, drugs need to be dosed so they will not interfere with lifestyle, which may enhance compliance and keep drugs effective. See Table 1-3 for a summary of administration routes.

FIGURE 1-9 Transdermal Patch Administration

(a) protective covering removed; (b) patch applied to clean, dry, hairless skin and labeled with date, time, and initials.

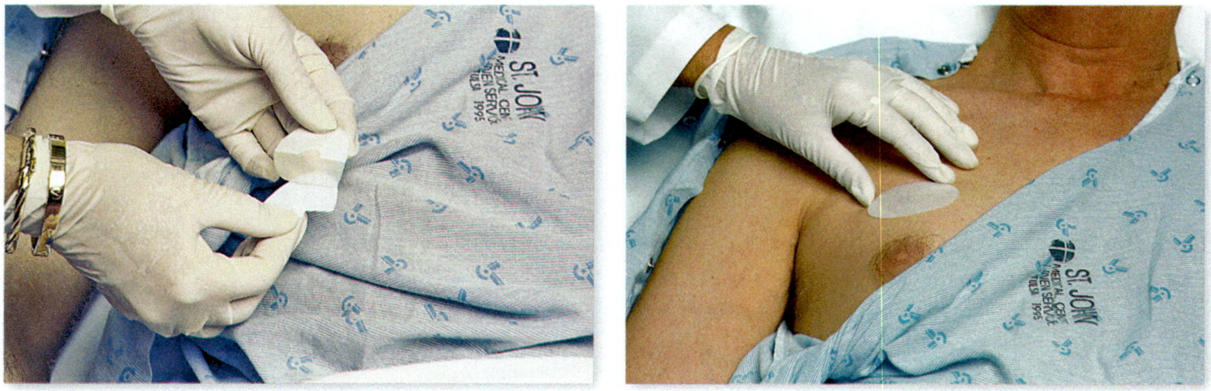

(a) (b)

Source: Pearson

TABLE 1-3 Examples of Drug Administration Routes

Route	Major Points	Examples
Oral (PO)	May be enteric-coated, sustained-release, tablet, or capsule; some are crushable, some lose their potency when crushed; this is the most convenient and economical route	Most prescribed drugs and over-the-counter (OTC) medications
Sublingual (SL)	Provides quick onset with good salivary flow	Nitroglycerin
Rectal (PR)	Can be more convenient when patients cannot swallow (nausea/NPO)	Antinausea medications
Nasogastric (NG) tube	Be careful of drug stability and clogging up the tube	Nutritional feedings
Percutaneous endoscopic (PEG) tube	More comfortable than NG tube	Nutritional feeding and liquid medication; tablets or capsules that are not sustained release dosage forms
Intravenous (IV)	Use in quick onset, emergency situations, and long-term infusions	Emergency medications
Intramuscular (IM)	Once injected, there to stay—even if side effects occur	Iron
Transdermal	Is easier to remember because dosing is less frequent	Nicotine or nitroglycerin patches
Inhalational	Has fewer systemic side effects, requires coordination	Metered-dose inhalers (MDIs), dry-powder inhalers (DPIs) Small-volume nebulizers (SVNs)

1.7 PHARMACOKINETICS

Pharmacokinetics means the movement (kinesis) of the drug throughout our body. Pharmacokinetics is the study of what happens to the drug from the time it is put into the body until it has left the body. Pharmacokinetic principles help determine drug dosage in terms of amount, duration, and frequency. Pharmacokinetics includes the following processes: *absorption, distribution, metabolism,* and *elimination* of a drug (ADME for short). Absorption occurs when the drug passes from its administration site into plasma. Distribution determines where the drug goes once it is within the body. For any drug to work, it must be absorbed and distributed to an active site. Metabolism refers to biotransformation, in which drugs are converted to a water-soluble form for elimination. Elimination of a drug occurs by hepatic metabolism or renal excretion. Each of these components of pharmacokinetics will be broken down and discussed in a different section.

Learning Hint

Pharmacokinetics is often confused with pharmacodynamics. Pharmacokinetics is what the body does to the drug. Pharmacodynamics, on the other hand, is what the drug does to the body and will be discussed shortly.

1.7a Absorption

A drug must first be disintegrated or dissolved before it can be absorbed into the systemic circulation. The rate-limiting step in absorption is disintegration. If a drug does not have to disintegrate and is already in a solution, it will begin to work more quickly. Most injections of drugs (IM, subcutaneous, and intradermal) are absorbed from body tissues; only intravenous injections completely bypass the absorption step and directly enter the bloodstream.

Not all of the drug may even reach the bloodstream. **Bioavailability** measures the amount of drug that is absorbed into the circulation. Bioavailability is influenced by drug solubility, dosage form, route of administration, pH values, and salt form, to name a few factors. One example of this concept is how the pH (a measure of the acidity or alkalinity) of different parts of the gastrointestinal (GI) tract can affect the absorption and thus the bioavailability of the drug. Some drugs are permanently charged, but most are weak acids or bases whose ionization is affected by pH. In other words, the drug can exist in either its ionized or its nonionized form, depending on the pH values of surrounding fluids.

The important aspect of ionization is that the nonionized (no charge or neutral) drug is absorbed through membranes, so it can be active, while the ionized (charged) form of the drug is not. The stomach is very acidic, at pH 1–2, whereas the intestines are about pH 4–5; farther along the GI tract, the alkalinity increases. This means that drugs such as aspirin, which are more in their nonionized form at an acidic pH, are better absorbed in acidic environments such as the stomach. Alkaline drugs such as quinidine become more nonionized in alkalinic environments and are therefore better absorbed as they progress through the GI tract.

Clinical pearl

Specially coated (enteric) tablets are designed to resist being absorbed in the stomach, where they may be irritating to the stomach lining.

Ultimately, drugs must be absorbed through membranes to reach their site of action. Drugs can pass through some membranes but not all. Mechanisms by which drugs pass through membranes include passive diffusion, facilitated diffusion, active transport, and passage through ion channels. These transfer processes will be discussed in chapters where they are pertinent. See Figure 1-10, which shows factors such as drug molecule size, ionization, and lipid solubility and their effects on membrane passage.

FIGURE 1-10 Variables That Affect Passage of Drugs Across Plasma Membranes

(a) size of drug molecule, (b) ionization of drug, (c) lipid solubility across the lipid cell membrane.

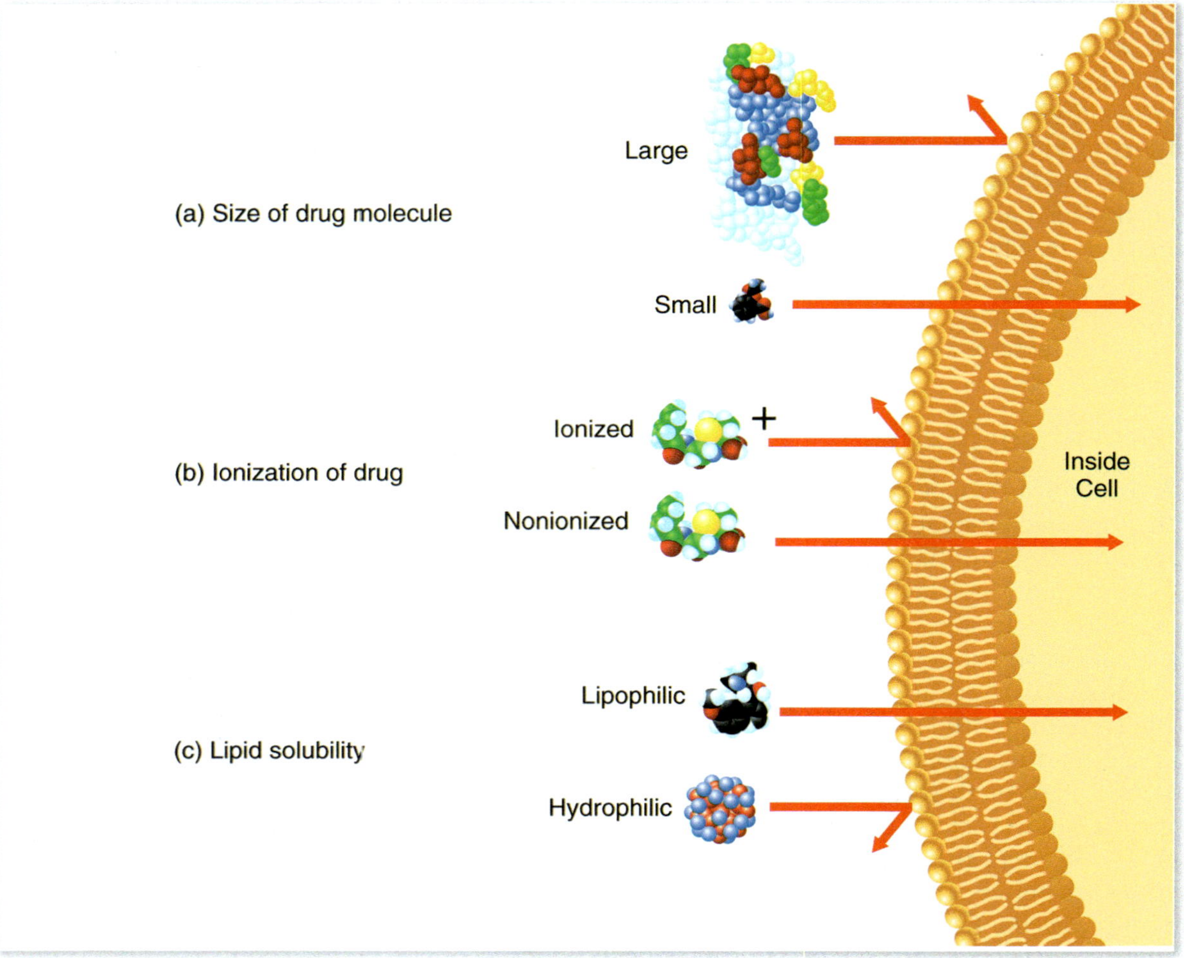

time for review

If you were in severe pain, would you rather have a morphine tablet or solution? Why?

Intravenous drug administration differs depending on whether the drug is given as a continuous infusion (IV drip) or as an intermittent dose (injected IV shot or bolus). A continuous infusion gives a regulated, consistent dosage over time without peaks and valleys in drug concentration. An intermittent intravenous dose has more peaks and troughs in drug concentration (see Figure 1-11).

FIGURE 1-11 Intermittent and Infusion Dosing

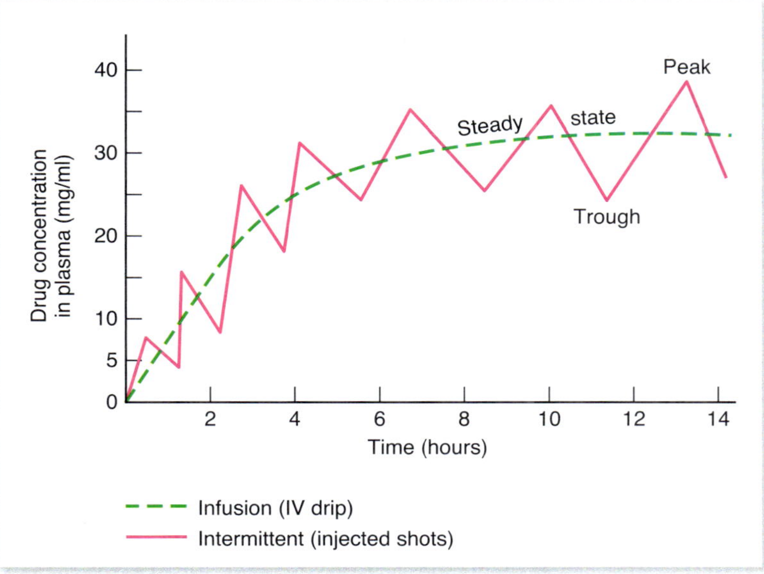

For some drugs, laboratory testing of blood levels is available to tell us whether an individual patient has enough drug in the blood to be effective or toxic. The effective blood level is considered the therapeutic blood level and has a defined **therapeutic range**. Below this level, the drug is likely less effective, and above this level, toxicity may result (see Table 1-4, which lists common drugs for which blood-level testing is available).

Clinical pearl

When testing blood levels, the timing of the blood draw relative to the dose is important for interpretation. Also, even if patients have identical serum drug concentrations, there may be different clinical responses among individuals.

TABLE 1-4 **Drugs with Blood-Level Tests and Therapeutic Ranges**

Drug Name	Therapeutic Range
theophylline	5–15 mcg/ml
digoxin	0.5–2 ng/ml
phenytoin	10–20 mcg/ml
lithium	0.6–1.2 meq/L
carbamazepine	4–12 mcg/ml
gentamicin	<2 mcg/ml
vancomycin	5–20 mcg/ml

Clinical pearl

The rate of absorption may be proportional to the rate of blood flow at the site. Sometimes drugs are administered in combination with epinephrine, which is a vasoconstrictor. When epinephrine is given with a local anesthetic, such as lidocaine, the decreased blood flow from vasoconstriction keeps much of the drug at the desired site; this may therefore decrease the risk of systemic side effects when just a local effect is desired.

1.7b Distribution

After absorption, the drug is distributed in the body. The major vehicle for distribution is via the bloodstream. As mentioned in the section on absorption, the drug must also distribute through membranes to reach certain active pharmacologic sites called receptors. Different drugs are able to distribute to different locations. The blood flow, fat, or water solubility of the drug and **protein binding** influence drug distribution.

Protein binding occurs when portions of the drug are bound to proteins in the bloodstream, such as albumin, and are thus unable to bind with active pharmacologic sites to have a desired effect. For example, if a person has low serum albumin (i.e., is malnourished), there is not as much protein for the drug to bind to; therefore, much of the drug will be free in the bloodstream. Because free, unbound drug is active drug, a patient with low albumin may have higher blood levels of free, active drug than someone with normal albumin and will show a greater drug response.

Drugs differ in their percentage of protein binding. The PDR includes information on protein-binding percentages. Knowledge of protein binding is important because protein-binding displacement is one mechanism by which drugs interact with each other. If there are only so many proteins for a drug to bind to and another drug is added to a patient whose proteins are already bound by a previous drug, the drugs will compete for placement on the protein. The one that is not bound will be free to find an active receptor site.

Volume of distribution (VD) describes the areas in the body where drugs can be distributed. Fat-soluble (lipophilic) drugs pass through fat more easily than through water. Fat-soluble drugs have an increased effect in patients with more fat, and water-soluble drugs have an increased effect in those with larger water compartments. Fat and water compartments change with age and are one explanation for why different doses may be needed in young and elderly patients. For example, the sedative diazepam (Valium®) is a fat-soluble drug. Obese patients may be sedated longer on a given dose of diazepam than lean patients.

1.7c Metabolism

After a drug has been absorbed and distributed, metabolism occurs because the body works to get rid of anything foreign. Before a drug can be excreted, it usually has to be metabolized so that it becomes more water-soluble and more able to leave the body via urine, feces, or sweat. The drug is broken down into several components or metabolites. Some metabolites of a drug are active and others are not. Metabolism may occur by means of chemical reactions, such as oxidation, conjugation, acetylation, or glucuronidation, to name a few.

One of the major organs for drug metabolism is the liver. The liver has a microsomal drug oxidation system called the cytochrome P450 system, which is responsible for metabolizing many drugs. These enzymes can be induced (increased in activity) or inhibited (decreased in activity). This is a common mechanism for drug interactions. Enzyme induction may explain why patients who drink alcohol frequently are more tolerant of the effects of alcohol—because the alcohol may be metabolized more quickly.

Drug doses can change depending on whether the liver enzymes are inducing or inhibiting, and there is no easy way to know other than to be aware of drugs that affect enzymes. See Table 1-5 for drugs that affect liver enzymes.

Clinical pearl

Some races have an increased frequency of a genetic deficiency of the enzyme that metabolizes alcohol and are therefore more susceptible to its effects. The field of research that studies genetic differences in drug response is called pharmacogenomics.

Table 1-5 Drugs That Affect Liver Enzymes

Inducers	Inhibitors
barbiturates	cimetidine
phenytoin	disulfuram
carbamazepine	allopurinol
rifampin	influenza vaccine

There is no good way to predict the liver's ability to metabolize drugs in a given patient. Some patients genetically lack enzymes to metabolize certain drugs. In addition, lab tests of liver function do not correlate with the body's ability to metabolize a drug, and elimination in the liver cannot be assessed quantitatively. Liver disease may indicate that a particular drug should not be used or should be dosed differently. Because the liver is a site of drug metabolism, it is also susceptible to drug-induced toxicity. More than 600 drugs have been associated with drug-induced liver toxicity. Alcohol and acetaminophen are two common ones, especially when used in combination.

LIFE SPAN CONSIDERATIONS

Age and Its Effect on Metabolism

Drug metabolism in children may be reduced at birth and mature along with age. The fetal liver has about one-third the drug metabolism capacity of the adult liver.

Drug metabolism in the elderly may be affected both by underlying diseases and by advancing age. Advancing age alone results in a reduction in liver mass by about 20%–30%. As a result of these changes, drug metabolism that depends on the liver may be reduced in the elderly. This may result in an exaggerated clinical response or intolerable adverse effects (e.g., propranolol causing severe bradycardia or an excessive feeling of tiredness). In general, this is why the dosages of drugs are usually reduced in children and the elderly.

1.7d Elimination

The last component of pharmacokinetics is elimination. Some drugs are eliminated after they are metabolized, and others are excreted unchanged in the urine. Still others are eliminated in feces or even through the skin or pulmonary system. Inhalation anesthesia requires that the gas pass from inspired air to the blood and brain. Drug action is terminated when the drug is eliminated in the lungs.

Renal excretion rate is affected by glomerular filtration, tubular secretion, and tubular reabsorption. Impaired renal function can prolong the effects of drugs eliminated by the kidneys because they will not be readily eliminated and will remain longer in the system.

Because drugs can be excreted in the urine, urine testing is becoming more common in the workplace. Urine testing can be used to screen patients for drug abuse or for poisoning identification. Whether the drug is fat- or water-soluble influences how long after ingestion it may be detected in the urine. Urine testing and even saliva testing are useful to monitor patients in drug rehabilitation programs. Tests differ in sensitivity and specificity.

Clinical pearl

The alcohol breath test is used to assess intoxication for DUIs because ethanol is excreted in expired air. Urine screens are used in the workplace to detect past and current medication use on the basis of excretion of drug metabolites (breakdown products) in the urine.

time for review

Why would patients with kidney disease or decreased kidney function, such as the elderly, be prescribed lower doses of a medication?

Now that we have completed the discussion of pharmacokinetics, see Figure 1-12, which relates its four phases.

FIGURE 1-12 Pharmacokinetics: The Whole Picture

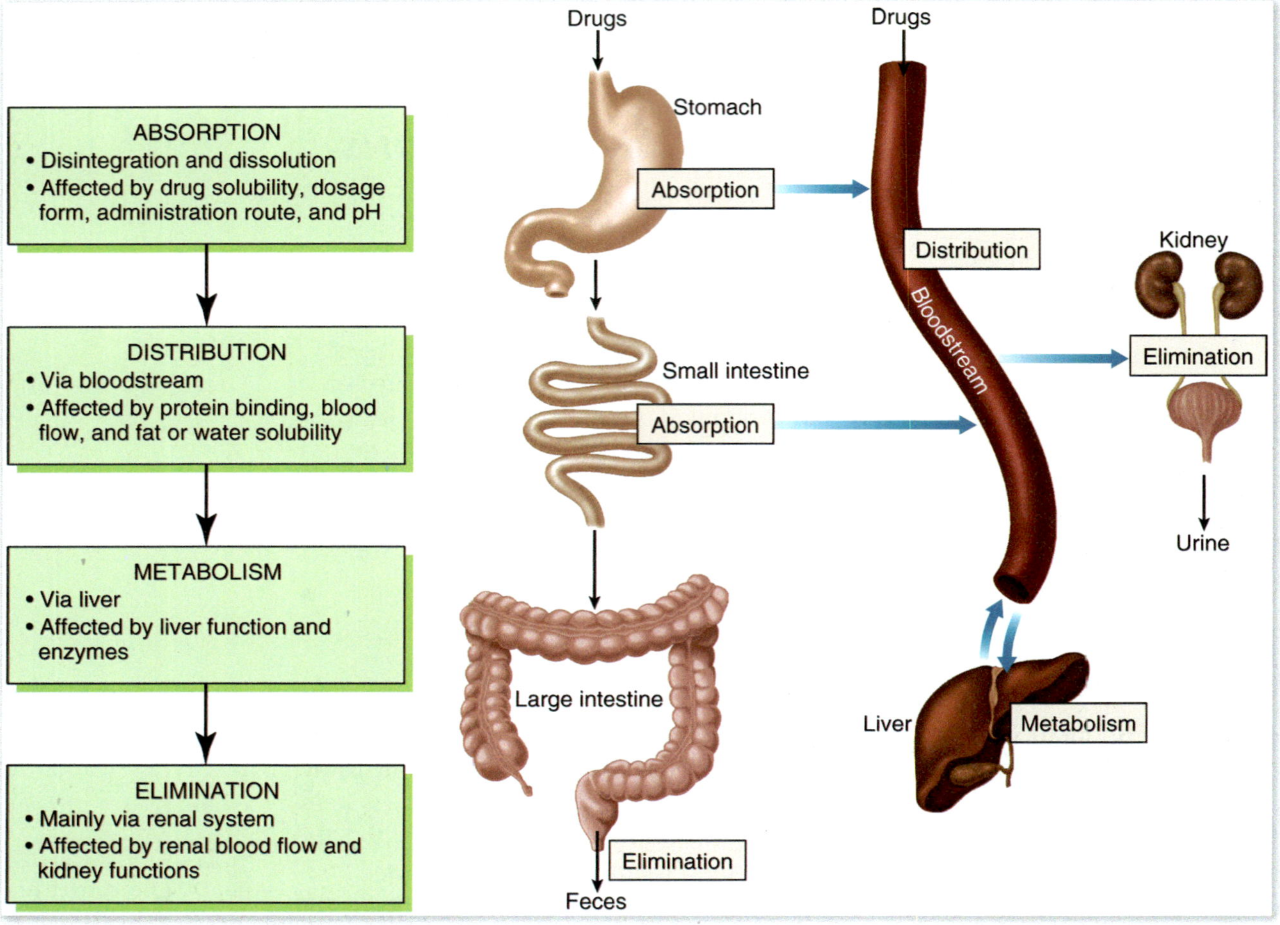

1.8 PHARMACODYNAMICS

As stated earlier, **pharmacodynamics** is what the drug does to the body. Once a drug is absorbed and distributed, drug action requires drug presence at a particular type of **receptor**. Receptors are targets for drugs; they are molecules located on the cell surface. This is where the action takes place. They are not, however, the only target for drugs; drugs also bind to carrier molecules and ion channels, for example—each of which will be discussed in upcoming chapters.

1.8a Selectivity

There are only so many receptors per cell and only certain kinds of receptors on different cells. Because most drugs produce several effects, **selectivity** refers to the extent to which a drug acts at one specific site or receptor. The more specific a drug can be on a particular cell or tissue, the more useful it is. Unfortunately, no drug acts with complete selectivity, which is why side effects occur. If you give a drug that kills a microorganism but it is not selective enough to avoid killing the patient, then the drug is not selective enough to be useful. Another example is the search for drugs that kill only cancer cells, not all living cells.

A drug produces a particular effect by combining chemically with a receptor on which it acts. When a drug binds to a receptor, one of the following can happen:

(1) An ion channel is opened or closed.

Example: Calcium-channel blockers inhibit excess calcium from entering myocardial tissue.

(2) Biochemical messengers are activated that initiate chemical reactions.

Example: Beta-adrenergic bronchodilators increase levels of cyclic 3,5-AMP, which causes smooth muscle relaxation.

(3) A normal cellular function is turned on or off.

Example: Antibiotics inhibit specific cellular functions that result in cell death.

1.8b Lock-and-Key Receptor Theory

A simplified description of interactions between drugs and receptors is the lock-and-key analogy. If the drug does not fit the receptor, no activity can occur. For example, current pain medications that have been derived from chemical variations of opium capitalize on this theory. Scientists worked with the lock-and-key theory to identify what parts of the chemical structure fit the receptor to cause analgesia and what parts cause side effects and dependence, and then they adjusted the chemistry to make more useful drugs. See Figure 1-13, which illustrates the lock-and-key theory.

FIGURE 1-13 The Lock-and-Key Receptor Theory: Which Drug Has Receptor Selectivity?

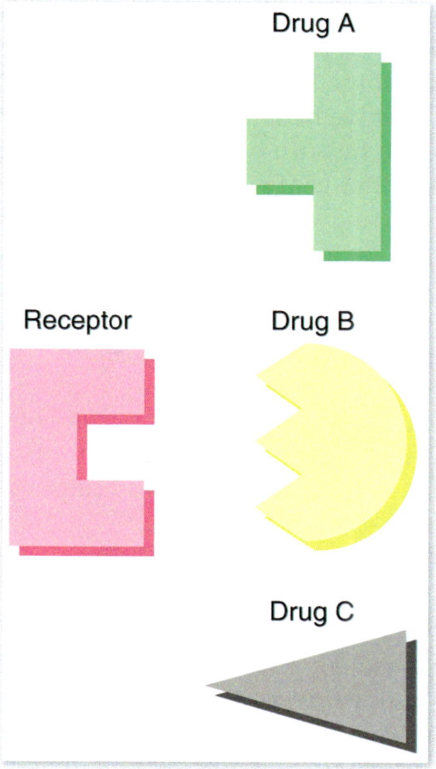

1.8c Racemic Mixtures

Many drugs are commercially available as a **racemic** mixture, meaning one that contains two different isomers. Isomers have the exact same chemical components, only bonded differently, and can be thought of as chemical mirror images. Another way of explaining this would be the fact that we have two hands. While they may not exactly be mirror images of each other, if you are right-handed, you can usually do more with this hand than your left. Each isomer usually has different activity or one is more potent than the other. An example is racemic epinephrine, which is made up of an L and a D isomer. The L isomer of epinephrine is 15 times more active than the D isomer. Isomer isolation is the target of a lot of pharmaceutical research, but the clinical importance is questionable—especially since the single-isomer products are more expensive. The single-isomer bronchodilator levalbuterol will be discussed further in Chapter 5.

1.8d Agonists Versus Antagonists

Learning Hint

The medical term *endo* means "within" and therefore refers to substances that are actually produced within the body, such as surfactants needed to keep the lungs open. *Exo* means "outside of"; exogenous surfactants are given to premature infants who are not producing endogenous surfactants.

The lock-and-key receptor theory explains the effects of chemicals on biologic systems. Drugs bind to cellular receptors according to their chemical structure, which starts biochemical reactions that can change cell physiology. The same explanation applies whether chemicals are endogenous (physiologically produced *within* the body) or exogenous (pharmacologically administered). However, drugs can bind with the receptor site and activate or block a response.

For example both **agonists** and **antagonists** can bind to a receptor; however, they differ in what they do once combined. Agonists are drugs with affinity for a receptor that cause a specific response. Affinity is the strength of binding between a drug and a receptor. Antagonists are also drugs with affinity for a receptor but have very little or no response when combined. Agonists activate the receptors. Antagonists combine at the same site but do not cause activation of the receptor. Drug antagonism can occur when the effect of one drug is lessened or blocked completely in the presence of another. An example of chemical antagonism is when protamine is used to neutralize the anticoagulant effects of heparin by forming an inactive heparin–protamine complex. This is desirable in cases of hemorrhage due to heparin overdoses for treatment of blood clots.

Drugs within a class differ in their affinity or likelihood of interacting with a receptor. If all drugs had to do was occupy a receptor to produce a pharmacologic effect, then all drugs acting on a receptor would produce the same effect. The reason this is not true is intrinsic activity, which can best be explained using numbers. Intrinsic activity is a measure of a drug's effectiveness in causing a response, or the **efficacy** of the drug at the receptor. For example, a drug with an intrinsic activity of 1 is a full agonist. A drug with an intrinsic activity of 0.5 is a partial agonist. An antagonist has intrinsic activity of 0 but does have affinity to bind. Both full and partial agonists want to bind to the receptor and thus have affinity, but a full agonist is more efficacious and causes a greater response.

1.8e Potency

Drug potency refers to the amount of drug required to produce the response desired. When the response is measured against drug concentrations, a dose–response relationship can be seen (please see Figure 1-14). Dose–response relationships are important for understanding how to titrate drugs to reach maximum efficacy. The lower the dose required to provide a certain effect, the more potent the drug is. Notice in Figure 1-14 that drug A and drug C are more potent (require less of a dose for the desired response) than drugs B and D.

FIGURE 1-14 Dose–Response Curves

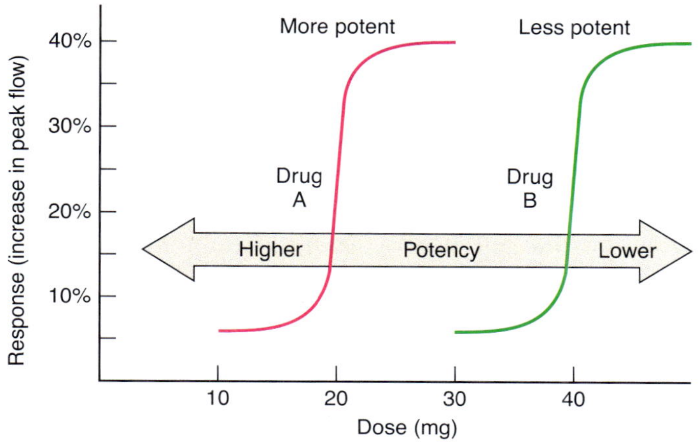

Drug A is more potent than drug B.
Drug A is equal to drug B's efficacy or response.

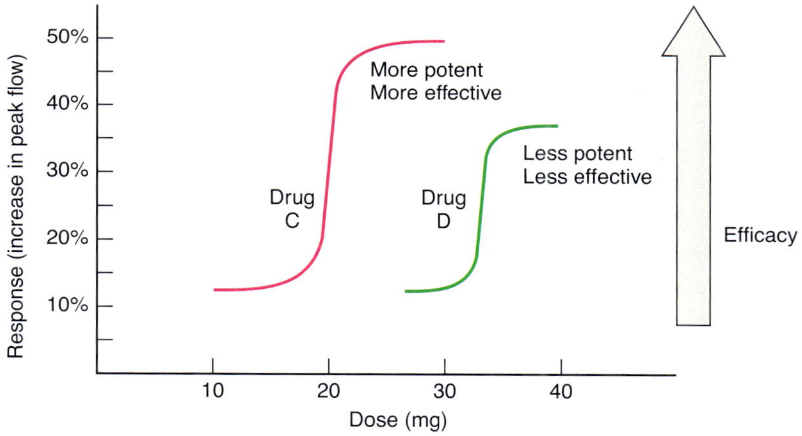

Drug C is more potent than drug D.
Drug C has greater efficacy than drug D.

Efficacy refers to the maximum effect a drug can produce. Unfortunately, the assumption that responses are directly proportional to occupancy at receptors is not valid. The fact that you are occupying a chair in class does not mean that you will learn something. Likewise, the fact that a drug is occupying a receptor does not mean that it will produce a therapeutic effect. Notice in Figure 1-14 that drugs A and B have equal efficacy, whereas drug C has greater efficacy than drug D.

1.8f Tolerance

Clinical pearl

Technically, *tolerance* is the term used for diminished responsiveness that occurs over time and repeated use, whereas *tachyphylaxis* is a more rapidly acquired tolerance after only a few doses.

Patients often ask, "Will this drug lose effectiveness with time?" The relationship between concentration and effect can change over time. Drugs can lose effectiveness because receptors change, are lost, are more readily degraded, or simply adapt. Receptor adaptation can be good and may explain why people become tolerant of side effects of drugs. However, receptor **tolerance** also means that an increased amount of the drug may be needed to produce the same therapeutic effect.

After a cell or tissue has been exposed to a drug for a period of time, it may become less responsive to further stimulation by that agent. This is called **desensitization**. An example of a drug class for which this occurs is the sympathomimetic drugs discussed in Chapter 5. The clinical significance is that desensitization may limit therapeutic response to sympathomimetic drugs when they are needed. Desensitization of beta-receptors to chronic beta-agonist use is a well-known phenomenon that will be discussed in Chapter 5.

Drug **dependence** is a related topic and can be physiologic or psychological. Do you need your coffee in the morning, or do you *need* your coffee in the morning? If patients have withdrawal symptoms when a drug is discontinued, they are dependent. Even laxatives can cause dependence, so that normal bowel movements may not occur after chronic stimulant laxative use.

1.8g Half-Life

Clinical pearl

Smoking can increase the metabolism of theophylline and thus decrease its half-life. Therefore, smokers may need higher theophylline doses than nonsmokers.

Once a drug is absorbed, attaches to a receptor, and is distributed, it is important to know how long it will remain in the body. Metabolism and excretion are two processes that are responsible for elimination of the drug from the body. By definition, the **half-life** ($T_{1/2}$) is the amount of time it takes for the concentration of the drug to decrease by half once it is administered. Some drugs have short half-lives and will not stay in the body long. Some drugs have long half-lives and remain in the body for longer periods of time. Dosing frequency may be different for drugs with short or long half-lives, and therefore half-life is also used to determine when a drug administered over time has reached **steady state**, or its maximum concentration in the body.

Learning Hint

Anything that slows the breakdown of a drug once it is in the body increases its half-life. For example, liver disease increases the half-life of many drugs, because the liver is a major organ for breaking down or metabolizing drugs.

Steady state means the amount of drug going in is the same as the amount being eliminated. Please again refer back to Figure 1-11. It takes approximately five to six half-lives to reach this steady state. For example if the half-life of a drug is 6 hours, steady state will be reached in 30 to 36 hours. These concepts are also useful in predicting how long it will take for most of the drug to be eliminated from the body. If the patient stops the drug today and it has a half-life of 5 to 6 hours, it will take about 30 to 36 hours (5 to 6 times the drug half-life) for most of the drug to be eliminated from the body. Liver disease may increase the half-life of some drugs that are metabolized by the liver, causing them to stay around longer and have greater-than-expected effects. Table 1-6 lists some common drug half-lives to show the variability that exists.

TABLE 1-6 Drug Half-Lives

Drug	Half-Life
digoxin	30–60 hours
aminoglycosides	2–4 hours
theophylline	7–9 hours
albuterol	2–5 hours
warfarin	0.5–3 days
heparin	1–2 hours

Because it can take a while to reach steady state and the patient may need immediate drug levels for therapeutic effect, a **loading dose** of such drugs as the antibiotic gentamicin or the antiseizure medication phenytoin are frequently used. Loading doses are given at a higher dose than a **maintenance dose** to achieve desired blood concentrations more quickly. Loading doses are used if a patient has not been on a drug before or when the receptors need to be saturated quickly for a quick response. After the initial loading dose is administered, smaller doses (maintenance doses) are needed to maintain adequate therapeutic levels.

1.8h Poisonings/Toxicity

All health-care professionals need to be aware of drug overdoses and poisonings. The study of drugs as they relate to poisonings and environmental toxins is called **toxicology**. It is estimated that there are 2 to 5 million poisonings a year in the United States, with the majority occurring in children younger than 6 years old. Adult poisoning may be intentional or occupational. Because reporting of poisonings is voluntary, the frequency of the problem is unknown.

Poison control centers operate regionally to provide information on poisonings with drugs, chemicals, household products, personal care products, and plants, as well as food poisonings and animal toxins. Information is usually provided on a 24-hour basis and includes management protocols. Childproof medication containers are one way to avoid poisonings.

Emetics (agents that induce vomiting) may be absolutely contraindicated, as in the case of ingestions of caustic agents, so they should not be used until advised by a medical professional. If a product such as a drain cleanser is caustic on ingestion, it can cause even more damage as it is brought back up through the esophagus or aspirated into the lungs. Another treatment of poisoning may include decreasing absorption by giving an adsorbent to bind with the toxic agent and inducing catharsis (bowel movements).

Activated charcoal is used to prevent absorption of some drugs, such as theophylline overdoses. While emesis can remove theophylline from the stomach if induced within 1 hour of ingestion, activated charcoal is effective any time after theophylline exposure. Other drugs have specific antidotes to antagonize the effects of poisoning, for example, *n*-acetylcysteine for acetaminophen (Tylenol®) poisoning and naloxone (Narcan®) for narcotic overdoses presenting as respiratory depression.

Clinical pearl

Often patients present with respiratory depression when central nervous system (CNS) depressants are taken in overdoses. Toxidromes are signs and symptoms consistent with toxic effects attributed to a particular class of drugs. For example, anticholinergic effects seen in toxicity include increased heart rate, decreased GI motility, pupil dilation, and altered mental status. If a patient presents with those symptoms, then anticholinergic toxicity may be suspected.

Learning Hint

Don't confuse absorption and adsorption. An *adsorbent* binds with a substance to prevent its *absorption.*

1.9 PHARMACOGENOMICS

Pharmacogenomics is a science that examines how genes can explain whether a drug will work or if it will be toxic to our bodies. Enzymes that metabolize drugs are genetically determined. Because of this, some patients may metabolize drugs faster or slower than the average person. This may cause the drug to have a greater effect in a slow or poor metabolizer, and possibly a poor effect—or no effect—in a rapid metabolizer, when compared to the average patient. There are many examples of how pharmacogenomics may help predict drug efficacy or toxicity, but we will provide an example pertinent to respiratory pharmacology.

There is a gene responsible for encoding the beta-2 adrenergic receptor located in the lungs. There are many different variants of this gene in the population. This may explain why some patients are less responsive to beta-2 agonists (bronchodilators) than other patients. The hope is that the science of pharmacogenomics will help optimize drug therapy in individual patients by increasing effectiveness, reducing toxicity, and avoiding unnecessary treatment.

1.10 PRESCRIPTION ORDERS

All drugs require a properly authorized prescription order. Hospitals may have protocols, standing orders, or established therapy guidelines for treating a particular disease. These protocols or guidelines exist to improve the quality of patient care and control costs. Please see Figure 1-15 for the components of a medication order.

FIGURE 1-15 Sample Medication Order.

Note that the DEA# represents the Drug Enforcement Agency number for prescribing controlled substances, as will be further explained in Chapter 11.

Name Jane Cleary Age 36

Address 3376 W. 141st St., Scottsdale Date July 1, 2015

This prescription will be filled generically unless physician signs on line stating "Dispense as written."

℞

Tetracycline 250 mg PO

Disp. #30

Sig. 1 qid take on an empty stomach

F. March

Dispense as Written Substitution Permissible

Frances March, M.D. 120 Madison Road Scottsdale, NY

DEA # ER639524 Ph. No. 685-9533

Frequently, medical abbreviations are used on medication orders. For a review of common medical abbreviations pertinent to drug therapy, see Table 1-7. It has been estimated that half of all medication errors occur at the stage of drug ordering. These errors include incorrect medication, dose, frequency, or route and are often compounded by illegible handwriting. Many jokes have been made about physicians' sloppy handwriting, but this problem is no laughing matter. A "do not use" list of commonly mistaken abbreviations exists due to this fact. Computerized physician order entry (CPOE) within hospitals and electronic transmission of outpatient prescriptions directly to pharmacies (called ePrescribing) should eliminate errors related to illegible handwriting. In addition, ePrescribing and CPOE can provide valuable assistance to the entire health-care team by integrating drug and patient information at the time of prescribing.

Most hospitals have formularies. This means that they only stock or dispense certain drugs from particular pharmacologic classes. A **formulary** is a list of drugs available in a particular health-care system. Committees (e.g., Pharmacy and Therapeutics Committee) that make decisions on what drugs to stock may also be involved in deciding what drugs should be prescribed and when. For example, some hospitals have eliminated levalbuterol from their formularies. They do not stock the medication, so it is not available to be prescribed by a physician. This is because levalbuterol is much more costly than albuterol and both drugs are thought to have equivalent bronchodilator efficacy and safety when prescribed as recommended.

Clinical pearl

The Joint Commission on Accreditation of Healthcare Organizations (JCAHO) has a website with a list of medical abbreviations that should *not* be used because they can be mistaken or confused with another abbreviation. For example, Q.D. (every day) and Q.O.D. (every other day) can be mistaken for each other, or the period between Q.D. can be mistaken for an "O." This can lead to too little or too much of a medication being administered. JCAHO suggests that "daily" and "every other day" be written out.

TABLE 1-7 Some Common Abbreviations

Abbreviation	Meaning
ac	Before meals
b.i.d.	Twice daily
cap	Capsule
cc	Cubic centimeter
$\bar{c}$	With
IM	Intramuscular
IV	Intravenous
L	Liter
ml	Milliliter
NPO	Nothing by mouth
pc	After meals
PO	By mouth
prn	As needed
q.	Every
q.h.	Every hour
q.i.d	Four times daily
q.2h.	Every 2 hours
q.3h.	Every 3 hours
q.4h.	Every 4 hours
Rx	Take
sig	Directions
stat	Immediately
tab	Tablet or tablets
t.i.d.	Three times daily
ut dict	As directed

Note: The abbreviation "cc" is on the JCAHO "do not use" list.

1.11 COMMONSENSE RULES

There are some classic safeguards that should be followed to ensure accurate medication administration. The basics are known as the six "rights"—the right drug, right dose, right patient, right time, right route, and right documentation. Before administering a drug, tell the patient the name and purpose of the drug. This is good patient education but also allows you to double-check the medication order if the patient gives you an unexpected response. The right dose may require calculations, or with the widespread use of unit doses, medications may be individually wrapped and labeled as a single dose. Although the right patient may seem obvious in the inpatient setting, the authors have seen confused patients in the wrong bed or answering "yes" to someone else's name. Therefore, *always check the patient's wrist tag*. Many hospitals have specific rules to follow when identifying patients, often requiring at least two reliable methods of patient identification. Medication timing may be routine at some institutions but sometimes may need to be individualized for patient response and application of pharmacologic principles. Route is important, because not all products have the same stability, and dose is influenced by route as well as speed of onset. Giving an IV injection of a product that is not soluble and is intended only for the IM route can be very dangerous.

It is wise to administer only medications prepared personally or by the pharmacist. Always check the drug stability and expiration date. Check for allergies and chart administration and results as promptly as possible. In this day and age, it is also important to be aware of your legal responsibilities in drug administration at the state and local or institutional level. Always remember to properly document drug administration according to your institution's policies.

time for review

Can you describe the six "rights" of medication administration?

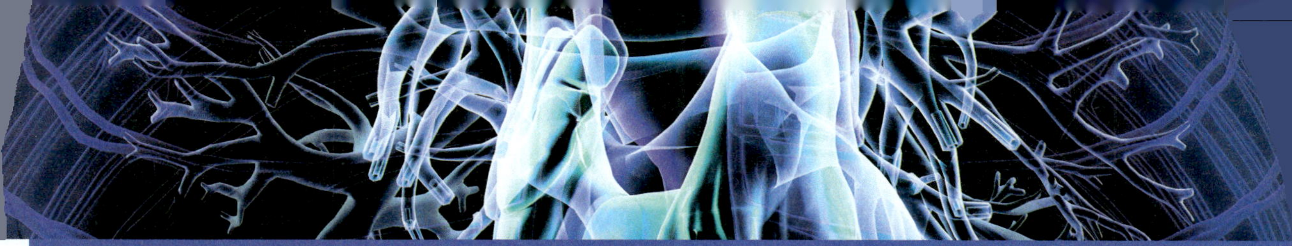

Summary

This chapter has two major goals. The first goal is to help you begin to feel comfortable reading drug information literature and to understand the organization and meaning of its contents. The second goal is to familiarize you with what the body does when a drug is introduced (pharmacokinetics) and what the drug does to the body (pharmacodynamics).

The earlier you are introduced to general principles of pharmacology, the more time you will have to apply them to drug classifications in the chapters that follow. It is never too soon to understand the risks of drugs and the responsibility that goes with drug administration. By being able to explain the rationale for drug use and possible side effects, you can be an effective member of the health-care team. This chapter has provided a sense of the need for lifelong learning about the dynamic topic of pharmacology.

REVIEW QUESTIONS

1. The drug name Proventil® HFA is a
   (a) chemical name
   (b) generic name
   (c) trade name
   (d) semiofficial name

2. The process of absorption, distribution, metabolism, and elimination (ADME) in the body is called
   (a) disintegration
   (b) bioavailability
   (c) pharmacokinetics
   (d) pharmacotherapy

3. A 42-year-old patient is in the hospital recovering from an asthma exacerbation. When the nurse brings him his oral medication, he says that it looks different than his white pill at home. What could explain this?
   (a) different manufacturer of the drug
   (b) drug error
   (c) patient confusion
   (d) change in dose
   (e) all of the above

4. After a drug is absorbed, which factors can affect drug distribution?
   (a) protein binding
   (b) fat solubility
   (c) water solubility
   (d) all of the above
   (e) none of the above

5. Match the following prescription abbreviations with their definition:

(a) q.i.d.	(1) as needed
(b) prn	(2) intramuscular
(c) IM	(3) nothing by mouth
(d) b.i.d.	(4) twice a day
(e) NPO	(5) four times daily

6. Define and explain the importance of the half-life of a drug.
7. Which route(s) of administration would you recommend in the following scenarios?
   (a) A home care patient has severe nausea.
   (b) A rapid onset is needed to treat an emergency in the hospital.
   (c) A patient is NPO.
   (d) A patient has a chronic respiratory inflammatory disease that requires corticosteroids that have many systemic side effects.
   (e) An executive smoker is trying to quit and needs nicotine replacement therapy.
8. Explain the relationship between pH and drug absorption.
9. Contrast agonists and antagonists.
10. What are the four phases of new drug testing and approval by the FDA?
11. Contrast the drug interactions of synergism, additive, and potentiation.
12. Explain this statement: "All allergies or hypersensitive reactions are ADRs, but not all ADRs are allergies."

Chapter 2

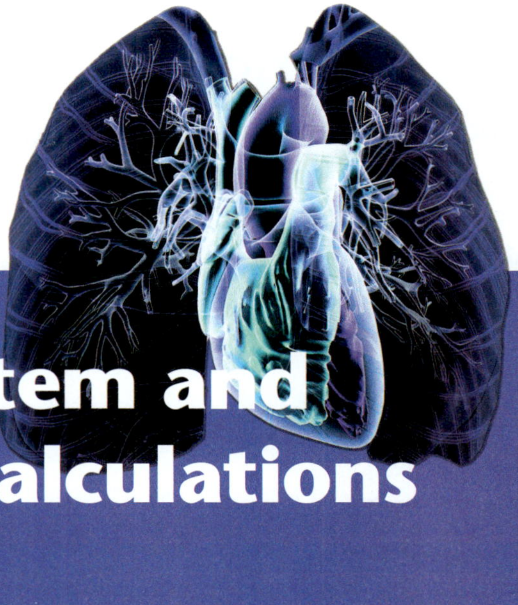

The Metric System and Drug Dosage Calculations

OBJECTIVES

Upon completion of this chapter you will be able to

- Define key terms relevant to drug dosage calculations.
- Perform conversions of units of measurement within the metric system.
- Perform conversions between units of measurement in the metric and English systems.
- Calculate strength of solutions in percentage forms.
- Perform drug dosage calculations.

KEY TERMS

base
cancelling units
English system of measurement
exponent
factor-label method or fraction method
gram
liter
meter
metric system of measurement
percentage of solution
proportion
ratio solution
scientific notation
solute
solution
solvent
volume/volume solution
weight/volume solution

ABBREVIATIONS

BSA	body surface area
c	centi-
cc	cubic centimeter
d	deci-
g	gram
gtt	drops
k	kilo-
kg	kilogram
l	liter
mc	micro-
m	meter
m	milli-
mcg	microgram
mg	milligram
ml	milliliter
SI	Système International
USCS	United States Customary System
v/v	volume/volume
w/v	weight/volume

Whereas Chapter 1 gave you the basics of the language of pharmacology, this chapter will give you the mathematical language of medicine. Many respiratory drugs form aerosols from various percentage strengths of solutions that are then administered via the inhalation route. In addition, many of the dosages are in milligrams or micrograms, and some conversions are necessary to other metric units. Therefore you need knowledge of strengths of solution and the metric system to perform drug dosage calculations.

Although most respiratory medications are packaged in *single-unit dosages* and are already premixed at a standard dose for you to aerosolize, occasions may arise when you will need to deviate from that standard premixed dose. You may have to adjust the dosage because of factors such as patient size or age, or the concentration of the medication on hand may be different than what is ordered. For example, a particular drug may be ordered to be given at 5 milligrams/kilogram (mg/kg) of body weight. To find the right amount to administer, you must be able to convert the patient's body weight in pounds to kilograms and then calculate how many milligrams need to be delivered from the strength of solution you have on hand. The process may seem complicated, but it really isn't if you have a basic understanding of the following concepts:

- Exponential powers of 10
- Systems of measurement
- The metric system
- Strengths of solution

This chapter will give you a solid understanding of each of these concepts so that you can perform drug dosage calculations. Make sure you understand each section and the example calculations completely before you move on, as each section builds on the ones before.

2.1 EXPONENTIAL POWERS OF 10

2.1a Exponents

The **metric system of measurement** is based on the powers of 10. Therefore understanding the powers of 10 will allow you to understand the basis of the metric system.

To understand the powers of 10, we need to review some terminology. Consider the expression b^n, where b is called the **base** and n is the **exponent.** The n represents the number of times that b is multiplied by itself. Please see Figure 2-1.

FIGURE 2-1 The Exponential Expression

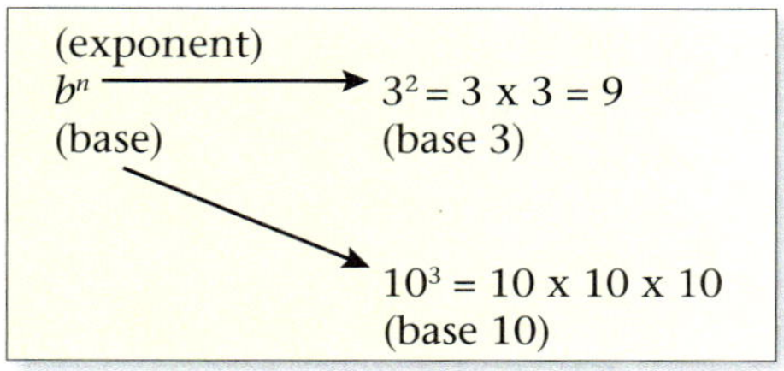

If we use 10 as the base, we can develop an exponential representation of the powers of 10 as follows:

$$10^0 = 1 \quad \text{(mathematically, any number that has an exponent of 0 = 1)}$$

$$10^1 = 10$$

$$10^2 = 10 \times 10 = 100$$

$$10^3 = 10 \times 10 \times 10 = 1{,}000$$

$$10^4 = 10 \times 10 \times 10 \times 10 = 10{,}000$$

$$10^5 = 10 \times 10 \times 10 \times 10 \times 10 = 100{,}000$$

$$10^6 = 10 \times 10 \times 10 \times 10 \times 10 \times 10 = 1{,}000{,}000$$

Thus far we have discussed positive exponents that result in numbers equal to or greater than 1. However, small numbers that are less than 1 can also be represented in exponential notation. In this case we use negative exponents. A negative exponent can be thought of as a fraction. For example:

$$10^{-1} = \frac{1}{10} = 0.1$$

$$10^{-2} = \frac{1}{10} \times \frac{1}{10} = 0.01$$

$$10^{-3} = \frac{1}{10} \times \frac{1}{10} \times \frac{1}{10} = 0.001$$

$$10^{-4} = \frac{1}{10} \times \frac{1}{10} \times \frac{1}{10} \times \frac{1}{10} = 0.0001$$

$$10^{-5} = \frac{1}{10} \times \frac{1}{10} \times \frac{1}{10} \times \frac{1}{10} \times \frac{1}{10} = 0.00001$$

$$10^{-6} = \frac{1}{10} \times \frac{1}{10} \times \frac{1}{10} \times \frac{1}{10} \times \frac{1}{10} \times \frac{1}{10} = 0.000001$$

Clinical pearl

In Chapter 1, we discussed JCAHO standards for medical abbreviations. This body also recommends that one never write a 0 by itself after a decimal point (write 1 mg, not 1.0 mg) and always use a 0 before a decimal point (0.1 mg). This helps prevent the decimal point from being missed.

Clinical pearl

In medicine we often use numbers that are extremely large (there are about 25,000,000,000 blood cells circulating in an adult's body) and extremely small (0.0000005 meter is the size of some microscopic organisms). It is often useful to write these numbers in a more convenient (or shorthand) form based on their powers of 10. This abbreviated form is known as ***scientific notation****. The rule is to move the decimal point to a place where you have one integer to the left of the decimal point and to note the appropriate power of 10 based on the number of spaces (powers of 10) moved. For example 25,000,000,000 becomes 2.5×10^{10} since you moved the decimal 10 spaces to the left. The number 0.0000005 becomes 5×10^{7}. Note that if the number is less than 1, the exponent is negative, and if greater than 1, the exponent is positive.*

2.2 SYSTEMS OF MEASUREMENT

2.2a United States Customary System

There are two major systems of measurement in use in the world today. The United States Customary System (USCS) is used in the United States and Myanmar (formerly Burma), and the Système International (SI) is used everywhere else—especially in health care (including in the United States). The SI system is also known as the International System of Units or metric system of measurement. The metric system is also the system used by drug manufacturers.

The USCS system is based on the British Imperial System and uses several different designations for the basic units of length, weight, and volume. We commonly call this the **English system of measurement**. For example in the English system, volumes can be expressed as ounces, pints, quarts, gallons, pecks, bushels, or cubic feet. Distance can be expressed in inches, feet, yards, and miles. Weights are measured in ounces, pounds, and tons. This may be the system you are most familiar with, but it is not the system of choice used throughout the world and in the medical profession. That is because the English system is very cumbersome to use because it has no common base. It is very difficult to know the relationships between these units because they are not based on powers of 10 in an orderly fashion, as in the metric system. For example how many gallons are in a peck? Just what the heck is a peck? How many inches are in a mile? These all require extensive calculations and the memorization of certain equivalent values, whereas with the metric system you simply move the decimal point by the appropriate power of 10.

Clinical pearl

The apothecary system, developed in the 1700s, included some measurements that are still used today. For example the pint, quart, and gallon are derived from this system. Apothecary measurements for calculating liquid doses of drugs include the minim and the fluid dram. Solids are measured in grams, scruples, drams, ounces, and pounds. Two unique features of the apothecary system are the use of Roman numerals and the placement of the unit of measure before the Roman numeral. However, the metric system is now used to calculate drug dosages because the apothecary system is less precise.

PATIENT & FAMILY EDUCATION

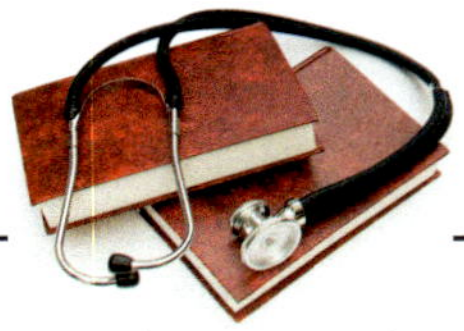

Health-care professionals need to be aware that families continue to use inaccurate devices, such as household spoons, for measuring liquid medications. They should encourage the use of more accurate devices such as the oral dosing syringe. Dosing errors should be considered when health-care professionals encounter patients who appear to be failing treatment or experiencing dose-related toxicity.

Learning Hint

Try to visualize the physical relationships between the metric and English systems. For example, a meter is a little more than a yard, a kilometer is about two-thirds of a mile, and a liter is a little more than a quart. This visual comparison becomes important if, for example, you are ordered to immediately withdraw an endotracheal tube 2 centimeters.

2.2b The Metric System

Most scientific and medical measurements use the metric system. The metric system employs three basic units of measure for length, volume, and mass; these are the **meter**, **liter**, and **gram**, respectively. In the sciences the term *mass* is commonly preferred (over *weight*), as mass refers to the actual amount of matter in an object, whereas weight is the force exerted on a body by gravity. In space or at zero gravity, objects have mass but are indeed weightless. However, because current health care is confined mostly to Earth, where there are gravitational forces, in this text we will use the term *weight.* Table 2-1 lists metric designations for the three basic units of measure, along with an approximate English system equivalent.

TABLE 2-1 Metric and English System Comparison

Type	Unit	English System Equivalent (approximate)
Length	meter	Slightly more than 1 yard
Volume	liter	Slightly more than 1 quart
Mass/weight	gram	About 1/30 of an ounce

Again notice that there are only three basic types of measure (meter, liter, and gram), and the metric system has only one base unit per measure. Because the metric system is a base-10 system, prefixes are used to indicate different powers of 10. Conversion within the metric system simply involves moving the decimal point the appropriate direction and power of 10 according to the prefix before the unit of measure. For example the prefix *kilo-* means 1,000 times, or 10^3. Therefore 1 kilogram is equal to 1,000 grams. See Table 2-2 for the common prefixes and their respective powers of 10.

TABLE 2-2 Common Prefixes of the Metric System

Thousands	Hundreds	Tens	Base Units			Tenths	Hundredths	Thousandths
kilo-	*hecto-*	*deca-*	*liter, meter, or gram*			*deci-*	*centi-*	*milli-*
(k)	(h)	(da)	(l)	(m)	(g)	(d)	(c)	(m)
10^3	10^2	10^1	10^0 or 1			10^{-1}	10^{-2}	10^{-3}

It can be seen from Table 2-2 that a kilometer is 1,000, or 10^3, meters. A centigram can be expressed as 0.01 gram, one-hundredth of a gram, or 10^{-2} gram. The ease of working with the metric system is that to change from one prefix to another, you simply move the decimal point to the correct place. In other words to convert within the system, simply move the decimal point for each power of 10 according to the desired prefix. For example to convert grams to kilograms, move the decimal point three places to the left. Therefore 1,000 grams equal 1 kilogram.

Learning Hint

The prefix deci- *can be associated with "decade," meaning 10 years;* centi- *can be associated with cents, there being 100 cents in a dollar; and* milli- *can be associated with a millipede, the bug with 1,000 legs. Biology note: Millipedes don't actually have 1,000 legs; it just seems like they do*

2.2c Example Calculation 1

In calculating drug dosages we often need to convert between grams and milligrams or between liters and milliliters. A common conversion might be something like "500 milliliters is equal to how many liters?" We know from Table 2-2 that 500 milliliters (ml) is equal to 0.5 liter (l) because we can simply move the decimal point three places (or powers of 10) to the left to find the equivalent value. Here we are starting with milliliters and going to the base unit of liters.

2.2d Example Calculation 2

How many grams are equal to 50 kilograms (kg)? Again, knowing the prefixes and powers of 10, we can move the decimal point three places (powers of 10) to the right to give the answer of 50,000 grams (g).

Refer to Table 2-3 for a more complete listing of prefixes that can be used in the metric system. This knowledge of the metric system will prove invaluable as you work in the medical profession—and even just if you travel outside of the United States. (That is, of course, unless you go to Myanmar.)

BVT Lab

Flashcards are available for this chapter at www.BVTLab.com.

Learning Hint

You should know the common prefixes in Table 2-2 and the micro- prefix in Table 2-3 because they are used frequently in medicine. Always check your result to see if it makes sense. For example a common mistake is to move the decimal point in the wrong direction. If you did that in Example Calculation 1, you would have erroneously said that 500 milliliters is equal to 500,000 liters. If you think about this, you would know that 500 comparatively very small units (milliliters) cannot possibly equal 500,000 comparatively larger units (liters).

Learning Hint

Yotta- is the prefix that means 10^{24} power—that is, 1 with 24 zeros after it. That certainly is a "yotta" zeros. The mass of the earth is 5,983 yottagrams.

TABLE 2-3 Metric System Prefixes and Abbreviation

Prefix	Power of 10	Meaning	Abbreviation
giga-	10^9	one billion	G
mega-	10^6	one million	M
kilo-	10^3	one thousand	k
hecto-	10^2	one hundred	h
deca-	10^1	ten	da
deci-	10^{-1}	one-tenth	d
centi-	10^{-2}	one-hundreth	c
milli-	10^{-3}	one-thousandth	m
micro-	10^{-6}	one-millionth	mc
nano-	10^{-9}	one-billionth	n

Note: Remember that the base units of liters, meters, and grams are equal to 10^0 or 1. Because the handwritten symbol *μ* looks almost exactly like the letter *m* and is therefore a frequent cause of overdoses, the abbreviation *mc* is preferred in the medical field for micro.

time for review

An IV solution of 1,500 ml is equal to how many liters?

One final note before we go on: It has been determined that 1 cubic centimeter (cc) is approximately the same volume as 1 milliliter (ml). Therefore, 1 cc = 1 ml (see Figure 2-2). You may hear someone say there is a 500-cc IV solution on hand, while someone else may say there is a 500-ml solution; they are both saying the same thing. JCAHO standards recommend the use of ml or milliliters because cc can be mistaken for other abbreviations when it is written carelessly.

time for review

What are some of the advantages of the metric system?

2.2e Conversion of Units

You should now be able to work comfortably in the metric system; but what if you need to convert an English unit to a metric unit? For example in the introduction to this chapter we said that a certain drug's dosage schedule was 5 milligrams per kilogram of body weight. What is the relationship between pounds in the English system and kilograms in the metric system?

FIGURE 2-2 **1 cc = 1 ml**

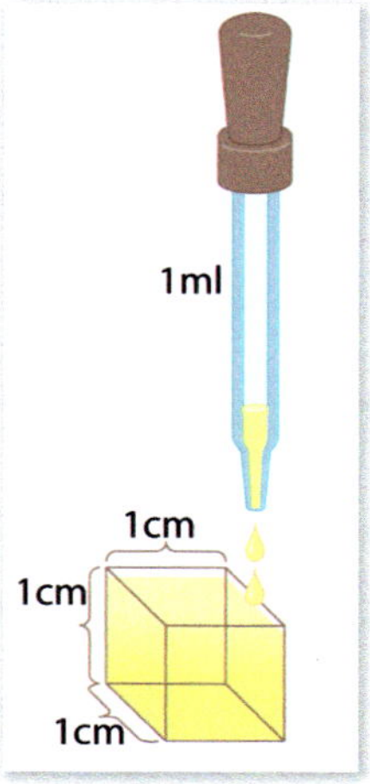

The following is a method for changing units or converting between the English and metric systems. This method is sometimes referred to as the **factor-label method** or **fraction method.** This method allows your starting units to cancel or divide out until you reach your desired unit. There are two basic steps. First write down your starting value, with its unit, as a fraction with the number 1 as the denominator. Because the denominator is 1, the numerical value is the same as the starting value itself.

The second step involves placing the units you started with in the denominator of the next fraction to divide or cancel out, and placing the unit you want to convert to in the numerator, along with the corresponding equivalent values. The quantities in the numerator and denominator must be equivalent values in different units! Because the values are equivalent, this is the same as multiplying by 1, which does not change the value of the mathematical expression. This allows you to treat the units as in the multiplication of fractions and "cancel" them out. Notice that by carefully placing the units so that **cancelling units** is possible, the units can be converted.

2.2f Example Calculation 3

How many inches are there in 1 mile?

First put your starting value, with its unit, as a fraction with 1 in the denominator.

$$\frac{1 \text{ mile}}{1}$$

Next put miles in the denominator and the desired unit in the numerator with equivalent values. You know that 1 mile = 5,280 feet, so

$$\frac{1 \cancel{\text{mile}}}{1} = \frac{5,280 \text{ feet}}{1 \cancel{\text{mile}}}$$

You have cancelled out miles, but you need to get to inches. Just continue the process until you reach the desired unit.

BVT Lab

Visit www.BVTLab.com to explore the student resources available for this chapter.

$$\frac{1 \text{ mile}}{1} = \frac{5,280 \text{ feet}}{1 \text{ mile}} \times \frac{12 \text{ inches}}{1 \text{ feet}} = 63,360 \text{ inches}$$

2.2g Example Calculation 4

How many seconds are there in 8 hours?

$$\frac{8 \text{ hours}}{1} \times \frac{60 \text{ minutes}}{1 \text{ hour}} \times \frac{60 \text{ seconds}}{1 \text{ minute}} = 28{,}800 \text{ seconds}$$

2.2h Factor-Label Method to Convert Between Systems

You could try to memorize the hundreds of conversions between the English and metric systems, but that would be nearly impossible. All you really need to memorize is one conversion for each of the three units of measure. This will allow you to "bridge" between the systems. The conversions you need to know are:

1 in. = 2.54 cm	used for units of length
2.2 lb = 1 kg	used for units of mass or weight
1.06 qt = 1 liter	used for units of volume

2.2i Example Calculation 5

One foot is equal to how many centimeters? There is an equivalency somewhere for feet and centimeters, but you don't need to know it as long as you know the factor-label method and the conversion for distance.

To answer the question of how many centimeters are in 1 foot,

$$\frac{1 \text{ foot}}{1} \times \frac{12 \text{ inches}}{1 \text{ foot}} \times \frac{2.54 \text{ cm}}{1 \text{ inch}} = 30.48 \text{ cm}$$

2.2j Example Calculation 6

If an individual weighs 150 lb and the drug dosage order is 10 mg/kg, how much drug should he receive?

First, you must change pounds to kilograms; therefore write the given weight as a fraction with 1 in the denominator. Then place the unit you want to cancel (pounds) in the denominator and the unit you want to convert to (kilograms) in the numerator of the next fraction.

$$\frac{150 \text{ pounds}}{1} \times \frac{1 \text{ kilogram}}{2.2 \text{ pounds}} = 68.18 \text{ kilograms}$$

Because the dose reads 10 mg/kg, this patient should receive 10 × 68.18 mg or 681.8 mg of the drug. You then have to be practical, working with the dosage units available; so round the dose appropriately—that is, to 682 mg.

time for review

A quart of blood is equal to how many milliliters?

2.3 DRUG DOSAGE CALCULATIONS

2.3a Solutions

Many drugs are given in **solution** form. A solution is a chemical and physical homogeneous mixture of two or more substances. Solutions contain a **solute** and a **solvent.** A solute is either a liquid or a solid that is dissolved in a liquid to form a solution. The solvent is the liquid that dissolves the solute. For example you can make the solution hot coffee by dissolving granules of instant coffee (solute) in hot water (solvent).

Drug solutions can be made by dissolving either a liquid or a solid solute, which represents the active drug, in a solvent such as sterile water or saline solution to form a solution that is delivered to the patient through various routes of administration. If the solute being dissolved is a solid, such as a powder, the resulting solution is termed a **weight/volume** (w/v) **solution**, where the *w* represents weight or amount of solute and the *v* represents the total amount of solution. One can also have a **volume/volume** (v/v) **solution**, in which the first *v* represents the volume of the liquid solute and the second *v* represents the volume of the solution (see Figure 2-3). A delicious nondrug example of this is mixing liquid chocolate syrup (solute) in hot milk (solvent) to form the solution hot chocolate. (Don't ask about the marshmallows.)

FIGURE 2-3 w/v and v/v Solutions

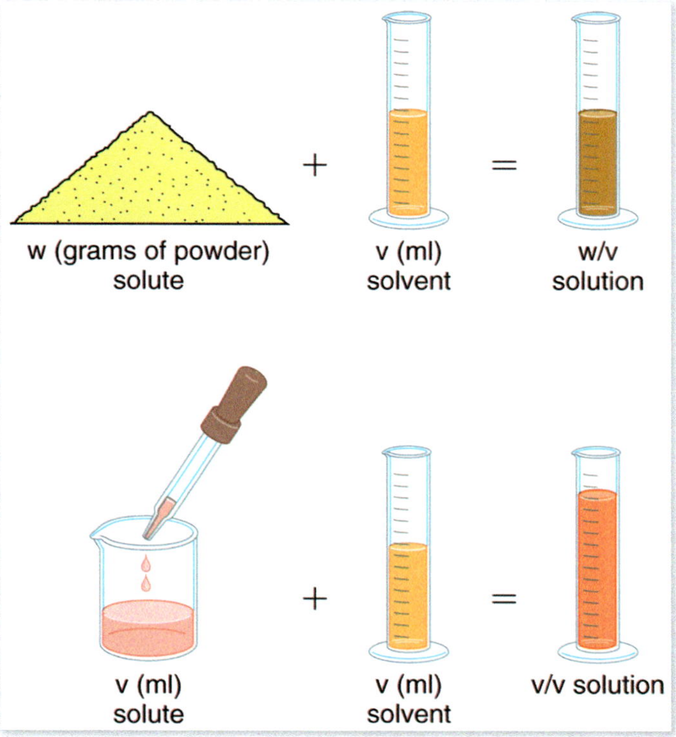

Learning Hint

The SOLVEnt is the one that disSOLVEs the solute.

2.3b Percentage Solutions

One way the potency of a drug can be described is by stating its **percentage of solution**, which is the strength of the solution expressed as parts of the solute (drug) per 100 ml of solution. After all that is what a percent is—some number related to 100. Remember that the solute can be either a solid or a liquid. If the solute is dissolved in a solid form, it will be expressed in grams per 100 ml of solution (w/v solution). If the solute is liquid, it will be expressed in milliliters (v/v solution).

For example a 20% saltwater or saline solution contains 20 g of salt (solid solute) dissolved in enough water (solvent) to create 100 ml of solution. We can use this information, coupled with proportions, to begin to solve drug dosage problems. The majority of drug dosage calculations can be solved by setting up simple proportions. A **proportion** is a statement that compares two conditions.

In general, the proportion

$$\frac{a}{b} = \frac{c}{d}$$

is equivalent to the equation $ad = bc$. Sometimes it is said that the product of the means (b and c) equals the product of the extremes (a and d). This is also known as *cross-multiplying*, so

$$\text{if } \frac{a}{b} = \frac{c}{d}, \text{ then } ad = bc$$

2.3c Setting Up Proportions

Armed with your previous knowledge from this chapter, you can solve drug dosage calculations with proportions in two basic steps. First set up a proportion of the *dose on hand* related to the *desired dose*. Second make sure all units are equal, then cross-multiply and solve the equation. See Figure 2-4, which illustrates these steps.

FIGURE 2-4 Steps to Solve Drug Dosage Calculations

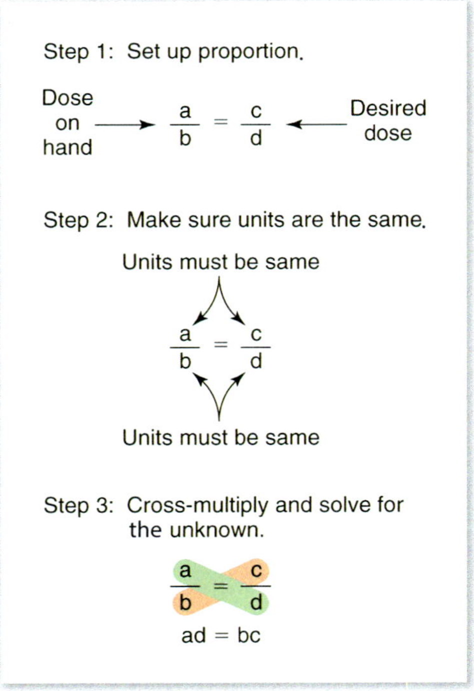

Several calculation examples follow. Notice that, although they all contain different information, they can all be solved using the same three-step process.

2.3d Example Calculation 7

How much salt is needed to make 1,000 ml of a 20% solution?

First, put down what you know, or your dose on hand:

$$20\%\text{ solution} = \frac{20\text{ g of salt}}{100\text{ ml of solution}}$$

Now place this into a proportion and relate it to your desired dose.

$$\begin{array}{ccc} \text{Dose on hand} & : & \text{Desired dose} \\ \dfrac{20\text{ g of salt}}{100\text{ ml of solution}} & = & \dfrac{x\text{ g of salt}}{1{,}000\text{ ml of solution}} \end{array}$$

The *x* g of salt represents how much salt is needed. The left side of the equation is what is known, or the dose on hand, and the right side is the unknown amount of the solute (in this case, salt) needed to make the final solution.

Solving by cross-multiplying,

$$\frac{20\text{ g of salt}}{100\text{ ml of solution}} = \frac{x\text{ g of salt}}{1{,}000\text{ ml of solution}}$$

$$20 \times 1{,}000 = 100x$$

$$20{,}000 = 100x$$

Divide both sides of the equation by the amount in front of *x* to find out what *x* is by itself:

$$\frac{20{,}000}{100} = \frac{\cancel{100}x}{\cancel{100}}$$

$$200 = x$$

$$x = 200$$

Learning Hint

After setting up the proportion, always ask yourself the catchy phrase, "Are my units congruent (equal or the same)?" This habit will help to ensure proper results.

So to make 1,000 ml of a 20% salt solution, you can take 200 g of salt and add enough water to fill a container to the 1,000-ml mark.

In this example 1,000 ml could have been given as the equivalent 1 liter. When that is the case, before cross-multiplying, you must make sure that all your units in the numerator and denominator are the same.

Clinical pearl

Normally the drug albuterol is mixed with a diluent such as saline solution or sterile water to allow it to be nebulized over a longer period of time. This diluent does not decrease the amount of drug or weaken the amount of drug given to the patient. In this example, there are 5 mg of the active drug albuterol in the solution, regardless of whether 3 ml or 5 ml of diluent are added. Only the nebulization or delivery time is increased. We will have more to say about this in Chapter 4, where we will discuss aerosol delivery devices.

2.3e Example Calculation 8

The bronchodilator drug albuterol is ordered to be given as 5 mg per aerosol dose. You have a 0.5% solution on hand. How many milliliters of drug solution should you deliver?

$$\text{What is known: } \frac{0.5\text{ g of albuterol}}{100\text{ ml of solution}}$$

$$\text{Proportion set up to what is needed: } \frac{0.5\text{ g of albuterol}}{100\text{ ml of solution}} = \frac{5\text{ mg of albuterol}}{x\text{ ml of solution}}$$

Before solving, convert the 0.5 g to 500 mg so the units are the same as the units in the denominator.

$$\frac{500 \text{ mg of albuterol}}{100 \text{ ml of solution}} = \frac{5 \text{ mg of albuterol}}{x \text{ ml of solution}}$$

$$500x = 500$$

$$x = 1$$

Therefore you need to draw up and deliver 1 ml of the drug solution to the patient.

2.3f Example Calculation 9

Clinical pearl

For some drugs, manufacturers have developed special systems for measuring doses. For example many types of insulin are available, but they are all measured in units.

Even if a drug such as heparin, insulin, or penicillin is given in units or international units, rather than grams or milligrams, you can solve the problem exactly the same way. If a solution of penicillin has 2,000 units/ml, how many milliliters would you give to deliver 250 units of the drug?

Dose on hand : Desired dose

$$\frac{2{,}000 \text{ U of penicillin}}{1 \text{ ml}} = \frac{250 \text{ U of penicillin}}{x \text{ ml}}$$

$$2{,}000x = 250$$

$$x = 0.125 \text{ ml}$$

Therefore 0.125 ml of the 2,000-unit solution can be given to deliver 250 units of penicillin to the patient.

time for review

You have a 10% drug solution on hand, and the order states to deliver 100 mg of drug. How many milliliters would you deliver?

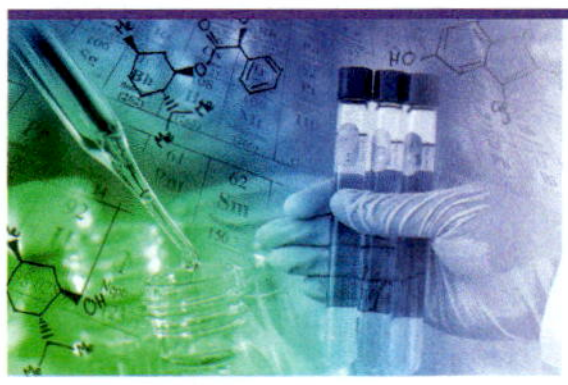

CONTROVERSY

It has been shown that many medication errors occur each year. Controversy exists over how many mistakes go unreported or unnoticed and what factors lead to these errors. What if you make a medication delivery or calculation error? What steps should you take? Whom should you notify? How can medication errors be prevented?

2.3g Ratio Solutions

Another possible means of expressing the strength of solution is by using a ratio instead of a percentage. A **ratio solution** represents the parts of the solute related to the parts of the solution. For example epinephrine is used in the treatment of anaphylactic shock and is usually administered IV in a 1:10,000 ratio. However, another route that can be used is the IM route; here a more concentrated 1:1,000 ratio solution is used since it is a lower volume to inject intramuscularly. A 1:1,000 solution of epinephrine contains 1 g of epinephrine in 1,000 ml (or, more practically, 1 mg of epinephrine in 1 ml) of solution. Confusing which ratio goes with which route can have serious consequences.

2.3h Drug Orders in Drops

Some orders for respiratory solutions to be nebulized used to come in the form of number of drops to be mixed with normal saline or distilled water. Now drops are ordered primarily for eye or ear medications; therefore a brief discussion is still warranted. The Latin word for drops is *guttae,* which is abbreviated gtt. It is helpful to know the following: gtt = drops, and it was previously accepted that 16 gtt = 1 ml = 1 cc. However, it should be noted that not all droppers are standardized, and this equivalency may change according to the properties of the liquid and the orifice size of the dropper.

FIGURE 2-5 **Nomogram for Determining Body Surface Area**

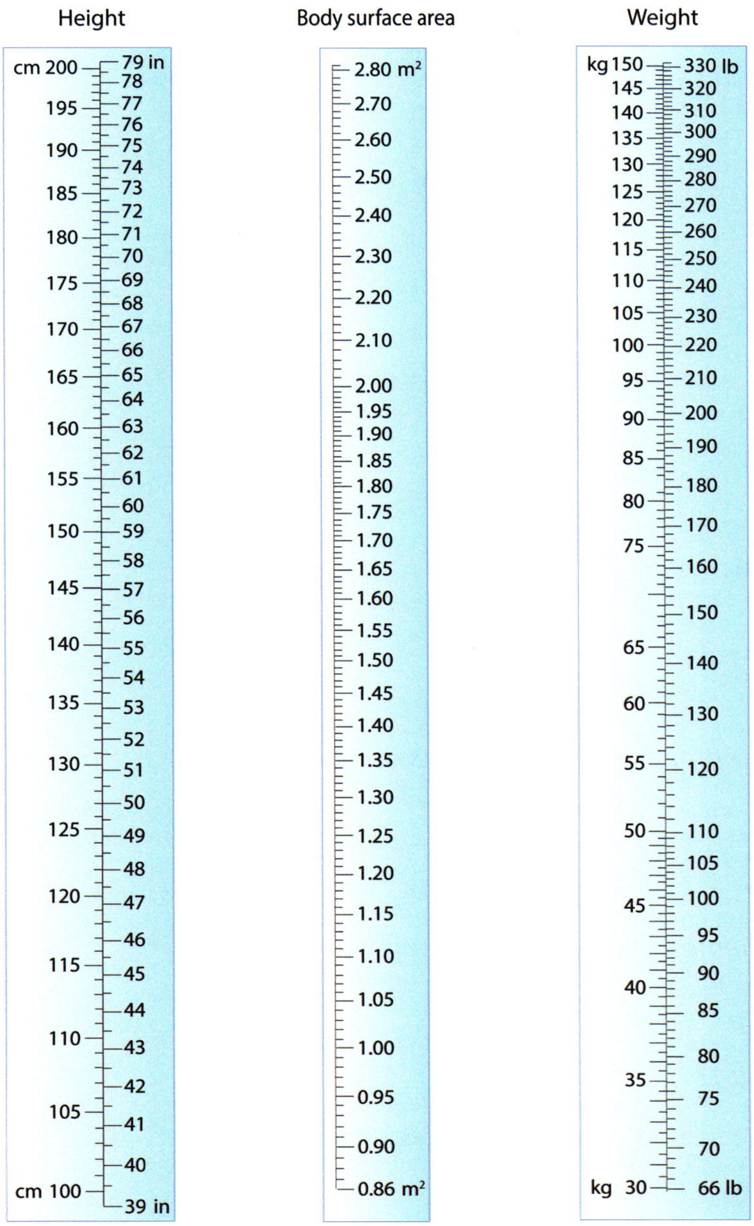

Clinical pearl

A 6-foot-tall man who weighs 240 lbs may require a different dosage than a 6-foot-tall man who weighs 150 lb. This is especially true with highly toxic agents such as those used in cancer chemotherapy. A method to determine the total body surface area (BSA) combines both height and weight in a single measurement to determine the true overall body size. Comparisons like this are called nomograms. *See Figure 2-5 for a nomogram used in determining BSA. Simply mark the patient's height and weight on the respective scales, then either draw a straight line or use a ruler to find the intersection point, which gives the BSA.*

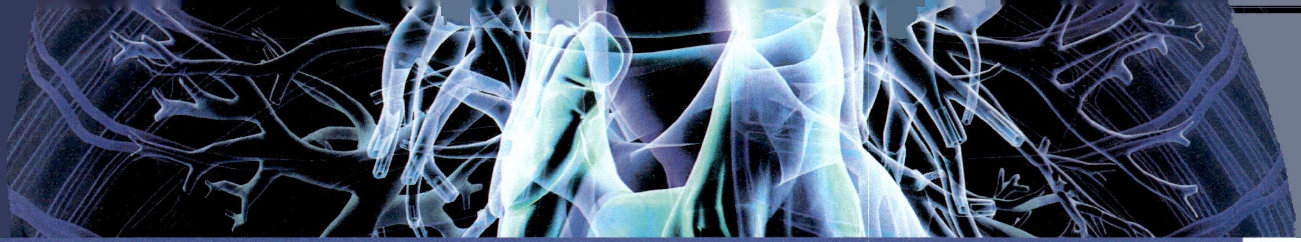

Summary

This chapter includes vital information that is necessary to understand the metric system and to calculate drug dosages accurately. You should feel comfortable making conversions between different systems of measurement and working within the metric system. Dosage measurements and calculations are a major responsibility because giving the wrong dose can be very dangerous to the patient.

REVIEW QUESTIONS

1. The metric system is based on exponential powers of
   (a) 100
   (b) 10
   (c) 2
   (d) 15

2. Which of the following is not a basic unit of measure in the metric system?
   (a) liter
   (b) gram
   (c) pound
   (d) meter

3. A cubic centimeter (cc) is equal to
   (a) 1 ml
   (b) 1 l
   (c) 1 mg
   (d) 10 kg

4. The body surface nomogram compares what two units of measure?
   (a) weight and sex
   (b) height and sex
   (c) surface area and length
   (d) height and weight

5. Which type of drug solution represents a powdered drug mixed in solution?
   (a) v/v
   (b) w/v
   (c) w/w
   (d) v/w

6. If a patient voids 3.2 l of urine in a day, what is the amount in milliliters?

7. Convert 175 lb to kilograms.
8. How many kilograms would a 3-lb baby weigh?
9. An order reads to deliver 200 mg/kg of poractant alfa, a natural surfactant, to a premature infant in the intensive care nursery. The infant weighs 500 g. You have a solution containing 80 mg of phospholipids per milliliter. How many milliliters will you administer to your patient?
10. If you give 6 ml of a 0.1% strength solution, how many milligrams are in the dose?
11. 500 cc of a solution is equal to how many liters?
12. Four milligrams of methylprednisolone is equivalent to 20 mg of hydrocortisone. Your patient is on 40 mg of hydrocortisone daily and the doctor wants to switch to methylprednisolone. What is the equipotent methylprednisolone dose?
13. If beclomethasone, an inhaled corticosteroid, is available in a device that delivers 42 mcg/puff, how many puffs per day will the patient need to get a dose of 336 mcg?
14. A patient is not controlled on 300 mg twice daily of theophylline sustained release. The doctor wants him to take 1,200 mg daily. How many 300-mg tablets should the patient take per day?

Chapter 3

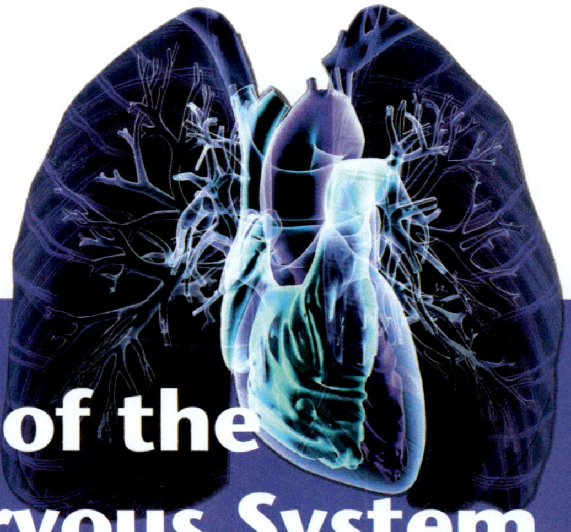

Pharmacology of the Autonomic Nervous System

OBJECTIVES

Upon completion of this chapter you will be able to

- Describe the divisions of the central and peripheral nervous systems.
- Define key terms relative to pharmacology of the autonomic nervous system.
- Describe the anatomy, neurotransmitters, and receptors of the autonomic nervous system.
- State four classifications of autonomic nervous system drugs on the basis of how and where they work.
- Relate the pharmacology of the autonomic nervous system to the specific chapters and drug classifications that are relevant.

KEY TERMS

acetylcholine
acetylcholinesterase
adrenergic
adrenergic receptors
afferent nerves
alpha-receptors
antiadrenergic
anticholinergic
autonomic nervous system
beta-receptors
central nervous system
cholinergic
dopamine receptors
efferent nerves
ganglion
muscarinic receptors
nicotinic receptors
norepinephrine
parasympathetic
parasympatholytic
parasympathomimetic
peripheral nervous system
reuptake
somatic nervous system
sympathetic
sympatholytic
sympathomimetic

ABBREVIATIONS

ACh acetylcholine
AChE acetylcholinesterase
ACLS Advanced Cardiac Life Support
ANS autonomic nervous system
CNS central nervous system
COMT catechol-O-methyltransferase
CPU central processing unit
GI gastrointestinal
LABA long-acting beta$_2$-agonist
LAMA long-acting muscarinic antagonist
MAO monoamine oxidase
NE norepinephrine
PNS peripheral nervous system
SABA short-acting beta$_2$-agonist
SAMA short-acting muscarinic antagonist

The nervous system and endocrine system represent the control systems of the body. These systems coordinate complex activities to maintain day-to-day functioning and a stable internal homeostatic environment. In times of stress, these systems must quickly integrate complex activities to combat the stress and maintain survival. The endocrine system will be discussed in Chapter 7 under the steroid classification of drugs.

This chapter discusses in general terms how the **central nervous system** (CNS) and the **peripheral nervous system** (PNS) receive and process information and how drugs can affect this activity. The nervous system is responsible for day-to-day functioning of both voluntary and involuntary activities throughout the body, and only by understanding how it works will you have the basis for understanding drug effects on various skeletal and smooth muscles, glands, and organs.

The pharmacology of drugs that affect the nervous system is admittedly difficult to understand. The majority of drugs discussed in this chapter work on the PNS. Only the basics of the PNS and CNS will be presented in this chapter, with specifics discussed later in appropriate chapters. For example drugs that work on the CNS, such as skeletal muscle relaxants and opioid medications for pain, are discussed in Chapter 11. PNS drugs that affect the heart rate and respiratory airway tone are addressed in the relevant chapters on bronchodilators and cardiovascular drugs. This chapter simply lays the foundation for understanding nervous system drug pharmacology; we will build on this foundation in upcoming chapters.

3.1 NERVOUS SYSTEM DIVISIONS

The nervous system consists of the *central nervous system* and the *peripheral nervous system*. The CNS is comprised of the brain and spinal cord. The brain is analogous to the central processing unit (CPU) of a computer, which handles information from a variety of sources. The spinal cord is the main branch that transmits messages to and from the brain.

The PNS is comprised of all the nerves "outside" of the brain and spinal cord. The anatomy and physiology of the PNS are more pertinent to cardiopulmonary pharmacotherapy than are those of the CNS, so this chapter emphasizes the PNS. Basically the PNS mediates between the CNS and external and internal body environments. Peripheral system nerves carry sensory information along **afferent nerves** from all parts of the body to the brain for processing. Therefore *afferent* and *sensory* are used synonymously in this context. Likewise the brain can send information along **efferent nerves** or motor pathways via the PNS and have "effects" on various parts of the body (see Figure 3-1).

Learning Hint

The flow of information into your brain, or sensory (afferent) input, is what helps you read this book. The output from the brain that controls the muscles (motor) is what helps you turn the pages in this book.

FIGURE 3-1 Major Components of the Nervous System

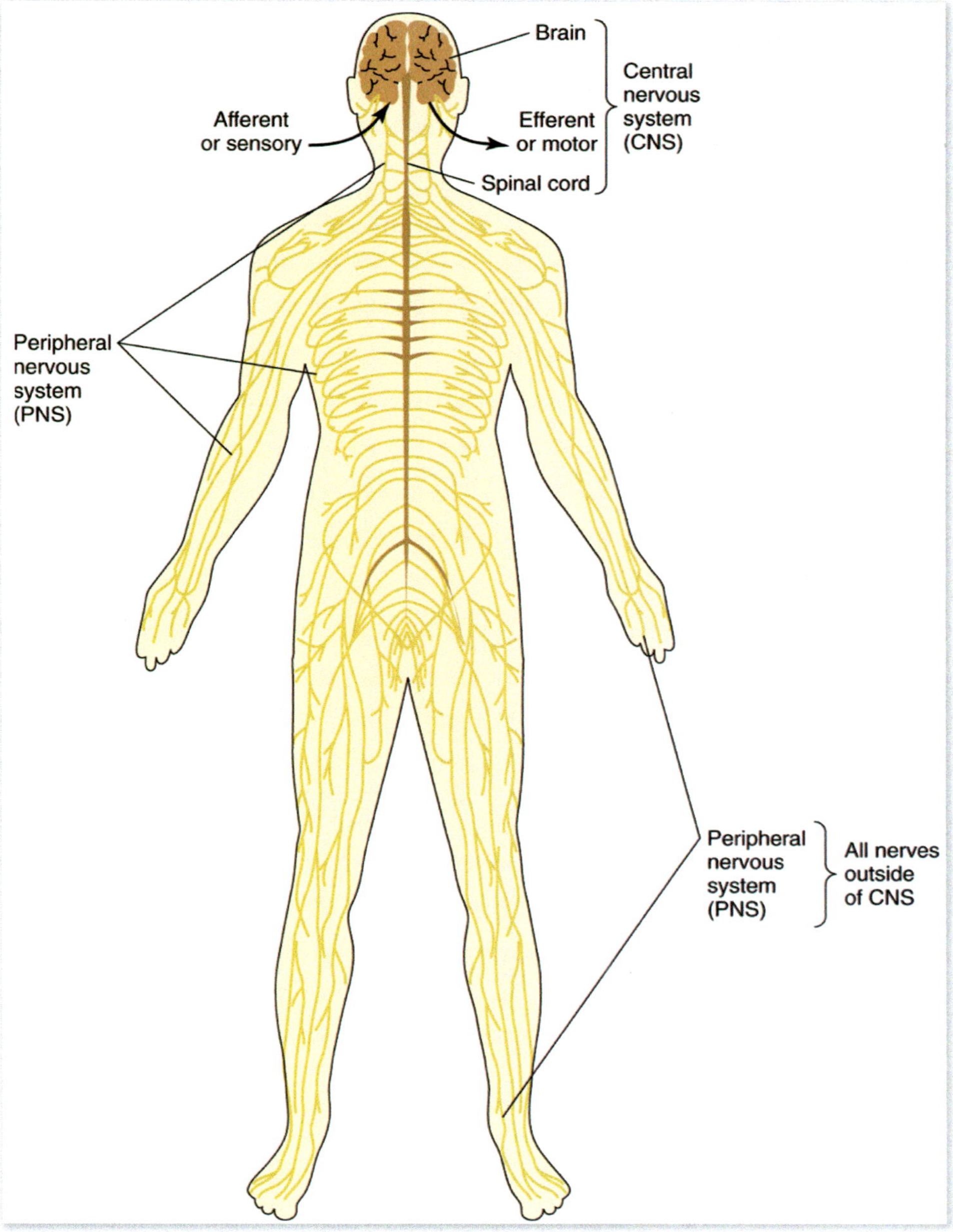

3.1a PNS Divisions

The peripheral nervous system is what connects the rest of your body, neurologically speaking, to your brain and spinal cord. The PNS is divided into two main divisions, the **somatic nervous system** and the **autonomic nervous system** (ANS). The somatic nervous system controls skeletal muscles during voluntary movement and therefore represents the voluntary portion of the PNS. An example of the somatic nervous system is the control of the muscles in your hand to turn the page of this book. We will focus on the somatic nervous system in Chapter 11, where we discuss skeletal muscle relaxants. The somatic nervous system also conducts sensory information such as pain and touch back to the brain via afferent nerves.

BVT *Lab*

Flashcards are available for this chapter at www.BVTLab.com.

Clinical pearl

If you have ever gone to the eye doctor and had to wear dark glasses after the doctor dilated your pupils, it was because a drug had temporarily blocked the autonomic pupil light reflex, which opens and closes the pupil during changing light conditions. Without the dark glasses, you could suffer retinal damage from too much light exposure.

The autonomic nervous system is the involuntary or automatic part of the PNS—we have little or no control over its action. An example of involuntary control is the reaction of the pupil to light on the retina: In bright light conditions, your pupil constricts to protect the retina from too much light exposure, which could be damaging. You do not consciously tell your pupil to constrict, and therefore this is an autonomic response of the PNS.

Other major organ systems in the body that are regulated by the ANS include the cardiopulmonary and digestive systems. Although you may consciously decide to eat a hamburger, using your voluntary or somatic system for this process, the rest of the digestive process is under autonomic control and goes on with little or no thought. In addition to glands and organs, the involuntary muscles controlled by the autonomic nervous system include the specialized cardiac muscles that control the heart and the smooth muscle found in airways, blood vessels, and the reproductive and gastrointestinal tracts.

time for review

What branch of the nervous system controls digestive actions?

The autonomic system is further divided into the **sympathetic** and **parasympathetic** branches. The parasympathetic branch is concerned with daily body upkeep and maintaining a homeostatic environment and thus is often called the "sleep-and-eat" system. The sympathetic system represents the alert system for stressful situations and is often referred to as the "fight-or-flight" system. Because the balance between these two systems is what controls our normal heart rate and the smooth muscle tone of our airways, this balance is of major pharmacologic importance. Please see Figure 3-2, which demonstrates the divisions of the nervous system.

It is important to note that the parasympathetic and sympathetic systems usually work in a coordinated but opposing fashion to regulate autonomic control. For example, if you were confronted by a stranger with a knife in a dark alley, several physiologic changes would occur because the sympathetic system would be alerted. Your pupils would dilate to bring in more light for the situation at hand. Your heart rate and force of contraction would increase to get much-needed oxygen to muscles for the impending "fight or flight." Your respiratory system would be stimulated to increase ventilation to bring in more oxygen. Certain vascular changes would occur to provide more blood flow to essential areas and constrict blood flow to nonessential areas such as the GI tract.

FIGURE 3-2 Organization of the Nervous System

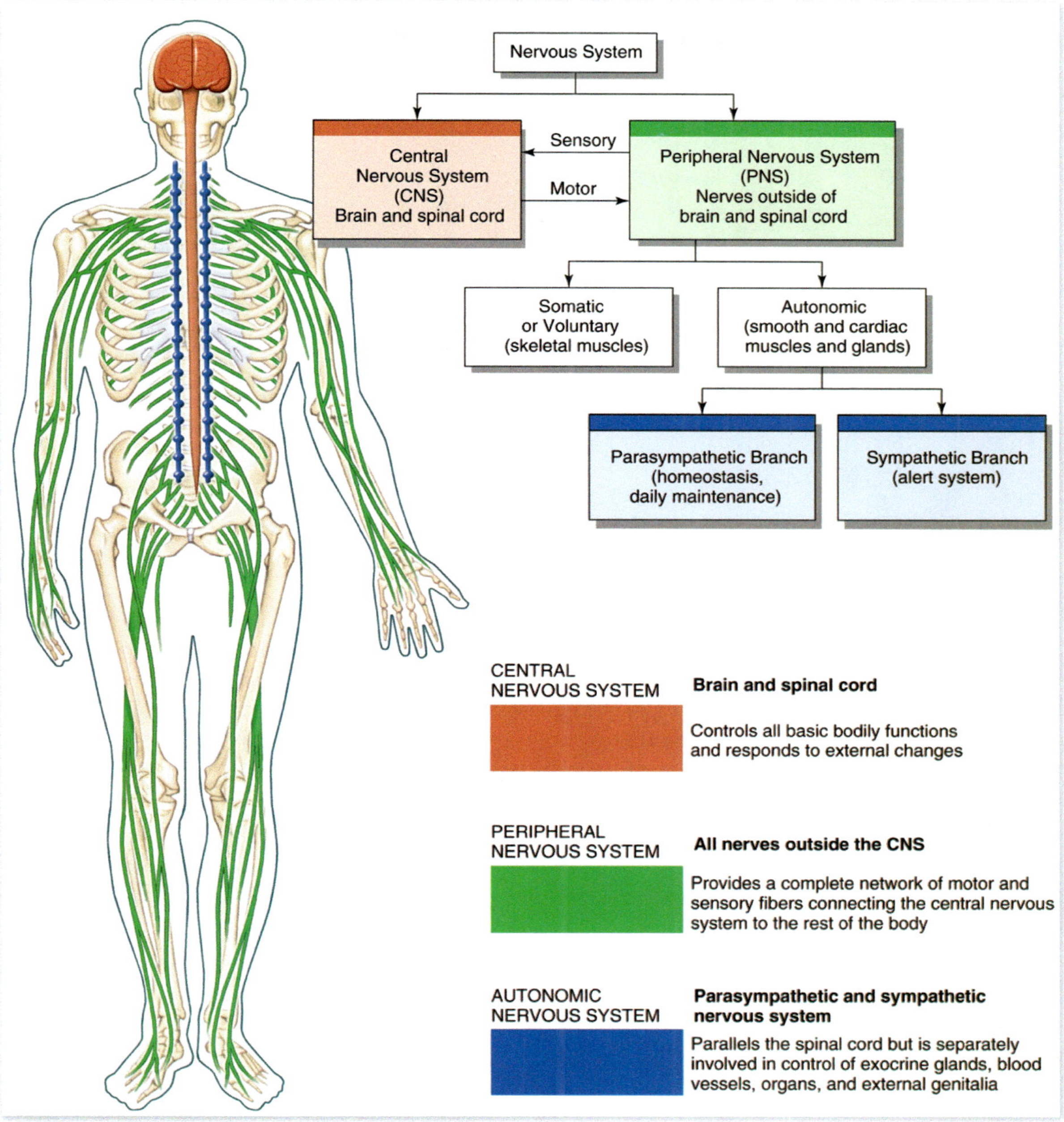

However, you cannot maintain this hypermetabolic state for long periods of time; once the danger is removed (hopefully by peaceful police intervention), you will eventually return to a homeostatic state, and then, we presume, you will wonder why you were ever in the dark alley in the first place. The parasympathetic system would then become dominant and bring your heart rate and respirations back toward normal resting levels. See Figure 3-3, which shows the effects of the parasympathetic and sympathetic nervous systems and their origins on the spinal column.

FIGURE 3-3 Effects of the Parasympathetic and Sympathetic Nervous Systems

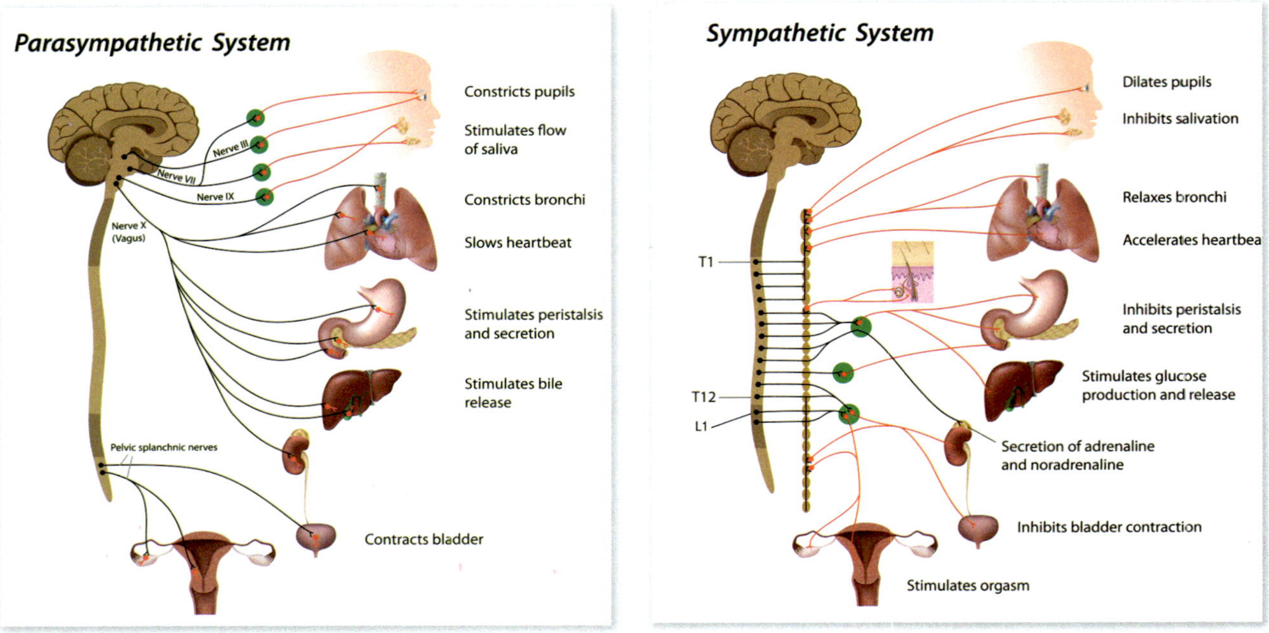

What was just described is a physiologic response to stress and a return to homeostasis via the two branches of the autonomic nervous system. The activity of each of these branches can also be altered by pharmacologic means. This is good because some pathologic conditions of the organs can be treated pharmacologically by capitalizing on the knowledge of these interactions. Please see Table 3-1 for actions of the parasympathetic and sympathetic nervous systems.

TABLE 3-1 Effects of the Parasympathetic and Sympathetic Nervous Systems

Organ or System	Parasympathetic Effect	Sympathetic Effect
Heart	Decreases rate and contractile force	Increases rate and contractile force
Lungs	Bronchoconstricts	Bronchodilates
Eyes	Pupil constriction	Pupil dilation
Hair muscles	Relaxes	Contracts and causes hair to stand on end (piloerection)
Gastrointestinal	Increases digestion	Decreases digestion
Urinary	Constricts bladder	Relaxes bladder

time for review

Have you ever heard the saying, "That made the hairs on the back of my neck stand up"? Would you consider this a sympathetic or parasympathetic response, and why?

3.2 NERVOUS SYSTEM CONDUCTION

To understand how drugs affect neurotransmission, you must know how messages are transmitted or conducted from one nerve (neuron) to another. When a resting nerve receives stimulation, an electrical impulse carries the signal along the nerve fiber or axon. At the terminal end of each axon is a small junction or synapse that may connect either to another nerve or to a muscle or gland. Regardless of where the connection leads, for the impulse to be carried on, a chemical neurotransmitter substance must now travel across the synapse. These chemicals are manufactured and stored at the terminal end of the axons and released upon stimulation by the electrical impulse. The two main neurochemical substances stored or manufactured at the ends of the nerve fibers are **acetylcholine** (ACh) and **norepinephrine** (NE). See Figure 3-4, which demonstrates the transmission of a nerve impulse with ACh as the neurotransmitter.

FIGURE 3-4 Transmission of a Nerve Impulse

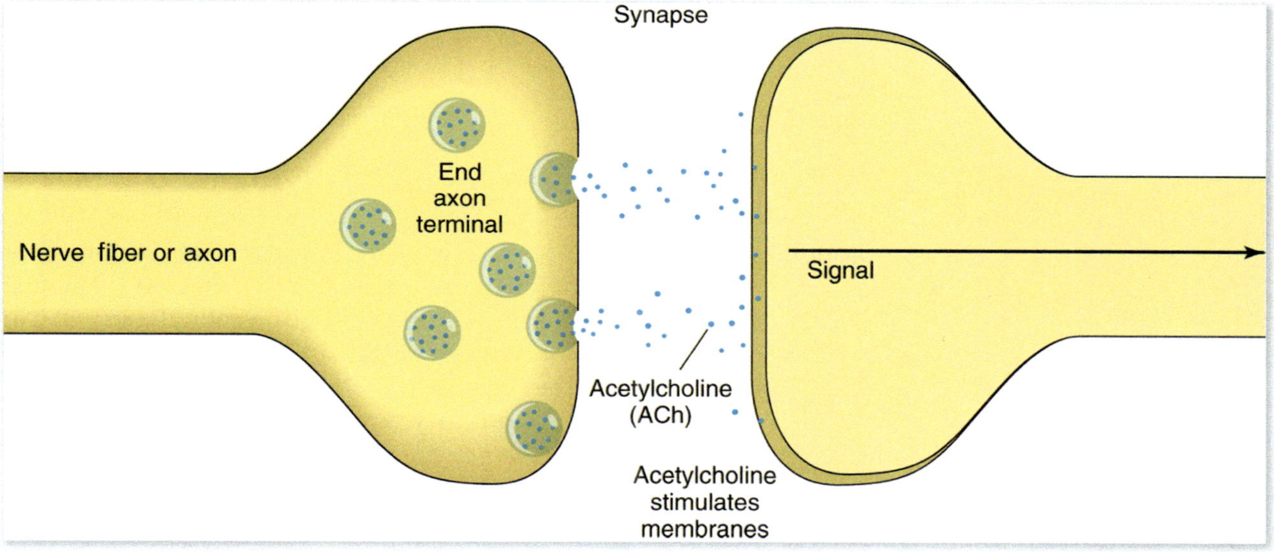

3.2a Types and Location of Neurotransmitters

The somatic nervous system, which controls the skeletal muscles, is a one-junction system in which the stimulus travels via a single nerve axon and then travels to one gap or synapse. The neurotransmitter must then pass the signal on to the brain for sensory input such as pain or on to the affected skeletal muscle for motor output to control the muscle (see Figure 3-5). Notice that ACh is the neurotransmitter substance found within the somatic system. The only kind of synapse in the somatic system is the neuromuscular junction that connects the nerve to the skeletal muscle or the synapse to the CNS, which brings in sensory information.

FIGURE 3-5 Somatic Nervous System Transmission

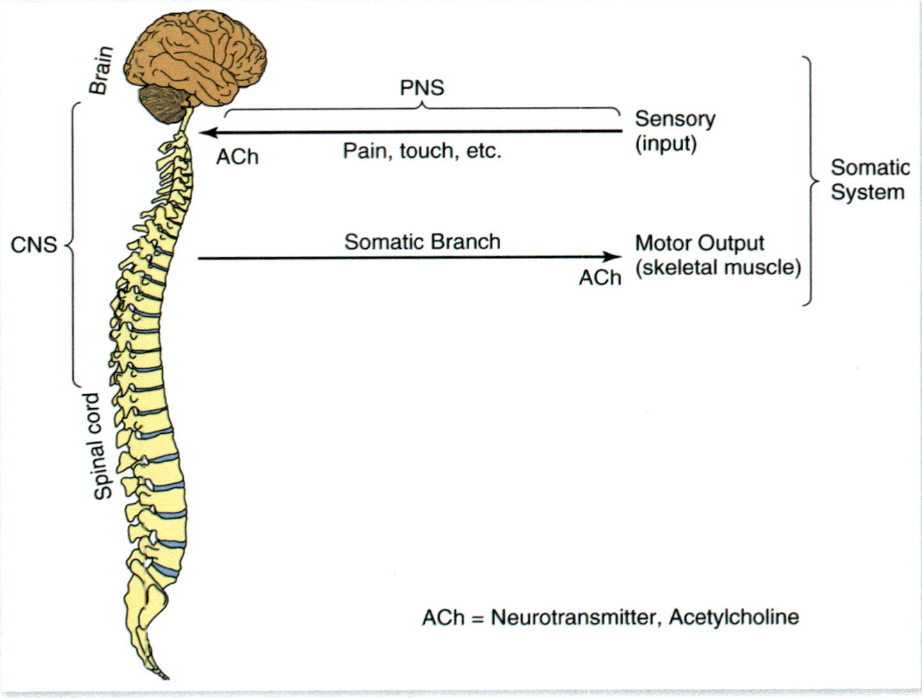

The autonomic branch of the PNS has two junctions to traverse in order for the signal to reach the intended site of an involuntary muscle or gland. The first neuron is a presynaptic or preganglionic neuron. A **ganglion** (plural, *ganglia*) can be thought of as simply a cluster of nerves that lie outside the CNS. Therefore the first part of the journey from the brain is to the first junction (synapse) and ganglia beyond. The second neuron is a postsynaptic or postganglionic neuron, and it travels from the ganglia to the target site of either an involuntary muscle (cardiac or smooth) or a gland.

Both the parasympathetic and the sympathetic system have preganglionic and postganglionic neurons. The neurotransmitter substance at both preganglionic sites is ACh. ACh is also found at the postganglionic site of the parasympathetic system. However, the neurotransmitter substance that carries the impulse to the involuntary muscle or gland at the postganglionic junction of the sympathetic system is norepinephrine. See Figure 3-6, which now adds the autonomic branches of the peripheral nervous system.

BVT Lab

Visit www.BVTLab.com to explore the student resources available for this chapter.

FIGURE 3-6 Synapses and Neurotransmitter Substances of the Autonomic Nervous System

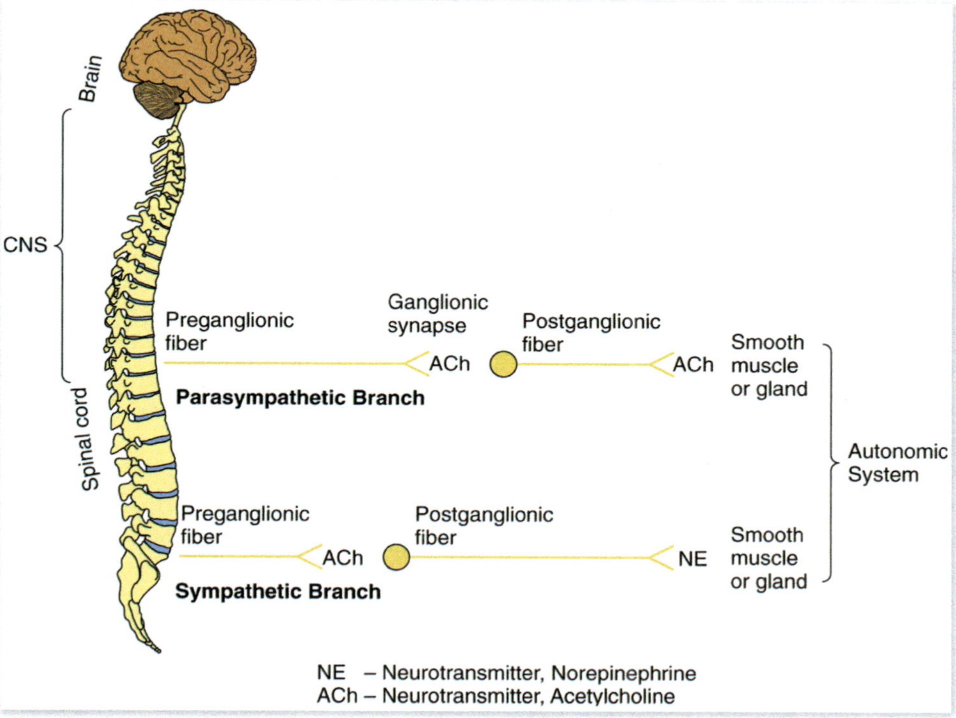

3.2b Receptors

In Chapter 1, we learned that receptor sites are "where the action is." Once the neurochemical transmitter substance is released, it binds to a receptor to elicit a response. If the stimulus begins in the ANS, it must first release ACh across the presynaptic junction and then diffuse and bind to postsynaptic receptors found on the postsynaptic nerve to pass the signal on. The receptors to which the neurotransmitter ACh binds as it diffuses across the presynaptic junction in either the parasympathetic or the sympathetic system are called **nicotinic receptors**. These receptors simply pass the signal on to the postsynaptic neuron and are then carried to the target gland, organ, smooth muscle, or cardiac muscle (see Figure 3-7).

Learning Hint

Remember that ACh is the neurotransmitter substance found everywhere (skeletal neuromuscular junction, sensory synapses, both preganglionic junctions, and the postganglionic junction of the parasympathetic nervous system), but NE is found only at the postganglionic junction of the sympathetic system.

FIGURE 3-7 Preganglionic Transmission in the ANS

This occurs in both parasympathetic and sympathetic systems, with only the length and location of the nerve fibers being different.

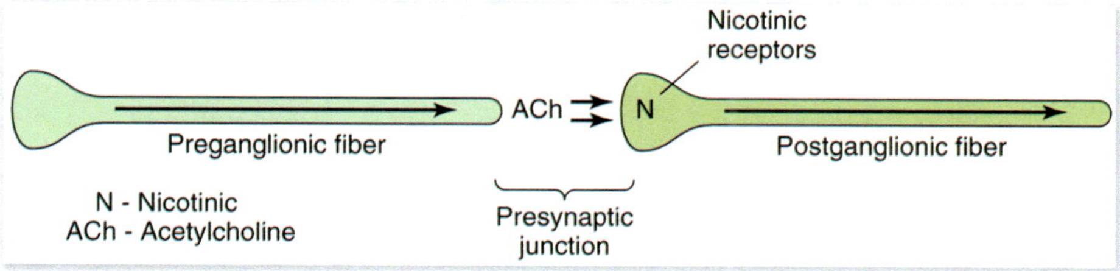

Learning Hint

Remember that the nicotinic receptors are found at preganglionic sites and help to pass the impulse along to the postganglionic neuron. The muscarinic receptors are at the actual effector site of the parasympathetic nervous system. In Chapter 5 you will learn about bronchodilator agents that work by blocking the muscarinic receptors and thus blocking the parasympathetic response of bronchoconstriction. Some are short acting and some are long acting and they are given the names SAMAs and LAMAs (for short-acting muscarinic antagonists and long-acting muscarinic antagonists, respectively).

Receptors are also found on the postsynaptic junction located on involuntary muscles or glands. This is where the "main" action is, so to speak, and it is referred to as the neuroeffector site. Once the neurochemical transmitter binds to receptor sites there, it initiates biochemical triggers that result in physiologic responses depending on what the nerve innervates (connects to). After the chemical transmitter has interacted with the receptor and initiated a response, its job is done and action is terminated. The neurotransmitter must be destroyed or removed after receptor activation. The neurotransmitters that do not bind are destroyed by enzymes or taken back into the synapse, or they diffuse away.

In the postsynaptic junction of the parasympathetic nervous system, the neurotransmitter substance is ACh. ACh binds with **muscarinic receptors** found on involuntary muscles or glands. For example, if the parasympathetic system is stimulated and muscarinic receptors innervating the heart bind with ACh, the physiologic reaction is the parasympathetic response of slowing heart rate.

However, if the sympathetic nervous system is stimulated and the impulse reaches the postsynaptic site, norepinephrine is released and binds with the **adrenergic receptors** found on the glands or smooth or cardiac muscle.

For example, if the sympathetic system is stimulated and adrenergic receptors found in the heart bind with NE, the physiologic reaction is the sympathetic response of increasing heart rate. The adrenergic receptors are further classified as alpha- or beta-receptors, which will be discussed further in Chapter 5. See Figure 3-8, which shows the synapses, neurotransmitters, and receptors of the ANS.

FIGURE 3-8 Synapses, Ganglia, Neurotransmitters, and Receptors of the ANS

Note: Adrenergic receptors are classified as alpha (α) or beta (β).

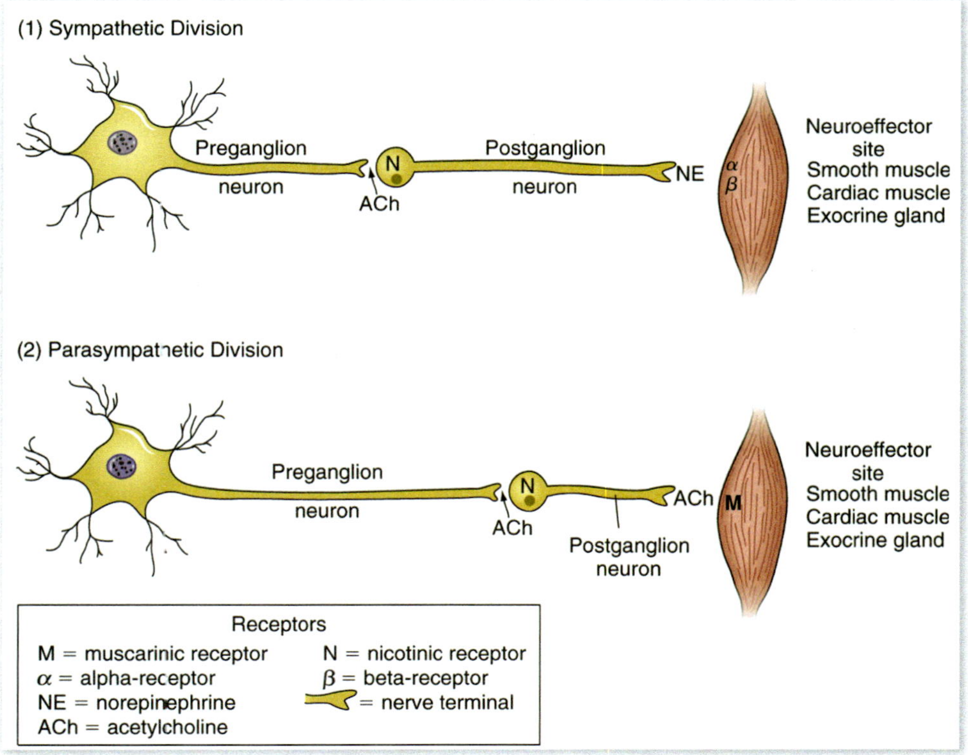

time for review

Identify where nicotinic and muscarinic receptors can be found in the parasympathetic and sympathetic nervous systems.

3.2c Receptor Classification

Receptors are classified by the type of neurotransmitter to which they respond at the various nerve endings. The receptors that bind with acetyl*choline* are termed *cholinergic receptors*. Cholinergic receptors are of two types, termed muscarinic or nicotinic depending on their location.

The receptors that bind with NE are called *adrenergic receptors*. Sympathetic agonists stimulate NE adrenergic receptors of either the **alpha-receptor** or **beta-receptor** type, depending on where they are found in the body. Alpha-receptors, found primarily in smooth muscle of blood vessels, can be of two types, either $alpha_1$ or $alpha_2$. Generally alpha stimulation causes vasoconstriction. Beta-receptors are termed either $beta_1$ or $beta_2$. $Beta_1$-receptors are found primarily in the cardiac muscle, where stimulation results in positive chronotropic (increase in rate), dromotropic (increase in conduction), and inotropic (increase in contraction) effects on the cardiac system. They are further discussed in Chapters 9 and 10. $Beta_2$-receptors are found abundantly within the smooth muscle of the airways and in certain blood vessels. $Beta_2$-receptor stimulation results in vasodilation and bronchodilation. $Beta_2$-agonists are the foundation for treatment of bronchospasm and are discussed further in Chapter 5, where you will learn about short-acting $beta_2$-agonists (SABAs) and long-acting $beta_2$-agonists (LABAs) and their role in bronchodilator therapy. See Figure 3-9 for the receptors found at nerve endings.

Learning Hint

We did not forget about the somatic branch of the PNS. Remember that this is a one-branch system innervating skeletal muscles, and nicotinic receptors are found at the receptor sites as shown in Figure 3-8. Again we will have more to say about this in Chapter 11.

FIGURE 3-9 Receptors Found at Nerve Endings

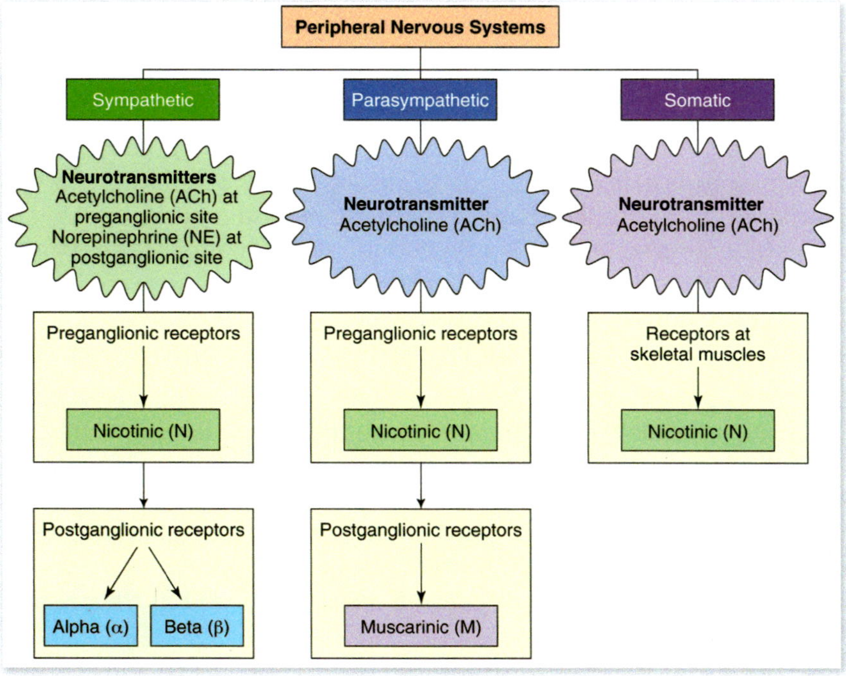

One other type of adrenergic receptor we have not yet mentioned are the **dopamine receptors** found in renal tissues. Their stimulation causes relaxation of the renal arteries and increases perfusion to the kidneys. See Table 3-2, which shows the various adrenergic receptor types, their locations, and their actions when stimulated.

TABLE 3-2 Types of Adrenergic Receptors (Adrenoreceptors)

Type	Tissue	Action
Alpha$_1$	Vascular smooth muscle	Contracts
	Pupil	Dilates (mydriasis)
	Pilomotor smooth muscle	"Goose bumps"
Beta$_1$	Heart	Stimulates rate and force
Beta$_2$	Respiratory	Bronchodilates
	Somatic motor (voluntary muscle)	Tremors
Dopamine	Renal	Relaxes arteries

Note: Beta$_3$-receptors have also been identified that enhance the breakdown of fat (lipolysis) in adipose tissue and help to generate heat (thermogenesis) in skeletal muscle.

time for review

State the effects on the heart, blood vessels, or lungs from stimulating the following receptors: alpha, beta$_1$, beta$_2$, and muscarinic.

3.3 ANS DRUG TERMINOLOGY

Physiologically the ANS acts as two major divisions: the parasympathetic and sympathetic. Again recapping the systems, one can think of the sympathetic system as a response system and the parasympathetic as a homeostatic or maintenance system. They work together to balance each other out. The sympathetic system is not essential for life, but it allows for adjustments to activity and stresses that occur in life. The parasympathetic nervous system controls essential activities and conserves energy for daily body maintenance and metabolic functioning. Each division of the ANS has a direct effect on organ systems such as the heart and lungs, and we will use these two organs as examples in the following classification system. Drugs that affect the function of the ANS are classified in four categories.

Learning Hint

Think of the medical terms *-lytic*, which means "to block or work against," and *-mimetic*, "to mimic or imitate."

1. Drugs that stimulate or mimic the parasympathetic receptors are called **cholinergics** or **parasympathomimetics**. Their responses include slowing the heart rate and causing bronchoconstriction. Remember from Chapter 1 that these drugs can also be called cholinergic agonists, because agonists stimulate a receptor. In addition they can be called muscarinic drugs because they stimulate the muscarinic receptors found in the parasympathetic system.

2. Drugs that block parasympathetic receptors are called **anticholinergics** or **parasympatholytics**. Their responses include speeding up the heart and causing bronchodilation—as opposed to what the parasympathetic system will do if stimulated. Remember that these drugs can also be called cholinergic antagonists or antimuscarinic agents. How do we use this information clinically? Airway obstruction in asthma and chronic obstructive pulmonary disease (COPD) is partly related to abnormally elevated parasympathetic tone. Anticholinergic medications, such as ipratropium bromide, reduce airway obstruction in these disease states by lowering parasympathetic tone.
3. Drugs that stimulate or mimic the sympathetic receptors are termed **adrenergics** or **sympathomimetics**. They include alpha- and/or beta-adrenergic drugs, depending on the receptor they stimulate. More specifically beta$_1$-adrenergics speed up the heart rate and beta$_2$-adrenergics cause bronchodilation.
4. Drugs that would antagonize the sympathetic response are called **anti-adrenergics** or **sympatholytics**. They are also referred to as blockers; therefore a beta-blocker blocks the expected effects of bronchodilation and increase in heart rate and thus causes bronchoconstriction and a decrease in heart rate.

Learning Hint

To connect *adrenergic* to *sympathetic,* when you think of the sympathetic nervous system being stimulated, think of the adrenalin rush.

Controversy

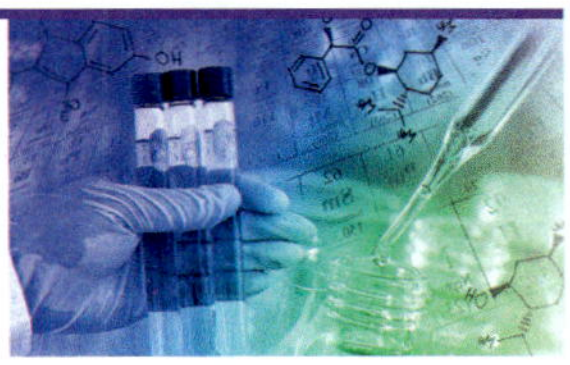

It certainly does get confusing when several terms can mean the same thing. For example a parasympatholytic can be called an anticholinergic or a parasympathetic antagonist or a vagolytic (after the major nerve, vagus, of the parasympathetic system). We can even throw in the term *antimuscarinic.*

Lung sounds also have several different terms that can mean the same thing because of carryover—such as a rale (an older term), which is the same thing as a crackle. Attempts have been made to standardize lung sound terminology to be less confusing. Do you think the same should be done for nervous system terminology?

As you can again see, functionally the sympathetic and parasympathetic divisions are opposing. Simulating one autonomic division may increase the activity of an organ, and stimulation of the other division may inhibit the activity. One easy way of remembering what each nervous system does to a particular organ is to recall the common names for each: the fight-or-flight (sympathetic) and the sleep-and-eat (parasympathetic) nervous systems. Stimulation of the sympathetic system causes an increase in heart rate and blood pressure (fight or flight), for example. Stimulation of the parasympathetic system would increase gastrointestinal motility (eat) and lower heart rate (sleep). Drug therapy can disrupt the balance of sympathetic and parasympathetic activity. For example sympathetic influences on the heart cause increased force of contraction and heart rate, and parasympathetic influences result in bradycardia and decrease in contractile force. Smooth muscles in the vessels are relaxed with a decrease in sympathetic activity and vasoconstricted with an increase in sympathetic activity.

time for review

Which of the four autonomic categories can cause bronchodilation? Which can cause a decrease in heart rate?

3.3a Direct- and Indirect-Acting Agents

Drugs can affect different steps in the neurotransmission process. Thus far we have talked about stimulating the receptors (agonists), which is a direct-acting agent. Indirect-acting agents that block the receptor site (antagonists) have also been mentioned. However, other indirect methods, such as increasing or decreasing transmitter substances by enhancing or inhibiting the enzymes that break them down, still need to be discussed. We will take one final look at the four classifications of autonomic drugs and further develop the concept of indirect-acting drugs.

Learning Hint

AChE can also be called cholinesterase. Remember that AChE is the "E"nzyme that breaks down ACh.

Clinical pearl

A potential antidote that soldiers carry with them when they might be exposed to nerve gas is, of course, a parasympatholytic agent such as the drug atropine, which can block the overstimulation of the parasympathetic system by nerve gas.

3.3b Parasympathomimetics

Acetylcholine is the main neurotransmitter in all autonomic preganglionic sites and at parasympathetic postganglionic synapses. Acetylcholine is synthesized from acetyl–coenzyme A (acetyl–CoA) and choline by the enzyme choline acetyltransferase. ACh is a simple molecule, yet it has activity at several different receptors. ACh is not a useful drug therapeutically because it is not specific enough at receptors and it is rapidly broken down in the body. As we discussed earlier, drugs that act on acetylcholine receptors are called cholinergic or parasympathomimetics.

Acetylcholine action is terminated when it is metabolized by **acetylcholinesterase** (AChE). Cholinergic drugs are subdivided according to whether they act directly at the receptor by increasing production of ACh or indirectly through inhibition of AChE, the enzyme that breaks down ACh. In either scenario, the action of ACh is enhanced either directly by increasing production or indirectly by preventing its rapid breakdown, thus allowing ACh to remain active longer.

Clinical pearl

The drug edrophonium (Enlon®) is used to test patients for the neuromuscular disease myasthenia gravis, which is a descending paralysis beginning with the facial muscles. It is caused by insufficient or ineffective ACh at the neuromuscular junction. Edrophonium works by inhibiting AChE from metabolizing ACh, so ACh accumulates and becomes more effective at the neuromuscular junction. A positive edrophonium test results in the return of facial tone after the medication has been administered.

AChE inhibitors are also widely used in agriculture as insecticides (malathion, parathion). In addition they have unfortunately been used as nerve gas in chemical warfare; overstimulation of the parasympathetic nervous system results in severe bradycardia, hypotension, and death.

Muscarinic agonists are direct-acting parasympathomimetic agents and therefore stimulate the parasympathetic nervous system by increasing ACh production at the effector site. Methacholine is a drug with muscarinic activity. Chemically it is close to acetylcholine, and it is used clinically as part of a bronchial challenge test to cause bronchoconstriction (parasympathetic response) and thereby diagnose asthma. Asthma, of course, is normally a contraindication for a parasympathomimetic drug, but here the drug is used in small doses for diagnostic purposes.

Drugs can also act specifically at the nicotinic receptor sites where ACh is the neurotransmitter substance. Remember, ACh transmits both sympathetic and parasympathetic impulses from preganglionic neurons to nicotinic ganglionic receptors on postganglionic neurons. Nicotinic receptors are also found at the skeletal muscles in the somatic nervous system. Nicotinic agonists are classified by whether they stimulate predominantly at the ganglionic level in the autonomic branch of the PNS or at the skeletal muscles of the somatic branch at the neuromuscular level. See Table 3-3 for sample cholinergic agonists and their indications.

TABLE 3-3 Sample Cholinergic Agonists and Indications

Drug	Indication
Direct-acting: directly stimulates cholinergic receptors	
bethanechol	Urinary retention
succinylcholine	Neuromuscular blockade—intubation
pilocarpine	Glaucoma
Indirect-acting: decreased AChE activity	
neostigmine	Myasthenia gravis
pyridostigmine	Reversal of neuromuscular blockade
Malathion	Insecticide
Nerve gas	Chemical warfare

time for review

Differentiate ACh and AChE. Now relate these terms to direct- and indirect-acting agents.

3.3c Parasympatholytics

Parasympatholytic drugs or anticholinergic drugs are pharmacologic antagonists of the parasympathetic nervous system. Cardiovascular effects from anticholinergics, such as atropine, include tachycardia, bronchodilation, and drying of secretions, which are all opposite to parasympathetic stimulant responses. Atropine derivatives such as ipratropium bromide, mentioned in Chapter 5, are used for their bronchodilation effects. In addition atropine is part of the Advanced Cardiac Life Support (ACLS) course for treatment of bradycardia.

Anticholinergic drug subgroups are antimuscarinic because the drugs block the effect at the postganglionic site where muscarinic receptors are found. They can also block the nicotinic receptors. Nicotinic blockers are further divided according to the two sites where nicotinic receptors are found: the ganglia and the skeletal muscles. Ganglionic blockers are not used clinically because they block both sympathetic and parasympathetic nerves. Neuromuscular blockers produce skeletal muscle paralysis and can be used for surgery or in critical care when patients need to be totally motionless or to facilitate mechanical ventilation. The significance of this will be discussed in Chapter 11. See Table 3-4 for some examples of anticholinergic drugs.

Learning Hint

A mnemonic used for atropine toxicity is "dry as a bone, red as a beet, mad as a hatter, and blind as a bat." "Dry as a bone" refers to decreased sweating, salivation, and lacrimation. "Red as a beet" refers to the vasodilation of arms, head, neck, and trunk that occurs with atropine overdoses. "Mad as a hatter" refers to CNS toxicity effects such as delirium. "Blind as a bat" refers to the pupil changes. You can see that excessive blockage of the parasympathetic system may not be tolerated well by patients.

TABLE 3-4 Anticholinergic Drug Class

Category and Function	Drug
Antimuscarinics—increase heart rate and bronchodilation	atropine ipratropium bromide
Nicotinic blockers At preganglionic sites—prevent nervous transmission	 hexamethonium

PATIENT & FAMILY EDUCATION

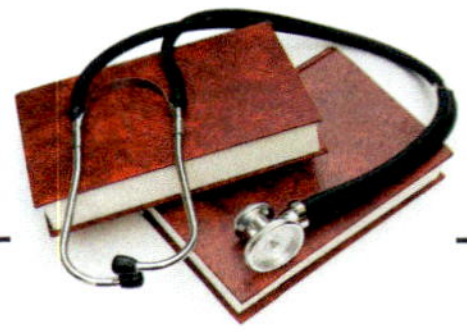

Certain common adverse effects of anticholinergic medications should be stressed when educating patients and/or their families. These include confusion, urinary retention, constipation, dry mouth, and blurry vision. These problems are more likely to occur in the elderly.

LIFE SPAN CONSIDERATIONS

Elderly patients are particularly susceptible to the adverse effects of anticholinergic medications. In general, these drugs should not be prescribed if alternative therapies are available. Aerosol use via the inhalation route is generally an exception due to its minimal systemic effects.

3.3d Sympathomimetics

To review, adrenergic drugs stimulate and therefore act like the sympathetic nervous system, which dominates in times of stress. It is a survival response that enables the body to prepare to face or flee from a perceived danger. The autonomic sympathetic nerves kick into high gear automatically, so you don't have to think before you act and precious life-or-death time isn't wasted. In danger, the heart rate increases, pupils dilate, blood flow increases in the vital organs where it is needed, and the lungs bronchodilate to take in more oxygen. At the same time some nonessential areas are shut down so energy can concentrate where it is needed the most.

Drugs that act on norepinephrine receptors are called sympathomimetic or adrenergic agonists and mimic sympathetic responses. In the sympathetic or adrenergic system, NE transmits most of the impulses in the sympathetic postganglionic synapse. NE synthesis is more complex than ACh synthesis. NE is released from the sympathetic nerve endings by the same mechanism as ACh, but the termination is different. Once it is released, NE crosses the synaptic cleft and binds to postsynaptic adrenergic receptors. There is not an enzyme that immediately breaks down NE to interfere or inactivate its action at the synaptic cleft. Instead of being metabolized immediately, NE is recycled back into the synaptic knob to be stored for future use. This process is called **reuptake**. Excess norepinephrine that does not participate in the reuptake process can eventually be metabolized by the enzymes monoamine oxidase (MAO) and catechol-O-methyltransferase (COMT) (see Figure 3-10). The reuptake and metabolism of NE by COMT and MAO will be important concepts in Chapter 5.

Sympathomimetics can also be either direct- or indirect-acting. Direct-acting sympathomimetics increase NE production and therefore bind with the adrenergic receptors found on the postsynaptic junction of the sympathetic nervous systems. These receptors can be either alpha- or beta-receptors, depending on location and action. Indirect sympathomimetics inhibit the reuptake and enzyme deactivation of NE, thereby preventing its breakdown. See Figure 3-11 for sympathomimetic drug subgroups.

Clinical pearl

What, no cheese, wine, or chocolate? There is a group of drugs called MAO inhibitors that interact with sympathomimetic amines and lead to hypertension. MAO is a digestive enzyme that normally breaks down catecholamines. Any food or cold medication that contains sympathomimetics, such as pseudoephedrine, should not be used with an MAO inhibitor. Wine, cheese, and chocolate have sympathomimetic components. This is one of the first drug–diet interactions that was ever recognized.

FIGURE 3-10 Life Cycle of Norepinephrine (NE)

(1) NE is synthesized from the amino acid tyrosine; (2) NE is released into the synaptic cleft; (3) NE binds to receptors on the postsynaptic membrane; (4) NE is taken back into the presynaptic neuron (reuptake); (5) NE is degraded by MAO; (6) Small amounts of NE enter the postsynaptic cell and are degraded by COMT.

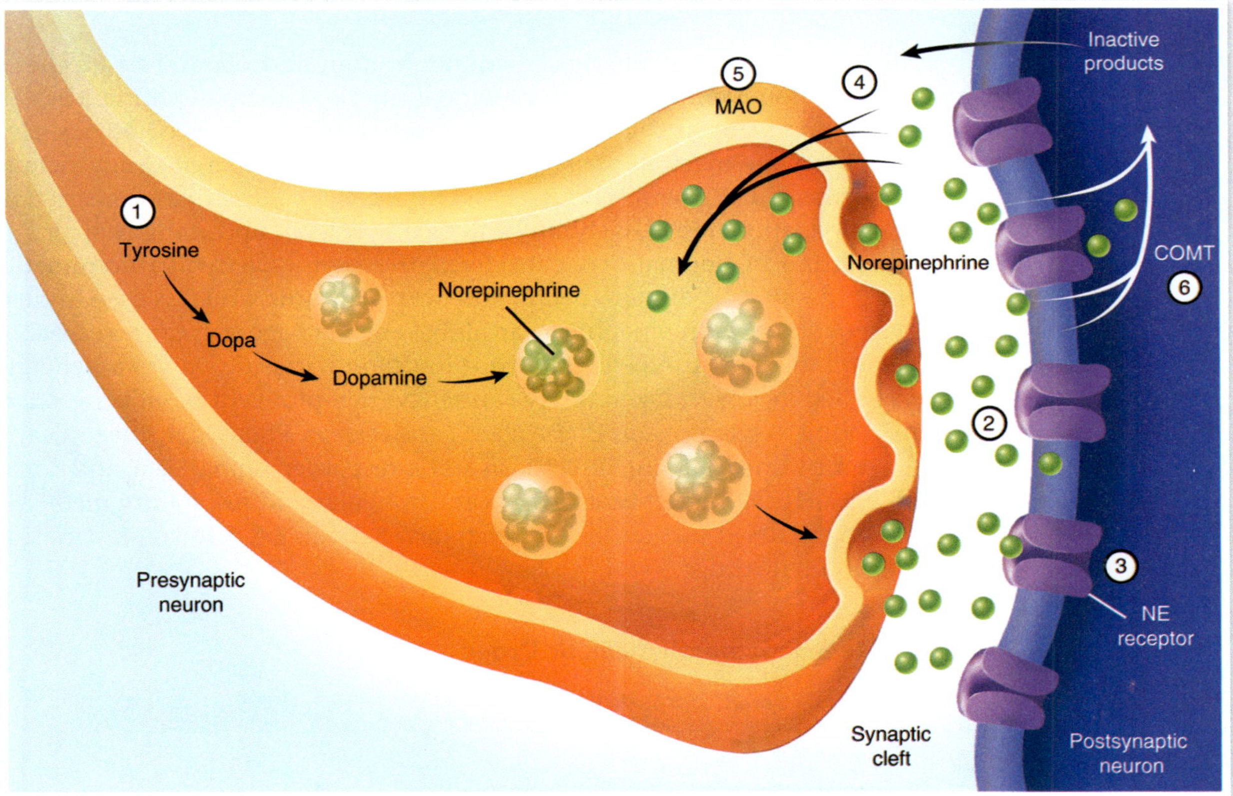

Enzymes that terminate the action of norepinephrine	MAO = Monoamine oxidase COMT = Catechol-O-methyltransferase

FIGURE 3-11 Sympathomimetic Drug Subgroups

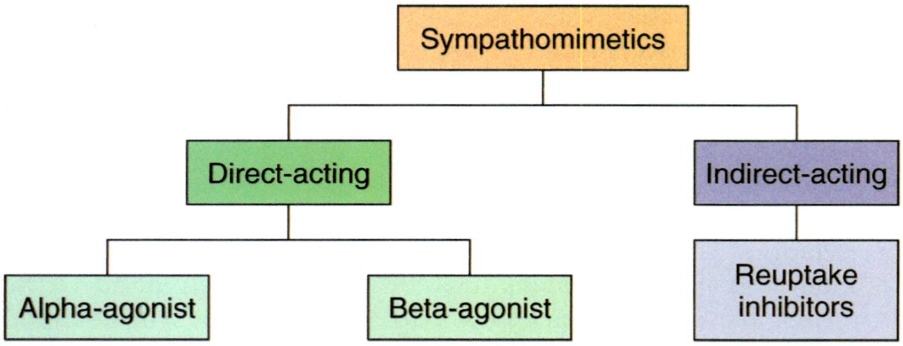

time for review

Contrast the mechanisms of neurotransmitter inactivation in the parasympathetic and sympathetic nervous systems.

BVT Lab

Improve your test scores. Practice quizzes are available at www.BVTLab.com.

Adrenergic agents may be catecholamines or noncatecholamines. Catecholamines include dobutamine, dopamine, epinephrine, and norepinephrine. They all have a common basic chemical structure, and they are all destroyed by digestive enzymes if they are ingested orally. Noncatecholamine adrenergic drugs include phenylephrine and albuterol. They are used for local or systemic vasoconstriction and bronchodilation, respectively, and will be discussed in upcoming chapters.

Epinephrine or adrenalin is considered the prototype sympathomimetic, with effects on alpha$_1$-, alpha$_2$-, beta$_1$-, and beta$_2$-receptors, and it is used to treat anaphylactic shock. Norepinephrine, an alpha- and beta-agonist, causes vasoconstriction and therefore can be used to treat low blood pressure. Alpha-adrenergic agents applied locally or taken orally can relieve symptoms of nasal congestion by constricting swollen vessels in the nasal passageways. Phenylephrine topically does the same thing by acting directly on alpha-receptors. Alpha, beta, and dopamine drugs are used for applications in cardiovascular and respiratory medicine and will be discussed further in later chapters. See Table 3-5 for representative sympathomimetic drugs.

Table 3-5 **Sympathomimetic Drugs**

Drug	Indications
Catecholamines	
epinephrine	Anaphylaxis
norepinephrine	Hypotension
dopamine	Shock
dobutamine	Shock, heart failure
Other sympathomimetics	
phenylephrine	Nasal decongestant, hypotension
albuterol	Asthma

3.3e Sympatholytics

Just like adrenergic agonists, sympatholytics or adrenergic blockers have many cardiovascular indications. However, their general effect is to block or slow the effects of the sympathetic system. These drugs consist of alpha- and beta-blockers used to treat tachyarrhythmias and hypertension. In addition to their cardiovascular indications, alpha-blockers have direct action on the urethral sphincter, reducing urinary hesitancy in prostate hyperplasia. Adverse effects of beta-blockers can include bradycardia, atrioventricular blockade, and exacerbation of asthma. However, there are more selective $beta_1$-blockers, which affect only the heart with minimal effects on the $beta_2$-receptors found in the lungs. This will be covered in more depth in Chapters 9 and 10. Subgroups of adrenergic-blocking drugs or sympatholytics are described in Table 3-6 along with sample drugs and indications.

Clinical pearl

Beta-blockers can mask the signs and symptoms of hypoglycemia such as tremor and tachycardia, so they are used cautiously in patients with diabetes.

Learning Hint

Have you ever experienced stage fright? Performing artists and public speakers have been known to use beta-blockers to control tremor, anxiety, and palpitations before appearances.

TABLE 3-6 **Sympatholytic Drug Subgroups**

Sympatholytic Subgroup	Drug	Indication
Alpha-blocker	doxazosin	Hypertension
		Benign prostatic hyperplasia
Beta-blocker	propranolol	Hypertension

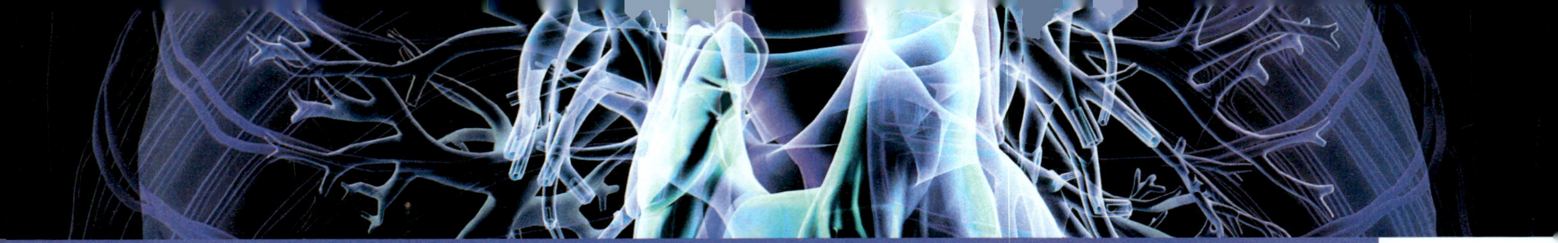

Summary

The autonomic nervous system (ANS) controls many of the activities of the heart and lungs; therefore, an understanding of this system is critical. The portions of the ANS that control the heart and lungs are the sympathetic (fight-or-flight) and parasympathetic (sleep-and-eat) branches. Stimulation of the sympathetic branch increases the rate and force of contraction of the heart and bronchodilates the lungs. The opposing parasympathetic branch, when stimulated, will decrease the rate and force of heart contractions and cause bronchoconstriction. Drugs given to "open up the airways" will either stimulate the sympathetic nervous system or block the effects of the parasympathetic nervous system.

REVIEW QUESTIONS

1. Which branches make up the peripheral nervous system?

I.	somatic	(a)	I and II
II.	parasympathetic	(b)	I, II, III, and IV
III.	sympathetic	(c)	IV only
IV.	central nervous system	(d)	I, II, and III

2. Indicate whether the following pertain to the sympathetic nervous system (S), parasympathetic nervous system (P), or both (B).

____ fight or flight
____ digestion
____ ACh at preganglion
____ NE
____ ACh at postganglion

3. Match synonymous terms in the autonomic nervous system.

____ sympathomimetic	(a)	cholinergic
____ parasympathomimetic	(b)	anticholinergic
____ sympatholytic	(c)	adrenergic
____ parasympatholytic	(d)	antiadrenergic

4. Bronchodilation can be achieved using which kind(s) of agent?

I.	parasympatholytic	(a)	I and II
II.	sympatholytic	(b)	II, III, and IV
III.	sympathomimetic	(c)	III only
IV.	parasympathomimetic	(d)	I and III

5. Skeletal muscles are found in
   (a) blood vessels
   (b) airways
   (c) heart
   (d) diaphragm
6. Contrast the two branches of the autonomic nervous system.
7. Differentiate afferent and efferent nerve impulses.
8. Give the physiologic responses to the following:
   $beta_2$ stimulation
   $beta_1$ stimulation
   $alpha_1$ stimulation
   $beta_2$ inhibition
9. What would be the anticholinergic response in the eyes, lungs, and heart?
10. What would be the adrenergic response in the eyes, lungs, and heart?

Chapter 4

Medicated Aerosol Treatments

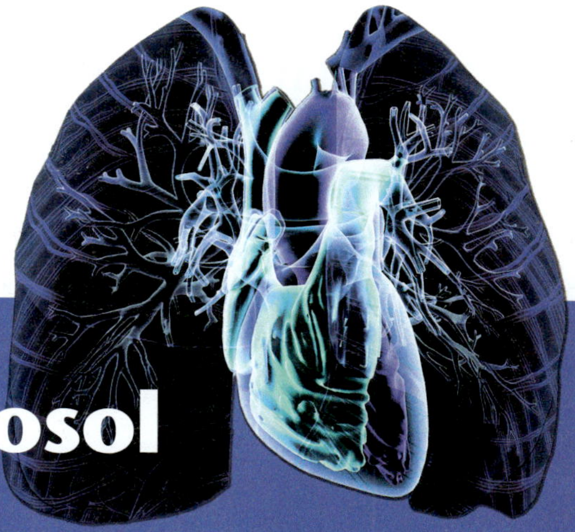

OBJECTIVES

Upon completion of this chapter you will be able to

- Define key terms related to aerosol therapy.
- Describe the main goals of aerosol therapy.
- State the advantages and disadvantages of the inhalation route of administration.
- Describe the factors that affect aerosol deposition.
- List advantages and limitations in using a metered-dose inhaler (MDI), a small-volume nebulizer (SVN), a breath-actuated nebulizer (BAN), and a dry-powder inhaler (DPI).
- Describe the proper technique for using an MDI, SVN, and DPI.
- State the advantages and limitations of using MDIs and SVNs in intubated and mechanically ventilated patients.
- Describe factors effecting aerosol deposition in mechanically ventilated patients.

KEY TERMS

aerosol
aerosol therapy
breath-actuated nebulizer
chlorofluorocarbons
deposition
dry-powder inhaler
hydrofluoroalkanes
inertial impaction
medicated aerosol
metered-dose inhaler
micron
penetration
small-volume nebulizer
spacer
stability
ultrasonic nebulizer

ABBREVIATIONS

AARC	American Association for Respiratory Care
BAN	breath-actuated nebulizer
CFC	chlorofluorocarbon
DPI	dry-powder inhaler
HFA	hydrofluoroalkane
HHN	hand-held nebulizer
HME	heat/moisture exchanger
MDI	metered-dose inhaler
OTC	over-the-counter
SVN	small-volume nebulizer
USN	ultrasonic nebulizer

The inhalation route is a very fast-acting and effective route for delivering humidification and/or medications directly to the respiratory system. Nonmedicated aerosols such as sterile water are referred to as bland aerosols. Bland aerosols are discussed in Chapter 6, in relation to bronchial hygiene and mucokinetic agents. In this chapter we focus on aerosolizing a medication that will be inhaled into the respiratory system and then absorbed into the rich capillary network of blood vessels within this system. Administering a drug via the inhalation route is very advantageous in that it delivers the medication to the needed site of action directly and thus minimizes systemic absorption. This, in turn, minimizes the occurrence—or at least the level of severity—of side effects that may be associated with the drug.

For example inhaled steroids are now a mainstay for treatment of moderate to severe asthma because they reduce the inflammatory response in the lung. An oral form of the steroid could be used, but a much higher oral dosage would be required to get high enough levels in the entire bloodstream that the drug would eventually travel to the lungs and produce the desired effect. Conversely, by inhaling an aerosol of the steroid, a much lower dose can be given because it will be delivered right to the needed site to reduce the inflammation. The side effects of steroids are numerous and dosage-dependent, so the inhalation route offers a way to minimize the serious systemic side effects yet maximize the effects on the lungs.

The inhalation route does present certain challenges to the practitioner. One challenge is to teach the patient to self-administer the medicated aerosol effectively. Another is to achieve consistent dosage delivery, considering that there are many variables that affect deposition within the respiratory system. This chapter provides the necessary background to understand the different delivery devices and the factors that will optimize medicated aerosol delivery to the respiratory system.

4.1 BASIC CONCEPTS OF MEDICATED AEROSOLS

4.1a What Is Aerosol Therapy?

An **aerosol** is a suspension of solid or liquid particles within a gas. For example, when we sneeze, we create an aerosol of liquid droplet particles that are suspended in the rapidly exhaled gas from our lungs. A dust storm also creates an aerosol, but in that case the aerosol particles are solid in nature. **Aerosol therapy** can deliver either solid or liquid aerosol particles into the respiratory tract for therapeutic purposes. According to Egan's *Fundamentals of Respiratory Care,* three main goals of aerosol therapy are the following:

1. To humidify inspired gas, which may be dry or humidity deficient: An example is an intubated patient, whose natural humidification system (upper airways) is bypassed.
2. To improve the mobilization and elimination of secretions: Examples include patients with thick tenacious secretions who are having difficulty expectorating, or patients who have a dry, nonproductive cough and need a sputum induction to obtain a sample for analysis.
3. To deliver medications to the respiratory tract.

Each of these indications is discussed in depth in later chapters. The first two indications are discussed in Chapter 6, which deals with mucokinetics. The third indication is discussed in various chapters covering specific categories of drugs that can be administered via aerosol therapy. This chapter will focus on the overall *principles* of effective aerosol delivery to the respiratory system.

BVT Lab

Flashcards are available for this chapter at www.BVTLab.com.

4.1b Advantages and Disadvantages

The advantages of delivering drugs via the aerosol route center around two major facts. First the lungs have a large surface area and rich corresponding vasculature for drug absorption. Recall from Chapter 1 that blood flow influences the extent and rate of absorption. Therefore medications delivered via the inhalation route act very quickly. Second the aerosol route can be used to deliver a medication locally to the lungs or for other purposes (e.g., inhaled insulin). Smaller doses are effective because the entire bloodstream is not being medicated and there is no first-pass effect in the GI tract. When the lungs are the intended site of action, medication is delivered directly using smaller dosages. This results in a rapid onset of action and reduces whole-body adverse effects. From a patient perspective, the inhalation route is effective and convenient if proper instruction and education are given.

As attractive as inhaled medication aerosols may be, there are also some disadvantages that we need to be aware of. Unlike oral or IV routes of drug administration, it can be difficult to deliver a precise dose to the lungs with each aerosol treatment. The exact amount of drug delivered by inhalation is affected by many factors, including properties of the drugs themselves, characteristics of the devices used to generate the aerosols, and the way the patient inhales the aerosol. These will be discussed more fully in the following paragraphs. Most of these problems can be minimized if the health-care practitioner understands the principles of aerosol medication delivery, knows the proper use of the various aerosol delivery devices, and can instruct and educate the patient properly. Good patient education is particularly important for patients who self-administer aerosolized medications. Patients must learn not only to administer aerosols to themselves but also to care for the specialized equipment that is used to deliver the aerosol in order to ensure proper function and infection control. See Table 4-1 for a list of advantages and disadvantages for medicated aerosols.

TABLE 4-1 Advantages and Disadvantages of Medicated Aerosols

Advantages	Disadvantages
Smaller required doses	Difficult to deliver consistent, precise dose
Quick drug response	Requires patient compliance and education
Fewer, less severe side effects	Equipment maintenance
Painless and convenient	

time for review

Why does the inhalation route provide a fast onset of action?

4.1c Technical Background

Let's return to the sneeze as an example of an aerosol. The liquid particles (the very small water droplets from the lungs) are suspended in a gas (the air expelled from the lungs). The aerosol particles can travel and settle out on inanimate objects such as the floor, or they can be breathed in by another individual and settle in that person's lungs. This is why the sneeze (or cough) represents a likely mode of transmission for certain pulmonary diseases. We certainly don't want the possibly contaminated aerosol particles of a sneeze to travel into someone else's lungs, and we hope the aerosol droplets will all hit a tissue and be properly discarded. While the aerosol produced by a sneeze is definitely not something you want to inhale, it can be very beneficial to deliver certain types of medication into the lungs in an aerosol form.

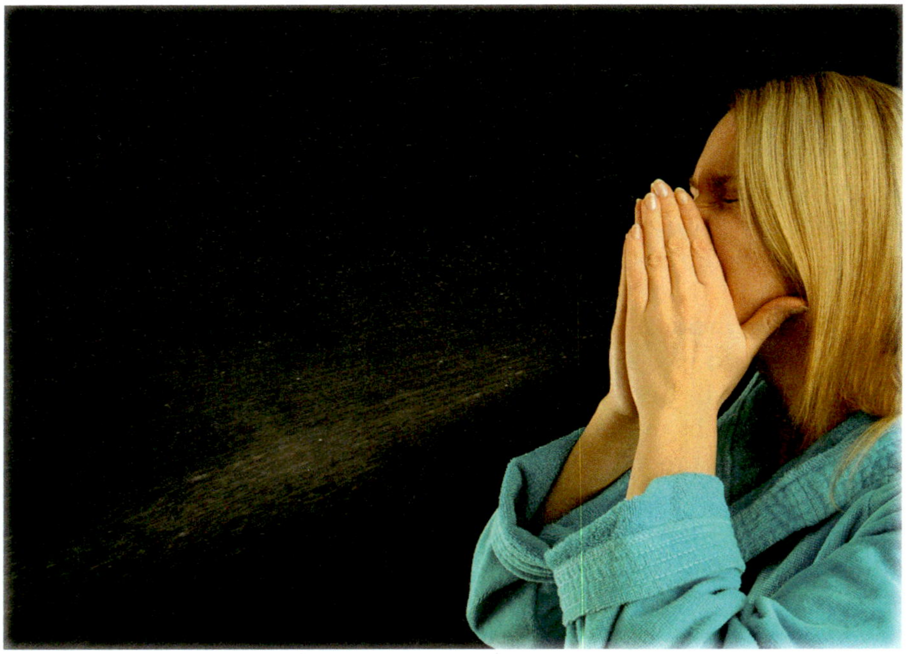

Source: Shutterstock

A **medicated aerosol** is simply a suspension of a liquid or solid drug in a carrier gas. As we mentioned earlier, numerous factors are involved in determining how medicine is delivered into the lungs. Let's start with four technical terms that are used in reference to medicated aerosols. These are all factors that influence drug delivery within the lungs. First, **stability** refers to the tendency of an aerosol to remain in suspension. Currently available delivery devices, particularly metered-dose inhalers, create very stable aerosols that are capable of reaching the lower airways. However, it is important for patients to hold their breath after inhalation so that the particles will "rain out" into the lungs rather than be exhaled.

Second, **penetration** refers to how far into the lungs the aerosol particles travel. Penetration is related to several factors, such as the size of the aerosol particle, the patient's breathing pattern, and the disease state. Optimally you want the aerosol to penetrate to the desired level of action. How you accomplish this mainly depends on the breathing pattern, which will be discussed shortly.

The third term is **deposition**, which refers to the aerosol particles falling out of suspension. Ideally we want them to fall out into the desired area of the lungs. Targeting aerosol therapy to specific regions of the airway can be difficult. The patient's disease state, breathing pattern (inspiratory flow rate, respiratory rate, tidal volume, ratio of inspiratory time to expiratory time, and breath-holding), and the particle size are all factors in determining where particles will be deposited in the lung.

The final term is **inertial impaction**. Even though these particles are very small, they nevertheless have weight and must obey the laws of physics. They will develop inertial energy depending on the speed of the delivery device and/or the rate of breathing. If something gets in their way, such as a bifurcation of the lung, and their inertial energy is such that they cannot negotiate the turn, they will impact on the airway wall.

time for review

What factors influence drug delivery in the lungs?

4.1d Aerosol Size Matters

One final technical aspect of aerosol particles is size. Size is one of the most important factors in determining whether the aerosol will get to the lung. Aerosol particles are measured in **microns**, which equal one-millionth of a meter. Critically small variances in size will determine how far the aerosol can penetrate.

For example 10- to 15-micron particles deposit in the upper airways (nose and mouth). Many nasal sprays produce particles in this range, because this is where we want deposition to occur. Slightly smaller particles, within the 5- to 10-micron range, penetrate to large bronchi. Particles that are 1 to 5 microns in size penetrate to the lower airways, where most bronchoactive drugs are needed. Most aerosol-generating devices therefore produce aerosol particles in this range. Particles smaller than 0.5 micron have so much stability that although they may penetrate to the alveoli, they may also be exhaled right back out. See Figure 4-1, which shows where various particle sizes will deposit.

FIGURE 4-1 Deposition of Various Sizes of Aerosol Particles in the Respiratory System

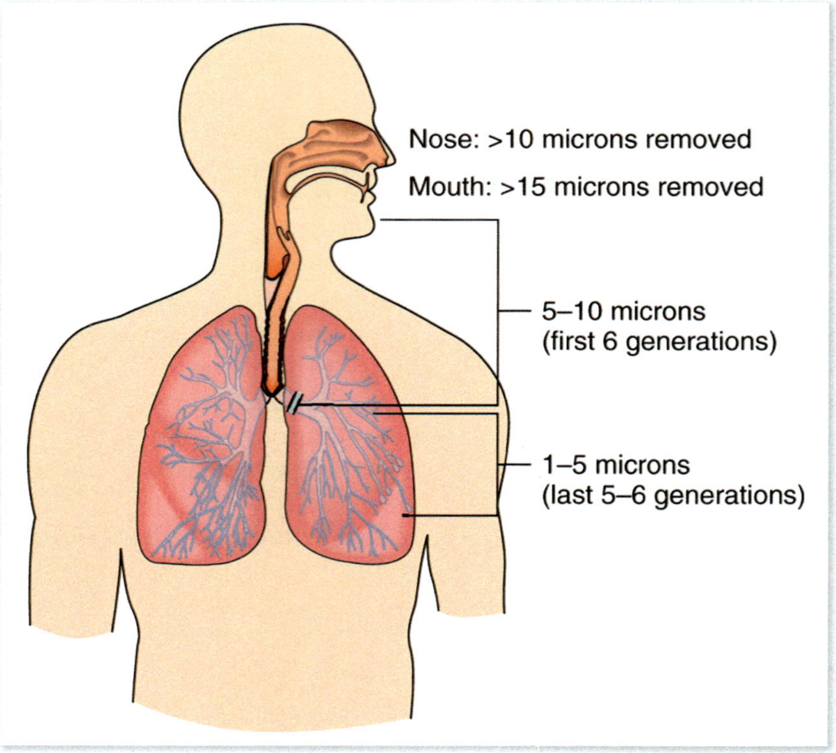

Learning Hint

If you were an aerosol particle and tried to reach the bottom of the tracheal bronchial tree, would it be better to travel very quickly or very slowly? Picture a fork in the road (not the kind you eat with); you need to take one of the roads to get deeper into the lungs. You must slow down in order to negotiate the curve of your choice.

Numerous factors determine particle size. Some of the most significant variables include the design of the nebulizer, the flow and density of gas powering the nebulizer, the dead volume of the nebulizer, and the volume of diluent used. Flow rates of 6 to 8 liters/minute are optimal when using air or oxygen to power a jet nebulizer. Nebulization time is usually not more than 10 minutes. The *dead volume* of the nebulizer is the volume of solution that cannot be nebulized. Adding a diluent such as saline increases the amount of drug that is nebulized because the volume of solution that remains in the nebulizer contains less medication. The dead volume usually ranges from 1 to 3 ml, depending on the design of the nebulizer. Increasing the fill volume would reduce the proportion of the dose lost as dead volume but would require an increase in the nebulization time. Therefore a fill volume of 4 to 6 ml is recommended.

Clinical pearl

Disease states can influence aerosol distribution in the lungs. In patients with chronic obstructive pulmonary disease (COPD), aerosol particles may distribute more centrally than in non-COPD patients, who have more particles in the peripheral portions of the lungs.

4.1e Breathing Pattern

If the particles are within the proper range, how much aerosol actually gets to the lung depends greatly on the patient's breathing pattern. Remember that one of the disadvantages of the inhalation route is imprecise dosing. Even if the aerosol-generating device is used properly, studies estimate that only around 10% to 50% may actually get into the lungs under optimal conditions. If poor technique is used, only 1% to 2% may actually deposit in the lungs.

If you visualize the tracheal bronchial tree, it is a maze of sharp turns that presents a great potential for inertial impaction that will interfere with even distribution of the aerosol in the lungs. Rapid inspiratory flows can cause turbulence that favors inertial impaction and deposition higher in the respiratory tract. Slow inspiration produces more laminar (layered) flow and results in deeper penetration of the aerosol particles.

Looking at all factors, one can see why the optimal breathing pattern for effective aerosol delivery to the lungs is a slow deep breath with a hold. Slow breathing minimizes the inertial impaction that can cause the medication to deposit in the upper airways. Deep breathing allows for maximum penetration within the lungs. A breath hold allows for these very small, stable particles to deposit out of the aerosol and onto the lung tissue. Therefore a slow deep breath through the mouth with an *inspiratory hold* is the optimal breathing pattern for maximal penetration and deposition within the lungs.

BVT Lab

Visit www.BVTLab.com to explore the student resources available for this chapter.

Occasionally you may want to deliver medicated aerosols to the upper airway. The upper airway includes the nasopharynx, oropharynx, larynx, trachea, and supraglottic area. You may want to deliver a topical anesthetic to the supraglottic regions before doing bronchoscopy procedures. As another example glottic edema can cause upper airway swelling, which could asphyxiate a patient, and vasoconstrictors can be given to shrink the swelling and maintain a patent airway. If your target for aerosol deposition is the upper airway, larger particles (of 5 microns or more) should be used along with a faster inspiratory flow rate to favor inertial impaction and deposition in the upper airways. In summary, in most situations, you are striving for deposition in the peripheral regions of the lung, so a *slow deep* breath through the mouth with an *inspiratory hold* is best. Table 4-2 provides general guidelines on breathing patterns for aerosol deposition.

Table 4-2 **Optimal Breathing Pattern**

Peripheral Distribution	Oropharynx, Larynx, Trachea, and First Six Airway Generations
Slow inspiratory flow (less than 30 liters/minute), deep breath, and a 10-second breath hold. If the patient can't hold his/her breath for 10 seconds, encourage slow breathing with an occasional deep breath. Aerosol particle size range should be 1–5 microns.	Fast inspiratory flow (more than 30 liters/minute) to increase deposition in the larynx and supraglottic area. Normal flow at 30 liters/minute increases deposition in the trachea and the first six generations of airways (larger airways) with aerosol particles in the range of 5–10 microns.

4.1f Types of Aerosolized Drugs

What types of drugs can be aerosolized and delivered into the respiratory system? The list may surprise you because many people are only familiar with over-the-counter (OTC) nasal decongestant sprays or the commonly prescribed bronchodilators used to treat asthma. In addition to steroids (which were mentioned in the introduction), several other drug classifications can be given via inhalation. More in-depth discussions will be included in the chapters that deal with each of these specific classifications. Following is a brief description of these drug classifications.

Nasal Decongestants

Nasal decongestants appear primarily as OTC metered-spray pumps that you spray into your nostrils. These produce larger particles, which settle in the nasal region. Basically, they are fairly powerful vasoconstrictors that decrease the blood flow to a stuffy nose. This, in turn, allows the nasal passageway to clear because the vessels shrink and the passageways open up. It should be noted that vasoconstrictors can increase blood pressure, which therefore should be monitored. A representative drug in this class is Neo-Synephrine® (generic name: phenylephrine).

Bronchodilators

Bronchodilators enlarge the diameter of the airway through a number of different mechanisms, most of which include relaxing the smooth muscle that surrounds the airways. Some representative drugs include albuterol (Proventil® HFA), ipratropium (Atrovent® HFA), pirbuterol (Maxair®), and salmeterol (Serevent® Diskus®). These and others are discussed in Chapter 5.

Mast Cell Stabilizers

This category of drugs desensitizes the allergic response and therefore prevents or decreases the incidence of asthma attacks. Representative drugs are cromolyn sodium and nedocromil sodium, which are discussed in Chapter 7.

Corticosteroids

Inhaled corticosteroids are used to control asthma and prevent or decrease the severity of an attack. These drugs are the backbone medications used to treat persistent asthma of varying severity. They help to control airway inflammation, resulting in improved lung function and a decreased need for short-acting bronchodilators. Representative drugs include beclomethasone (Qvar®), fluticasone (Flovent® HFA), and budesonide (Pulmicort®). These and others are discussed in Chapter 7.

Clinical pearl

We have included both generic and brand drug names because you will encounter both in your practice. Examine the generic names carefully because they often will give you a clue about the drug's mechanism of action or pharmacologic classification. For example note that most corticosteroid generic names end in *-one.*

Mucolytics

Mucolytics break down the secretions in the lungs to make it easier to expectorate and clear the lungs. Besides nebulization, sometimes these medications are instilled directly into the lungs in liquid form via an endotracheal tube or bronchoscope. A representative drug is acetylcysteine. This drug and others are discussed in Chapter 6.

Antimicrobials

Much promise lies in this new area in which aerosolized antibiotics and antiviral agents have been, and continue to be, developed to fight both bacterial and viral infections involving the respiratory system. Representative drugs include gentamicin, amphotericin B, ribavirin, and pentamidine. These and others are covered in Chapter 8.

4.2 AEROSOL DELIVERY DEVICES

4.2a Metered-Dose Inhaler

The most common type of aerosol treatment is the **metered-dose inhaler** (MDI). MDIs are small, portable, aerosol-delivery devices that can effectively deliver medication to the respiratory system. They basically consist of a propellant inside a canister filled with medication (see Figure 4-2). Because MDIs are usually self-administered, they require patient education and cooperation.

FIGURE 4-2 Schematic and Photo of MDI Delivery Systems

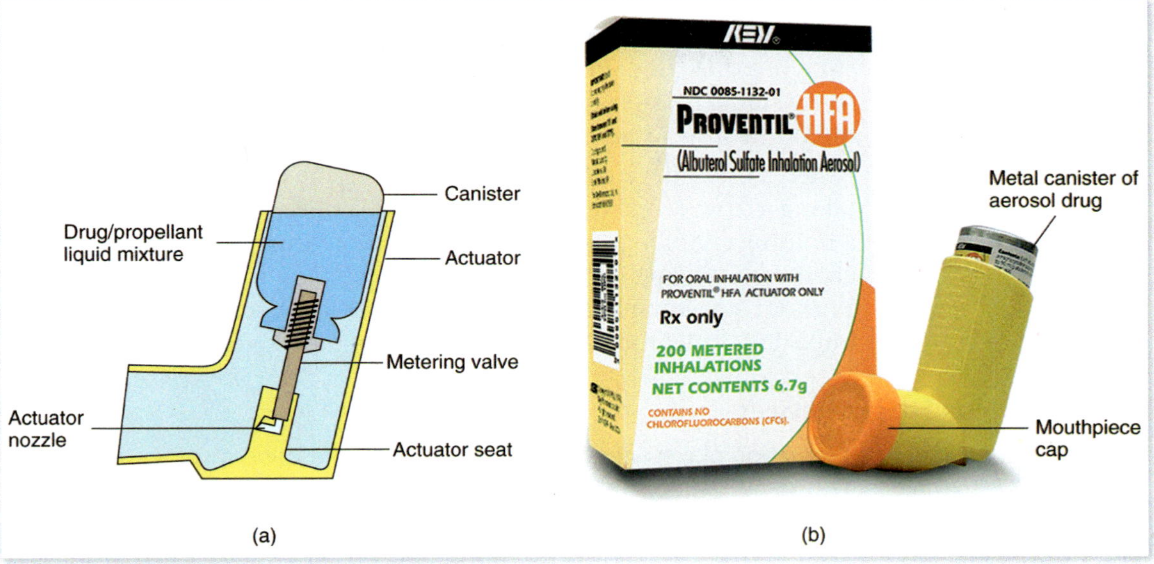

Source: Merck Archives; Merck, Sharpt & Dohme Corp., 2015

CONTROVERSY

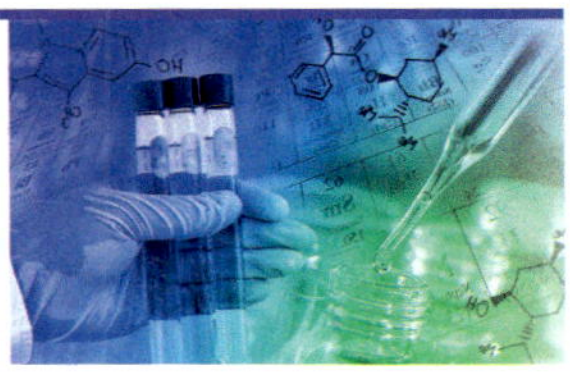

The propellants used in MDIs are blends of liquefied gas **chlorofluorocarbons** (CFCs; Freon™), which are bad for the environment because they damage the Earth's ozone layer. In addition some patients are sensitive to these propellants and may experience bronchospasm. Therefore the United Nations Environment Program has stopped the manufacture of CFCs. Pharmaceutical companies have developed **hydrofluoroalkanes** (HFAs) to take their place. HFA propellants are safer for the ozone layer as well as for patients. The change from CFC to HFA propellants was complex. It required reformulation of the medications and reengineering of the inhalers, including both internal and external components such as the actuator and mouthpiece.

The HFA formulations of albuterol and ipratropium bromide have been shown to be equivalent to their respective CFC formulations in terms of safety and bronchodilation effect. However, the delivered dose of the HFA formulation of beclomethasone dipropionate (a corticosteroid) is five times greater than with the original CFC formula.

Spacers and Special Considerations

The administration of aerosols by MDI can be facilitated by the use of a reservoir device. A reservoir is an extension tube with a mouthpiece added to the MDI. There are two types of reservoirs: spacers and holding chambers. A **spacer** is a simple extension placed between the MDI and the patient to contain the aerosol as it travels to the patient. Holding chambers are spacers with one-way valves that hold the aerosol until the patient inhales and therefore assist in the coordination and timing of the aerosol delivery (see Figure 4-3). These devices provide three major advantages.

1. The particles that exit the MDI have a very high flow rate because of the pressurized delivery system. Therefore inertial impaction in the oropharynx is a likely occurrence. The reservoir slows the particles down and gives the patient time to coordinate inspiration. In addition many of the initial

Clinical pearl

There are some inexpensive alternatives that patients can use temporarily as a spacer. Examples include a 6-inch piece of corrugated aerosol tubing. However these are temporary solutions, and we recommend a proper spacer, which can be reused and cleaned properly. According to the American Association for Respiratory Care (AARC) clinical practice guidelines, an MDI with a spacer device and face mask is appropriate for patients (usually younger than 3 years) who are unable to use a mouthpiece.

particles are larger than 5 microns, and the reservoir allows enough time to vaporize them to the size of 1 to 5 microns, so lung deposition is better.

2. Some patients, as they depress the canister, may move the MDI and end up spraying their nose or eyes. The spacer device allows them to have something stable in their mouth as they depress the canister; the spacer will direct the flow of aerosol into the oral cavity and eventually into the lungs.
3. Patients often have difficulty coordinating the activation of the device and taking a slow deep breath. A spacer with a one-way valve (also known as a holding chamber) makes this a more forgiving process. With a holding chamber, if the patient lags behind in breathing in, it is of little consequence. Without a holding chamber, if the patient lags behind, the aerosol is already impacted in the mouth—or, if the patient moved, on the nose or eyes.

FIGURE 4-3 **Various Spacer Devices**

A schematic representation of a spacer device along with a child using a spacer device with a mask and a female patient using a spacer device with a mouthpiece.

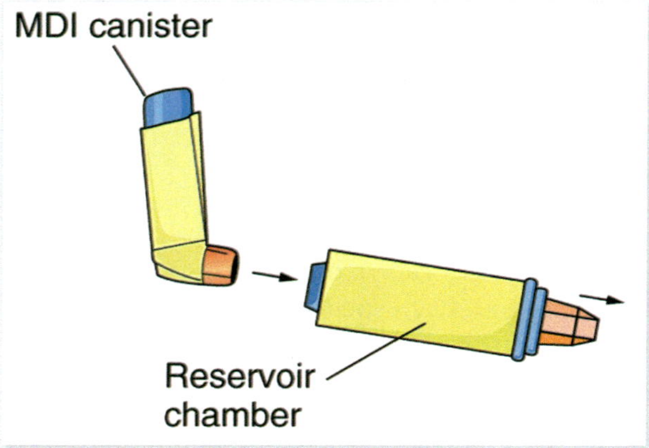

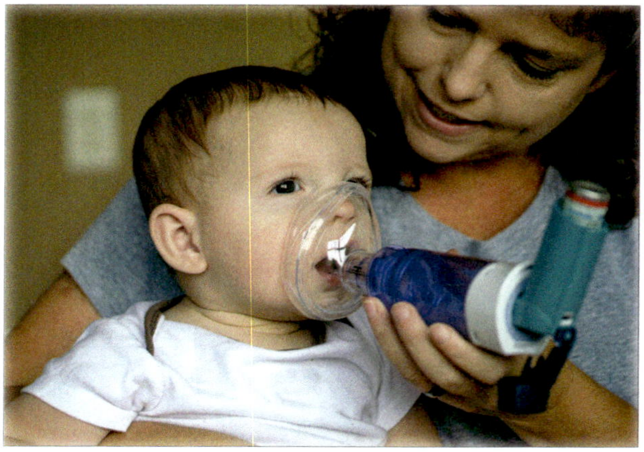

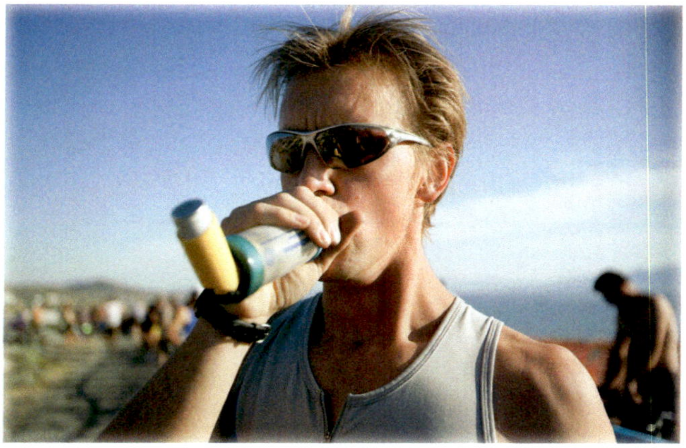

Source: Shutterstock, Thinkstock

Administering an MDI Treatment

Some studies have shown that up to 60% to 70% of patients do not use their MDIs correctly. Therefore we will discuss the steps and the factors involved in administering an MDI treatment and follow up with a simplified and streamlined set of specific steps.

If the MDI has not been used for days or weeks, the propellant may be lost or the first dose may not be properly charged. Therefore shake the MDI first and discharge three to four waste doses to prime the valve with drug and propellant. Please check the MDI manufacturer's instructions since the time period of inactivity prior to repriming the inhaler is different depending on the medication.

The next step is to exhale and place the spacer device in your mouth. If you don't have a spacer device, you may need to either hold the MDI 3 to 4 cm (two finger widths) away from your open mouth or place the mouthpiece fully into your mouth and close your lips around it. Take a slow deep breath in through your mouth as you depress the canister, continuing until your lungs are filled, to allow for maximum distribution throughout the lungs. Hold this breath for up to 10 seconds to allow for deposition of the medicated aerosol, and then breathe out normally.

Often a second dose is needed or prescribed, but it is important to wait a few minutes to allow the first dose to work. Most of the short-acting bronchodilators work very rapidly, and waiting a minimum of 1 to 2 minutes allows the airways to open and the next dose to deposit in lower generations.

Clinical pearl

If you are administering a short-acting bronchodilator and any other inhaled medication, there are additional considerations. The bronchodilator should be given first, to open the airways so that the additional medications can be widely distributed in the lungs. In addition, inhaled steroids can deplete or wipe out the normal bacteria in the mouth, and therefore it is critical to rinse the mouth after inhaling steroids to prevent an opportunistic oral infection.

Patient & Family Education

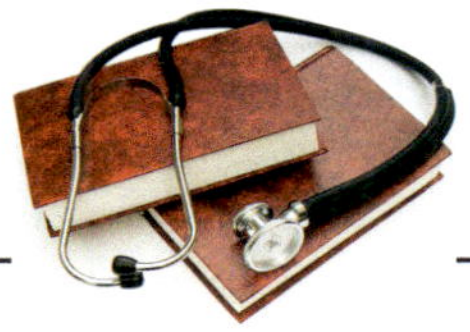

MDI Instructions

Using an MDI requires several steps and is most often self-administered. Proper use of an MDI is critical for effectiveness of medication delivery and requires excellent patient and family education. Here are some suggested steps in the process to facilitate patient education. Keep in mind that a return demonstration by the patient is critical to ensure proper and complete understanding.

1. Assemble the inhaler and hold it upright. Don't forget to take off the cap and inspect the canister for foreign materials such as lint or coins. One author treated a patient who aspirated a small steel pellet that had been in his pocket along with his MDI (which didn't have its cap on)!
2. Shake the MDI well. (Remember to discharge a waste dose if it has been more than 2 weeks since you last used the inhaler.)
3. Exhale normally.
4. Place the spacer device in your mouth, keeping your tongue down so it doesn't obstruct flow. If no spacer device is available, use the open-mouth technique and position the inhaler about 4 cm (two finger widths) away from your mouth. Some newer MDIs instruct patients to insert the mouthpiece in the mouth and close the lips around it. It is important to check the instructions for use with each MDI device.
5. Begin to take a slow deep breath through your mouth, pressing down on the canister as you continue to inhale.
6. Breathe in until your lungs are full; then hold your breath for up to 10 seconds.
7. Breathe out normally.

Clinical pearl

Having the patient tip his or her head backward slightly, as if sniffing, produces maximal opening of the airway and can improve drug delivery to the lungs.

(Continues)

8. Wait 1 to 2 minutes before taking the next puff in the same manner. If a third puff is prescribed, wait another 1 to 2 minutes before taking the third puff.
9. Reassemble and store the inhaler (put the cap back on).

NOTE: If you are using an inhaled steroid, follow the same procedure as for a bronchodilator, with the following considerations.
1. Use the bronchodilator first (if both are to be used).
2. Rinse your mouth and throat with mouthwash or water after finishing.

time for review

Instruct a classmate on the proper use of an MDI. If possible, obtain a placebo (containing no drug) MDI for optimal practice.

Clinical pearl

Shakespeare asked, "What's in a name?" The answer may be "plenty" when there are various names to describe the same thing. Some hospitals call SVNs *hand-held nebulizers* (HHNs), or spontaneous nebulizer treatment, or jet nebulizer treatment. Others use the brand name of the nebulizer device.

4.2b Small-Volume Nebulizer

The term **small-volume nebulizer** (SVN) covers a variety of devices that are used to administer liquid medications as aerosols. Whereas the MDI forms an aerosol only when it is activated, the SVN can aerosolize medication continuously via a flow of compressed air or oxygen. The most common SVNs are small-volume jet nebulizers, but these are not particularly efficient. They deliver only about 10% to 20% of the dose to the lungs. Their inefficiency is related to several factors, including the type and flow of gas powering the nebulizer, medication lost during exhalation, and the dead-space volume of the nebulizer, which is the portion of the dose that cannot be nebulized. The dead volume can be as little as 1 to 3 ml. This is the reason for using diluent: to increase the total volume of the dose to about 4 to 6 ml (see Figure 4-4).

4.2c Newer Nebulizer Designs

One newer type of jet nebulizer is breath-actuated, which nebulizes only on inspiration. It has a low dead volume, and waste during exhalation is essentially eliminated. The delivered dose can be more than three times greater than with continuous nebulization. The AeroEclipse® nebulizer is an example of a **breath-actuated nebulizer** (BAN). Another nebulizer design routes exhaled gas through an expiratory valve in the mouthpiece. This results in the release of more aerosol during the inhalation due to containment of the aerosol in the nebulizer chamber during exhalation. Finally some nebulizer designs add a storage bag with a one-way valve to the mouthpiece connector. This results in collection of the aerosolized medication during exhalation with subsequent delivery to the patient during inhalation. Small-volume **ultrasonic nebulizers** (USNs) are also quite efficient. They have a very low dead volume and may not need diluent, which shortens treatment time. However they are very expensive.

FIGURE 4-4 Schematic of SVN Device

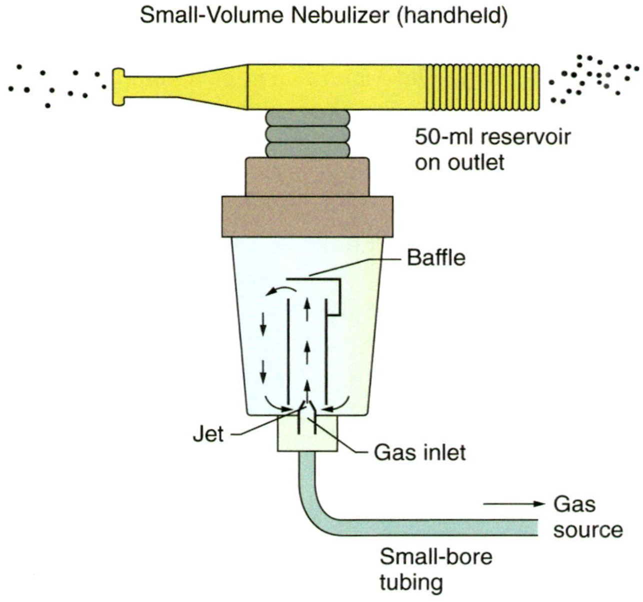

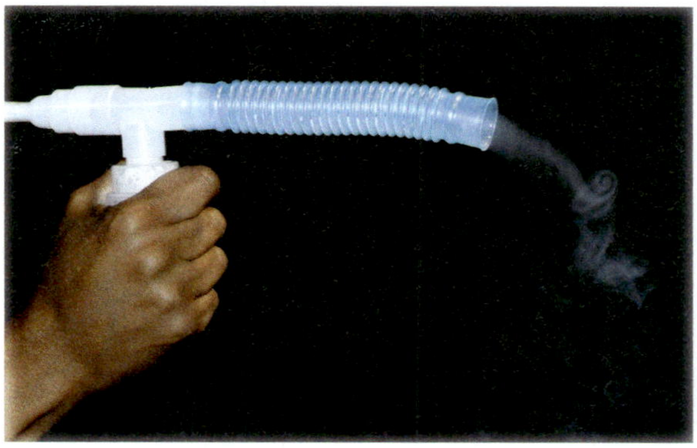
Source: Shutterstock

The newest type of SVN is the Aeroneb® or Aeroneb® Pro by Aerogen. The Aeroneb® uses a vibrating-mesh technology to nebulize liquid medication. Both the USN and the Aeroneb® are highly efficient, have low dead volumes, and can be either AC- or battery-powered. Up to 60% of the dose is actually deposited in the lung, compared to 10% to 20% of the dose using a jet nebulizer. Mesh nebulizers may be cost-effective for delivering precise doses of expensive or toxic medications. The I-neb® is an example of a nebulizer developed specifically to deliver precise doses of iloprost (Ventavis®) for the treatment of primary pulmonary hypertension. Widespread use of these types of SVNs is limited due to their high cost.

A spontaneous aerosol treatment can be given with a mouthpiece or a mask. A mask is not preferred because it reduces deposition in the lung. Much of the medication is deposited on the face—or, in the case of one of the authors, the beard. However situations that involve, for example, an obtunded or comatose patient, or a child who cannot maintain a good seal around a mouthpiece, may necessitate the use of a mask to deliver the aerosol. Another possible disadvantage is that the SVN is bulkier to use than the MDI because it requires an external pneumatic (gas) power source. Care and cleaning of the SVN is also more involved than for the MDI.

Some medications may require a specific form of aerosol delivery device. This is mainly because the type of drug may affect the performance of the nebulizer. See Table 4-3 for examples of medications that require a special delivery device.

TABLE 4-3 Medications That Require a Special Delivery Device

Medication	Nebulizer
budesonide	Jet or mesh
iloprost	Jet or mesh
pentamidine (Respirgard II®)	Jet
tobramycin (Pari LC Plus®)	Jet

4.2d Continuous Bronchodilator Therapy

More frequent dosing of bronchodilators may be necessary in cases of severe bronchospasm, such as status asthmaticus. When traditional dosing strategies fail to control bronchospasm, continuous nebulization of albuterol may also be considered. The *2007 Guidelines for the Diagnosis and Management of Asthma,* released by the National Heart, Lung, and Blood Institute Panel of Experts 3, recommends 2.5 to 5 mg of albuterol by nebulizer every 20 minutes for three doses or 10 to 15 mg of albuterol per hour by continuous nebulization. Specialized large-volume jet nebulizers such as the HEART® and HOPE® nebulizers are designed for this purpose. Patients who require such high doses of albuterol must be monitored continuously for further deterioration of their condition and for side effects such as tachycardia, arrhythmias, hypokalemia (low potassium), hyperglycemia, and tremors.

A review of the literature finds continuous nebulization to be safe if very closely monitored, but the reported dosages used in different studies vary, as do the results when continuous nebulization is compared to dosing every 20 minutes with a small-volume nebulizer. Overall the results suggest that continuous nebulization may be superior, but that lower doses may be just as effective as the recommended 10 to 15 mg/hour, and there is less toxicity.

Clinical pearl

Patients should be instructed not to exhale into the DPI, as this may blow out the powder and therefore reduce the dose. In addition, the added humidity from the breath may wet the powder and reduce delivery.

4.2e Dry-Powder Inhaler

From the definition of an aerosol, we can see that an aerosol can also contain solid particles suspended in a gas. **Dry-powder inhalers** (DPIs) are devices that actually deliver the drug in powder form to the lungs (see Figure 4-5). DPIs have no propellant or external power sources and are small, self-generating devices. According to the *2002 AARC Clinical Practice Guidelines,* the patient must generate sufficient inspiratory flow rates (equal to or greater than 50 liters/min) for the device to aerosolize the dry powder properly. This may be difficult to achieve in acute respiratory distress or with small children, especially during an asthma attack (see Table 4-4).

FIGURE 4-5 Examples of DPI Devices

(a) This Diskus® inhaler device contains the broncodilator drug salmeterol (Serevent®) in the form of a powder and in a dose strength of 50 mcg per actuation. The small dose indicator window shows the number of doses remaining in the Diskus®. Pulling the lever releases a premeasured dose of powdered drug, which is inhaled through the mouth and into the lungs. Copyright GlaxoSmithKline. Used with permission.

(b) The bronchodilator drug tiotropium (Spiriva®) is administered through a HandiHaler® device that crushes a capsule that contains the powdered drug. The powder is then inhaled through the mouth and into the lungs.

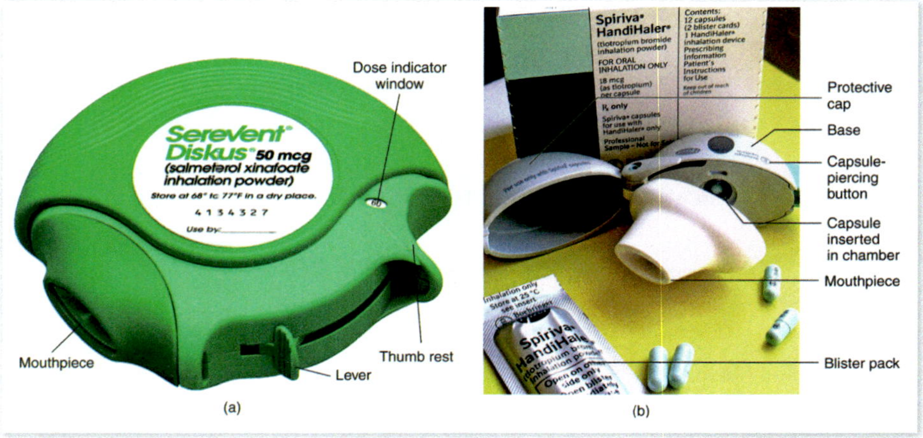

Copyright: GlaxoSmithKline. Used with permission.

TABLE 4-4 Advantages and Disadvantages of Dry-Powder Inhalers

Advantages	Disadvantages
Relatively small and easy to use	Fewer drugs available in powder form
Contains no harmful propellants	Some patients may react to the carrier substance
Easy to tell how much drug is left	Inspiratory flow of at least 50–60 liters/min is required
Eliminates timing and technique problems with MDIs	May not be appropriate for patients with altered mental status or neuromuscular weakness
Can be used in cold environments (e.g., on ski slopes), where propellants will not work	

4.2f Choosing the Appropriate Delivery Device

How do you choose among the MDI, SVN, and DPI? The choice depends on several factors. Generally, if a patient is able to follow instructions and demonstrates correct use of an MDI with a holding chamber, it is the preferred form to use. However the patient must have an adequate inspiratory capacity and be able to hold his or her breath. This is very important because the patient gets only two or three chances at good aerosol deposition. MDIs work well for patients in mild distress or who are taking a drug for prophylactic treatment. An unstable breathing pattern or respiratory distress will limit the effectiveness of an MDI.

Clinical pearl

SVNs may require unit-dose drug packaging if the patient is unable to prepare the correct dosage using a dropper.

An SVN is indicated if the patient is unable to follow the instructions to complete an effective MDI treatment or if the respiratory pattern is unstable. For example the patient may be in distress, tachypneic, and unable to take a slow deep breath with a hold. The SVN allows for numerous breaths over time, which provides more deposition in cases of acute respiratory distress. SVNs may make more sense in an acute asthma attack, although the research is not conclusive. The SVN with a mask is an option for disoriented or comatose patients who are breathing spontaneously.

DPIs are used less frequently because fewer drugs are available in this form and high inspiratory flow rates are needed. However, because of their portability (they are easy to keep in a pocket) and ease of use, they may be prescribed for children who have adequate inspiratory flow rates to use the device properly. DPIs also work well in cold weather conditions, where the MDI propellants may be hampered. The AARC guidelines do not recommend DPIs for children younger than 6 years of age.

In summation, if the patient can follow instructions and has a stable breathing pattern, and if the prescribed drug is available in that form, the MDI is the best device. We strongly recommend using a spacer with an MDI (even in these cost-containment days), because spacers help coordinate a better and more effective dose into the lungs and minimize the amount that is deposited in the mouth. However, for patients who are unable to use an MDI for whatever reason, or for patients with an unstable breathing pattern (fast rate, unable to hold breath or to deep-breathe), an SVN is a better choice. Remember, SVNs are bulkier and require an outside gas source and more meticulous cleaning, but if a patient cannot use a MDI, this is the best way to deliver medication into the lungs. Since the patient will ultimately be responsible for using the device, and all devices are effective when used properly, another way to select the best device is patient preference, taking into account such factors as convenience and cost.

4.2g Aerosol Delivery in Intubated Patients

Clinical pearl

According to the AARC guidelines, aerosol deposition from SVN nebulizers during mechanical ventilation is from 1.2% to 15% in adults and about 0.22% in infants. Aerosol deposition from MDIs during mechanical ventilation ranges from 6% to 11% in adults and is about 0.9% in infants

Many patients who require mechanical ventilation also need aerosol therapy. Both MDIs and SVNs are commonly used, but administration of aerosols to mechanically ventilated patients does require some special considerations. There are technical and patient safety issues to be considered, especially when administering SVNs to patients on ventilators. The complications associated with SVNs result mostly from the flow used to carry the aerosol into the ventilator circuit.

Getting an effective dose delivered to the lungs of a mechanically ventilated patient can also be quite a challenge. We will not provide a comprehensive discussion of aerosol delivery in mechanical ventilation because this requires a thorough understanding of how ventilators work. However, we do want to give a brief overview of some of the major issues involved, as well as the basic technique used, in the delivery of SVNs and MDIs in this particular setting.

Clinical pearl

The patient should be monitored for a buildup of pressure (Auto-PEEP) when prolonging the inspiratory time.

Factors that affect aerosol deposition in mechanical ventilation include the ventilator settings, the ventilator circuit, and the aerosol device used. Ventilator factors are related to the type of breath or breathing pattern of the patient. A patient-triggered breath tends to increase aerosol deposition in the lungs more than a breath triggered by the ventilator, probably because of the slight negative pressure generated by the patient's use of his or her diaphragm. As with spontaneous breaths, a slow deep breath with a hold is best, but it may be difficult to provide and may require several ventilator parameter changes to be made during the administration of the treatment. Some patients may not tolerate the changes that are ideal for aerosol deposition. Tidal volumes of 500 ml or more and slow inspiratory flow rates, which produce longer inspiratory times, increase aerosol deposition. In summary:

Requirements for Use of Ventilators in Intubated Patients

Patient-triggered breath

Tidal volume greater than 500 ml for adults

Slower respiratory rate

Slow inspiratory flow rate (30 liters/min or less)

Long inspiratory time

Some other factors that affect aerosol delivery are related to the ventilator circuit itself. The aerosol particles must pass through right-angle turns and narrow openings (including the endotracheal tube), which results in further losses as a result of impaction of aerosol particles. Endotracheal tubes that are 7 mm in internal diameter or larger are associated with better aerosol deposition than smaller tubes. Many ventilator patients are also receiving heated, humidified gas through their circuits. This causes the aerosol particles to become larger and increases the likelihood that they will be baffled or filtered out.

Finally characteristics of the aerosol-generating devices themselves affect the efficiency of aerosol deposition. These include the type of nebulizer used, where in the circuit it is placed, and whether it nebulizes continuously or only upon inspiration. When MDIs are used, the use of a spacer and the timing of the actuation with the beginning of inspiration are critical.

Technique for Delivering Drugs by SVN to Mechanically Ventilated Patients

1. Establish the initial dose (possibly 2 to 5 times the normal dose).
2. Add diluent to a total fill volume of 4 to 6 ml.

3. Place the nebulizer 30 to 45 cm (12 to 18 in) back from the endotracheal tube.
4. Turn off flow-by, flow trigger, or bias flow.
5. Remove the heat/moisture exchanger (HME) if one is being used.
6. Set the nebulizer flow at 6 to 8 liters/min.
7. Adjust ventilator settings and alarms as necessary to compensate for the added flow.
8. When possible, use a flow rate of 30 liters/min and a tidal volume of 500 ml.
9. Nebulize as much of the dose as possible.
10. Remove the SVN, rinse with sterile water, and dry.
11. Store the SVN in a clean, dry place.
12. Reconnect the HME.
13. AARC guidelines recommend changing the nebulizer every 24 hours.

Technique for Delivering Drugs by MDI to Mechanically Ventilated Patients

1. Establish the initial dose to be given (e.g., albuterol, 4 puffs).
2. Shake the MDI canister and warm to hand temperature.
3. Place the MDI into the spacer/holding chamber on the inspiratory limb of the ventilator circuit.
4. Remove the heat/moisture exchanger (HME) if one is being used.
5. Coordinate actuation with the beginning of inspiration. If the patient can take a spontaneous breath of at least 500 ml, coordinate firing with the beginning of inspiration and encourage a 4- to 10-second breath-hold.
6. Wait at least 15 to 30 seconds between doses.
7. Assess response to therapy.
8. Reconnect HME if one is being used.
9. Titrate dose to achieve desired effect.

Even under ideal conditions, aerosol deposition is hampered by mechanical ventilation. On average, pulmonary deposition ranges from 1.5% to 3%. However, deposition can be optimized by good technique and by using larger doses. Careful attention to ventilator parameters, aerosol devices, and their application can result in pulmonary deposition as high as 15%.

Ideal conditions are not always possible to achieve, so increasing the dose may become necessary. The dose may need to be increased by two to five times the normal dose for an SVN, and four puffs or more may be needed for an MDI.

time for review

Name at least one clinical setting for each form of medicated aerosol treatment—MDI, SVN, and DPI—in which that form would be preferred.

Life Span Considerations

Pediatrics and Aerosol Therapy

The dose delivered by aerosol drug delivery is reduced in children. This is thought to be due to their lower tidal breaths, faster respiratory rates, and smaller airways. Aerosol drug delivery does not work well in crying children but may be necessary depending on the clinical situation. The aerosol can be delivered by either a face mask or a mouthpiece since both methods tend to provide similar clinical responses. However, when a face mask is used with either a nebulizer or a spacer, it should be placed snugly around the child's face. Ill-fitting masks can result in large reductions of the delivered aerosol dose. Nose breathing should be discouraged since this will result in greater drug delivery to the upper airways, leading to more whole-body (systemic) adverse effects.

4.3 THE FUTURE

The future holds promise for the aerosol route. New or proposed uses for aerosol therapy include inhaled insulin for diabetics and gene replacement therapy, in which a defective gene is replaced to treat certain genetic diseases such as cystic fibrosis. You can find updates on specific new aerosolized drugs in the chapter that addresses their respective drug category.

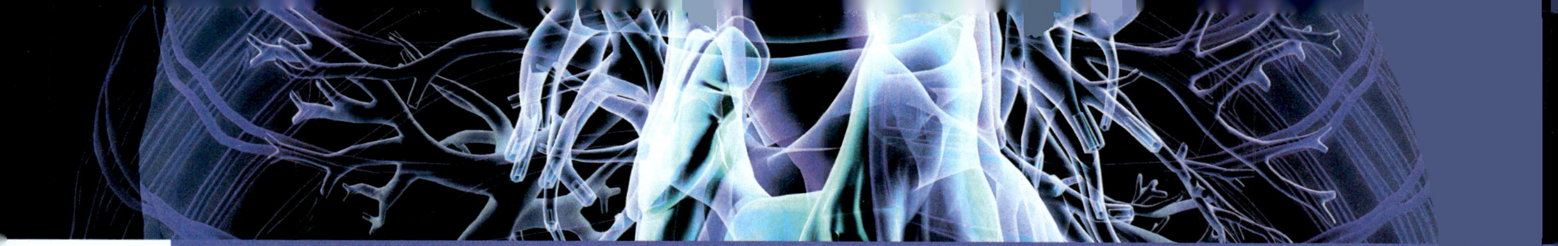

Summary

Aerosol drug delivery is used for a wide range of drug classifications. Like any pharmacologic therapy route, aerosol therapy has both advantages and disadvantages. To make clinical decisions about different methods of aerosol delivery, apply general pharmacologic principles introduced previously and reinforced in this chapter. You will achieve effective therapy only with careful attention to technical factors such as stability, penetration, deposition, inertial impaction, and breathing pattern. No other route of therapy is so dependent on the patient and the delivery technique.

REVIEW QUESTIONS

1. To deliver a topical anesthetic to the supraglottic tissues before bronchoscopy, which of the following techniques would be best?
   (a) Using an MDI that delivers particles in the range of 1 to 5 microns and slow mouth breathing with a breath-hold
   (b) Giving an oral medication and waiting for the systemic effects
   (c) Using a nebulizer that delivers particles in the range of 5 to 10 microns, high inspiratory flow rates, and mouth breathing
   (d) Using a nebulizer that delivers particles of 10 to 15 microns, high inspiratory flow rates, and nose breathing

2. Slow inspiratory flow rates
   (a) decrease penetration
   (b) enhance deposition in the upper airways
   (c) increase inertial impaction
   (d) maximize delivery to the lung periphery

3. The ideal particle size for aerosol delivery to the small airways is
   (a) 10 to 15 microns
   (b) 1 to 5 microns
   (c) 0.5 micron
   (d) 100 microns

4. What is the ideal pattern for DPI administration?
   (a) fast and deep
   (b) slow and deep
   (c) fast and shallow
   (d) slow and shallow

5. Chlorofluorocarbons were phased out as MDI propellants because they
   (a) tend to be unstable
   (b) are expensive
   (c) have an unpleasant smell
   (d) damage the ozone layer
6. List and describe the three main goals of aerosol therapy.
7. Contrast the advantages and disadvantages of aerosol therapy.
8. You are asked to evaluate several patients for aerosolized bronchodilator therapy. Which delivery device would you recommend for each of the following patients?
   (a) a 16-year-old cooperative and alert male with exercise-induced asthma
   (b) an 88-year-old female with dementia
   (c) an 18-month-old infant
   (d) a 58-year-old with COPD who is in the emergency department in acute respiratory distress
9. Describe the steps in the proper technique of administering a bronchodilator MDI treatment. What additional steps would be taken if an MDI corticosteroid were also ordered?
10. Describe the role of continuous nebulization aerosol therapy.

CASE STUDY 1

Mr. Blue

Chief Complaint

Mr. Blue is an anxious-appearing, 60-year-old male who was diagnosed with COPD 6 months ago. He was discharged from the hospital a week ago and now complains that the new inhaled medications are "not working." He also complains of a white tongue and throat and a strange taste in his mouth.

Past Medical History

His last hospitalization was for pneumonia; he was diagnosed at that time with congestive heart failure and prescribed home oxygen. Family history revealed positive for lung cancer in his mother. Social history: He is a 50 pack/year smoker.

Medications

Albuterol (bronchodilator) MDI 2 puffs q.i.d. and PRN
Beclomethasone (corticosteroid) MDI 2 puffs b.i.d.

What supports the statement that Mr. Blue is not using his MDIs correctly? What specific instructions would you emphasize during your patient education session? Are there any other suggestions you would make at this time to improve his health?

PART 2

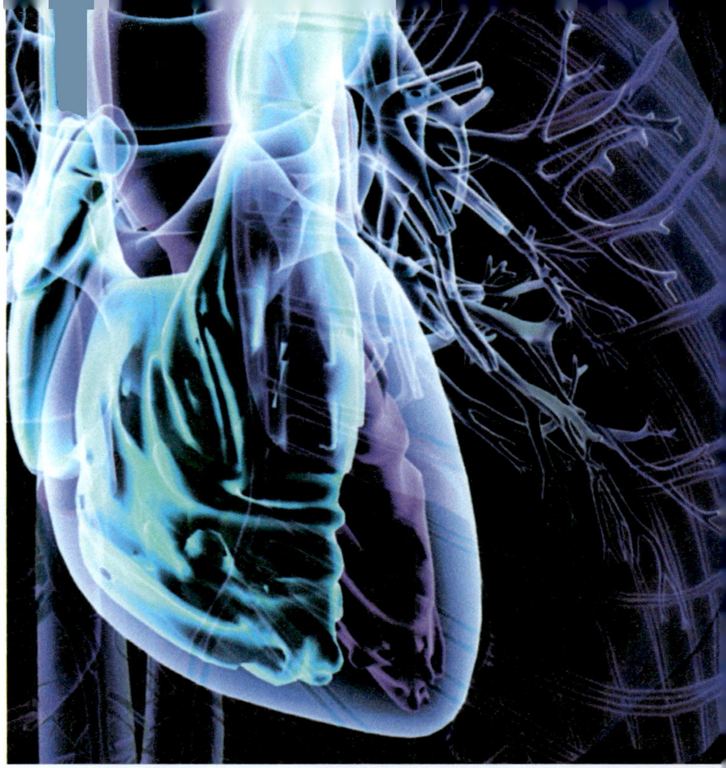

The Specific Drug Categories

Chapter **5**

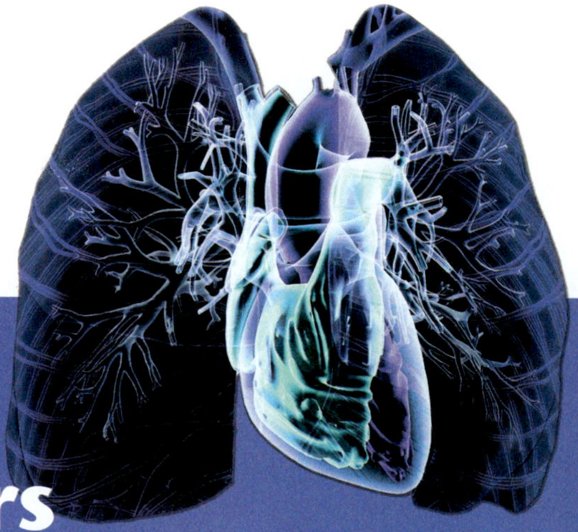

Bronchodilators

OBJECTIVES

Upon completion of this chapter you will be able to

- Define key terms relative to bronchodilator pharmacotherapy.
- Describe the neurologic control of bronchial smooth muscle, including the sympathetic and parasympathetic nerves, their chemical mediators, and how bronchodilation is achieved.
- Differentiate bronchospasm and bronchoconstriction.
- Describe three pharmacologic methods for bronchodilation (sympathomimetic, anticholinergic, and methylxanthine) and the mode of action of each.
- State the indications, contraindications, adverse reactions, onset of action, and dosage range for each bronchodilator.
- Recommend appropriate bronchodilator therapy for various patient situations, including drug, dosage, frequency, and route of delivery.
- Describe appropriate techniques for monitoring the patient's response to bronchodilator therapy.

KEY TERMS

asthma paradox
beta-agonist (β-agonist)
bronchoconstriction
bronchospasm
cyclic adenosine monophosphate
cyclic guanosine monophosphate
downregulation
dyspnea
epinephrine
forced expiratory volume in 1 second
maintenance therapy
peak expiratory flow rate
premature ventricular contraction
rescue therapy
ventilatory drive

ABBREVIATIONS

α	alpha-receptor
AMP	adenosine monophosphate
β_1	beta_1-receptor
β_2	beta_2-receptor
cAMP	cyclic AMP
cGMP	cyclic GMP
CHF	congestive heart failure
FEV_1	forced expiratory volume in 1 second
GMP	guanosine monophosphate
GTP	guanosine triphosphate
LABA	long-acting beta-agonist
LAMA	long-acting muscarinic antagonist
OH	hydroxyl
PEFR	peak expiratory flow rate
PVC	premature ventricular contraction
REMS	risk evaluation and mitigation strategy
SABA	short-acting beta-agonist
SAMA	short-acting muscarinic antagonist

Imagine you have been called to the emergency department to treat an asthmatic who is struggling to breathe. The treatment needs to be safe and work quickly. The administration of inhaled bronchodilators is the most important aspect of treating such emergencies. With the prevalence of asthma, COPD, and respiratory disease in general, bronchodilators are one of the most commonly prescribed drug classifications. The practitioner must be thoroughly knowledgeable about the actions, adverse reactions, dosages, onset of action, and duration of action of the various agents. In addition the practitioner must be knowledgeable about the mechanisms of bronchoconstriction in various disease states to be able to select the most beneficial agent for individual patients. The practitioner must also be able to select the best delivery system, instruct patients to develop techniques that ensure optimal delivery of the medication, and assess the patient's response to the treatment.

5.1 AIRWAY ANATOMY AND PHYSIOLOGY

Before discussing the specific agents, a brief review of airway anatomy and physiology is needed. The conducting airways of the lung are made up of three layers, the mucosa, the submucosa, and the adventitia. The *mucosa layer,* or respiratory epithelial layer, contains the ciliated cells that move the mucus toward the pharynx to keep the lumen of the airway cleared of debris. The *submucosal layer* contains bronchial glands, smooth muscle, capillary network, and elastic tissue. The smooth muscle of this layer plays a very important role in bronchospasm. Much of this chapter concerns the mechanisms by which various drugs relax the bronchial smooth muscle. Finally, the *adventitia* is a sheath of connective tissue that surrounds and supports the airways.

The large airways begin with the trachea, which divides to form bronchi. Between the submucosa and the adventitia of the large airways are plates or incomplete rings of cartilage that provide support to prevent the airways from collapsing. Somewhere between the 5th and the 14th generation below the subsegmental bronchi, the bronchi become bronchioles. The term *bronchioles* means small bronchi or small airways. They are 1 to 2 mm in diameter and lack the supporting cartilage of the large airways. The smooth muscle of the submucosa changes from sheets of muscle surrounding the bronchi to long strands that spiral and crisscross around the bronchioles. This configuration of muscle fibers reduces the diameter and length of the airway when the smooth muscle contracts (see Figure 5-1).

FIGURE 5-1 Cross-Sectional Anatomy of Bronchus, Bronchiole, and Alveolus

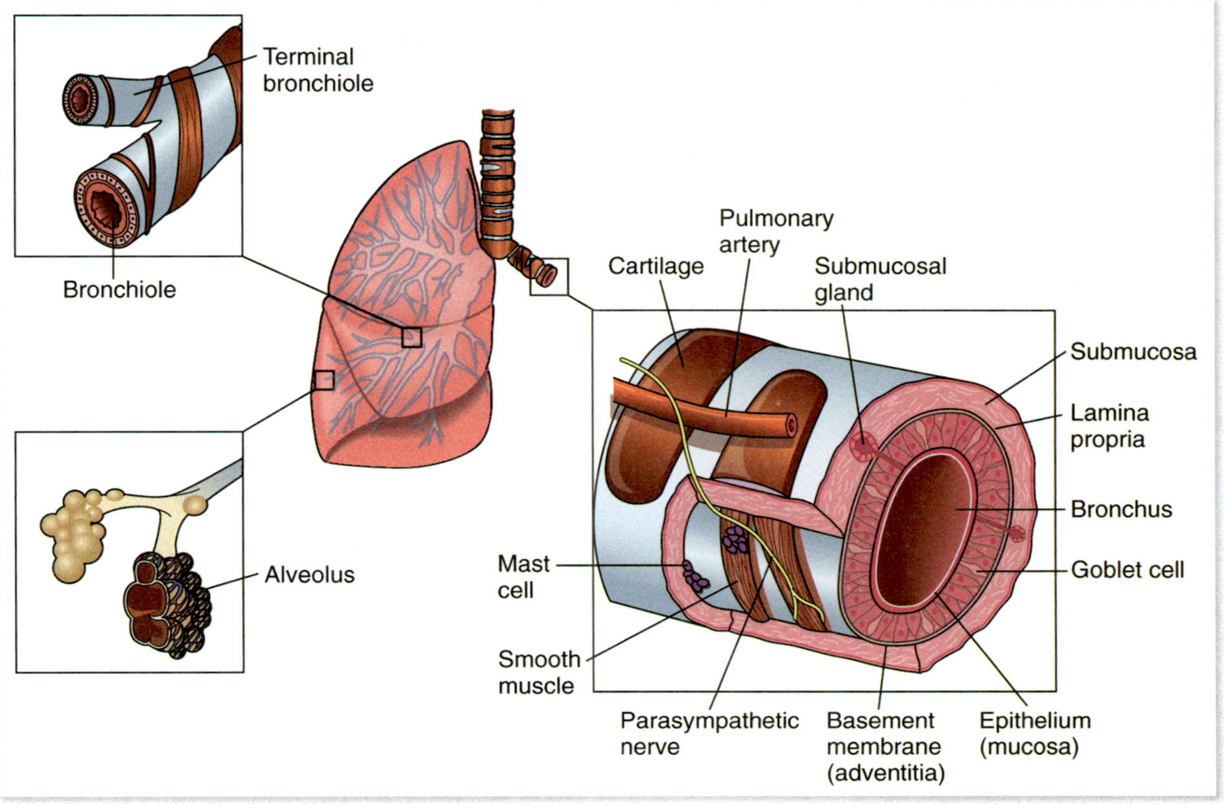

5.1a Bronchoconstriction Versus Bronchospasm

The term **bronchoconstriction** refers to a decrease in the diameter of the airway. This may be the result of three distinct mechanisms: **bronchospasm**, airway edema, or secretions. See Figure 5-2, which illustrates these three types of bronchoconstriction. Sometimes all three may be contributing factors in a patient's bronchoconstriction.

- *Bronchospasm* is the actual spasm or contraction of the smooth muscle in the bronchial wall. The airway diameter is reduced, which causes a reduction in airflow and increased work of breathing. Bronchodilating drugs are indicated for treatment of this problem.
- *Airway edema* occurs when insult or injury to the mucous membranes causes dilation of the blood vessels and accumulation of fluid in the tissues. The swollen tissue reduces the diameter of the lumen of the airway, and breathing becomes more difficult. In this case, treatment should be aimed toward constricting the blood vessels to reduce swelling or toward administration of steroids to block the inflammatory response. These agents will be discussed in Chapter 7 under anti-inflammatory agents.
- *Secretions* in the airway reduce the airway diameter. This is often the result of impairment of the normal mucociliary clearance mechanism of the lungs. Effective bronchial hygiene techniques coupled with wetting agents and mucolytics may be indicated for this process, and they are discussed in Chapter 6 under mucolytics.

Learning Hint

To get a feel for a reduced airway diameter, while seated and with nose clips on, mouth breathe through a straw and note the difficulties you experience in breathing. You can remove the nose clips and straw and easily return to normal; the bronchoconstricted patient must rely on appropriate medical treatment to return to normal breathing.

FIGURE 5-2 Types of Bronchoconstriction

(a) Normal Bronchi, (b) Bronchospasm,
(c) Mucosal Edema, and (d) Mucus Narrowing the Airway

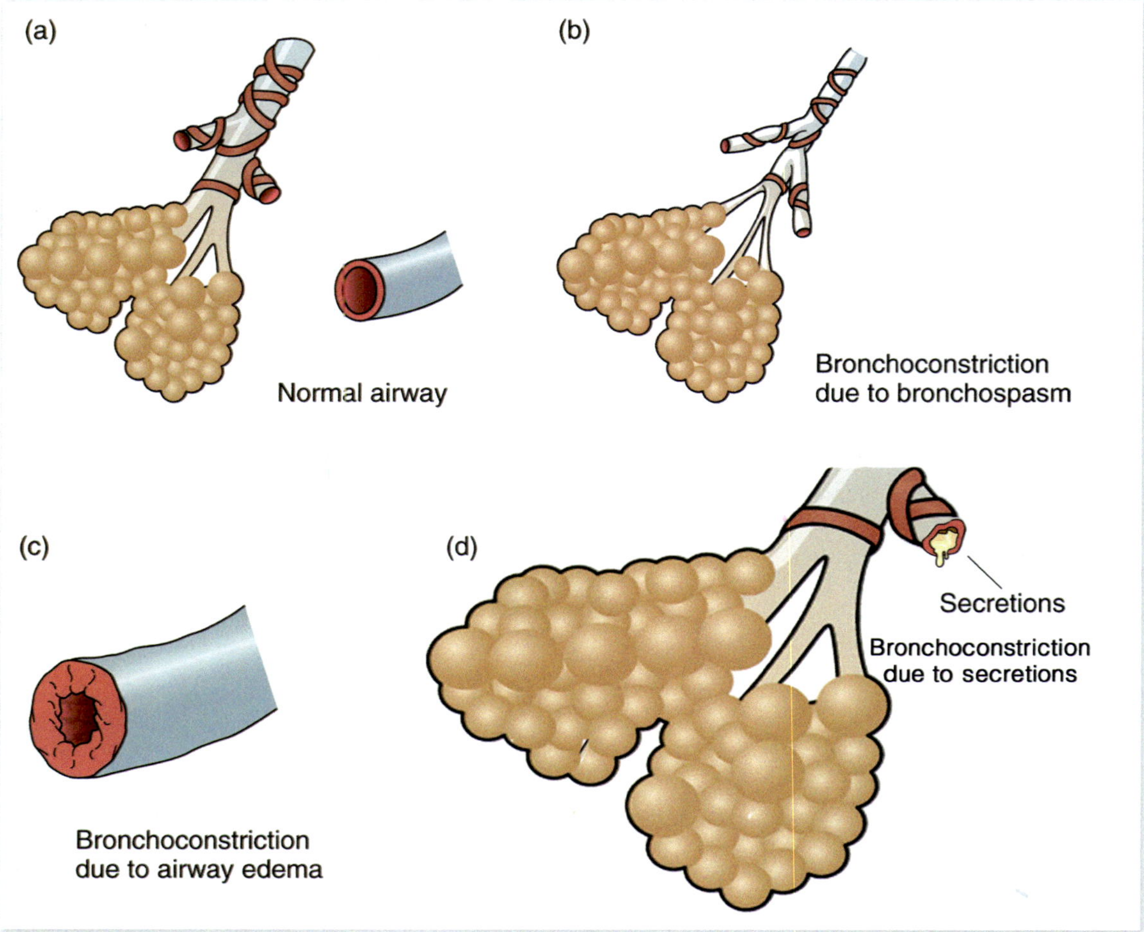

Regardless of the cause of the reduction in airway diameter, a bronchoconstricted patient experiences increased airway resistance, increased work of breathing, and dyspnea. To select the best bronchodilator, the practitioner must understand the pathophysiology of the disease and the mechanism of the bronchoconstriction. This chapter focuses on treating bronchoconstriction that results from bronchospasm.

time for review

Explain the statement, "Bronchospasm always results in bronchoconstriction, but not all bronchoconstriction is caused by bronchospasm."

5.2 NEUROLOGIC CONTROL OF BRONCHIAL SMOOTH MUSCLE

The bronchi are innervated by the autonomic branch of the peripheral nervous system as discussed in Chapter 3. Because the nervous system plays such an important role in maintaining airway diameter, it will be reviewed again briefly. These concepts are central to understanding the pharmacologic treatment of bronchoconstriction.

The autonomic nervous system is comprised of two divisions, the sympathetic nervous system and the parasympathetic nervous system. It was once thought that a balance between these two opposing branches of the autonomic nervous system was *solely* responsible for autonomic airway control. Drugs such as anticholinergics and beta-agonists, the two major classes of respiratory medications, were discovered based on the theory that diseases such as asthma produced an improper balance between parasympathetic and sympathetic control over the airways. The reader should be aware that numerous neurotransmitters, such as prostaglandins and hormones, have also been discovered that play a role in autonomic airway control.

5.2a Sympathetic Nervous System

The sympathetic nervous system dominates the body's reaction to stressful circumstances. This "fight-or-flight" response to sympathetic activation stimulates the heart, increases cardiac output and blood pressure, dilates the pupils, increases metabolism, and enhances alertness. The response mediated by the sympathetic nervous system also relaxes the bronchial smooth muscle to dilate the airways and lower airway resistance, facilitating increased ventilation. The increased rate and depth of breathing increase ventilation. Ultimately this results in increased carbon dioxide removal and increased oxygen delivery to the lungs and blood. Heart rate and blood pressure increase to supply more blood to carry oxygen from the lungs to the tissues. These physiologic changes provide the body with the energy to mount a maximum physical effort.

Learning Hint

If the balance is tipped to favor the parasympathetic system, bronchoconstriction will result. Conversely, if the scales tip toward the sympathetic system, bronchodilation results. Keep this visual picture in mind as you learn what factors tip the scales.

5.2b Parasympathetic Nervous System

The parasympathetic ("sleep-and-eat") nervous system dominates the body's maintenance functions, such as increased salivation and mucus secretion, increased blood flow to the gut, and increased peristalsis, defecation, and urination. It also decreases heart rate and blood pressure and increases bronchoconstriction and mucus secretion. Normally, the sympathetic and parasympathetic nervous systems are in balance, creating normal airway smooth muscle tone, but circumstances and certain medications can shift the balance in favor of one system over the other (see Figure 5-3).

FIGURE 5-3 Balance Between the Sympathetic and Parasympathetic Nervous Systems That Maintains Normal Bronchial Smooth Muscle Tone

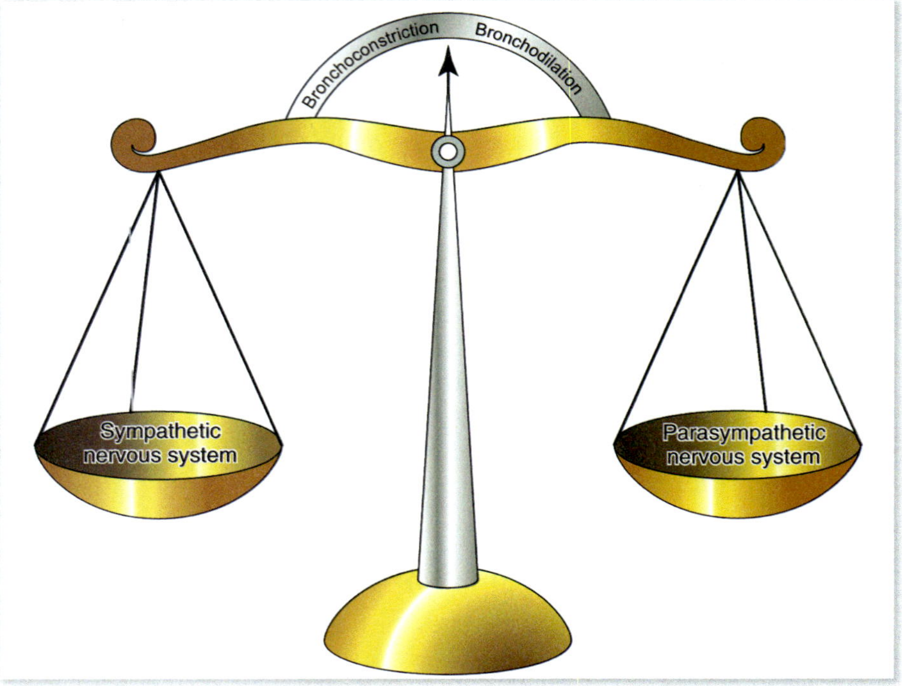

5.2c Chemical Mediators of Neural Transmission

Reviewing from Chapter 3, the impulses of the nervous system are transmitted from nerve to nerve and to the muscles or organs by chemical substances such as norepinephrine (NE) and acetylcholine (ACh). Both systems use ACh to transmit impulses from neuron to neuron. However, at the synapse where the neuron meets the smooth muscle, the chemical transmitter for the sympathetic nervous system is NE, and for the parasympathetic nervous system it is ACh. The action of ACh is limited by an enzyme called acetylcholinesterase (or cholinesterase; abbreviated AChE), which quickly metabolizes ACh. The synaptic junctions of the sympathetic nervous system have no such enzyme, so the effects of NE take longer to dissipate. The receptors for the parasympathetic nervous system are referred to as muscarinic and nicotinic. The receptors that are important in the lung are called muscarinic. When they are stimulated, they cause constriction of bronchial smooth muscle and increased mucus secretion (see Figure 5-4).

BVT Lab

Flashcards are available for this chapter at www.BVTLab.com.

FIGURE 5-4 Stimulated Parasympathetic Nerve Causing Bronchospasm

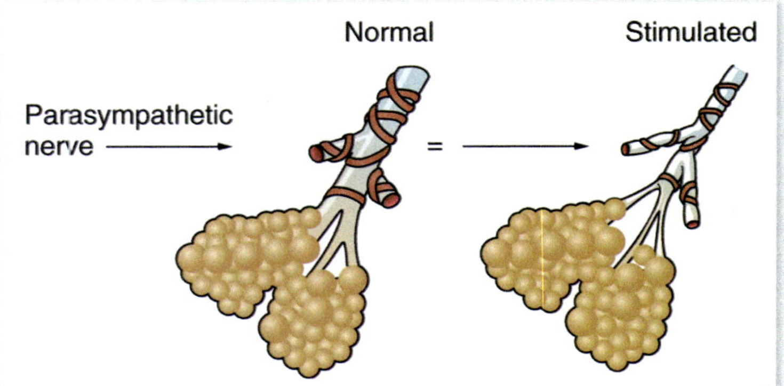

Because the parasympathetic system uses ACh at the transmitter between the nerve and the muscle, it is also called the cholinergic system. The sympathetic system's action is based on NE as the transmitter. **Epinephrine**, also called adrenaline, is a drug that is very similar to NE, so the sympathetic nervous system is sometimes referred to as the adrenergic system. Figure 5-5 contrasts a parasympathetic neuron with a sympathetic neuron.

FIGURE 5-5 Impulse Transmission in the Sympathetic and Parasympathetic Nervous Systems

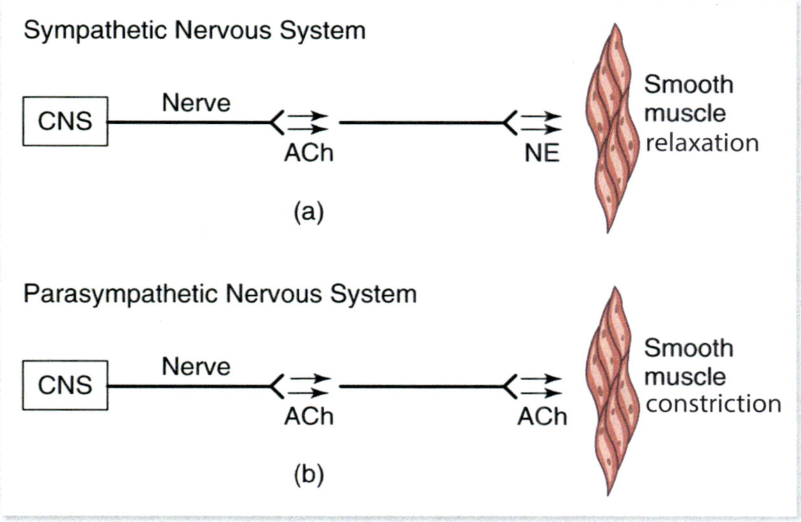

Learning Hint

The cardiopulmonary system is interrelated at many levels. Notice that β-receptors can affect both the heart and the lungs. To remember that β_1-receptors affect primarily the heart and β_2-receptors affect primarily the lungs, think of how many hearts you have and how many lungs you have.

5.2d Sympathetic Nervous System Receptors

The sympathetic nervous system has essentially three types of receptors. They are referred to as alpha (α)-, beta$_1$ (β_1)-, and beta$_2$ (β_2)-receptors. (Actually, there are alpha$_1$- and alpha$_2$-receptors, as well, but they will not be differentiated for the purposes of this discussion.) Each of the three receptor types is distributed to different parts of the body and produces different effects when stimulated. The α-receptors are found mainly in arteries and veins throughout the body, including the blood vessels in the lungs. They are distributed evenly in the large and small airways, and their stimulation results in vasoconstriction.

The β_1-receptors are found mainly in the heart, where they increase both the rate and the force of contraction of the heart when stimulated. The β_2-receptors are found in the bronchiolar smooth muscle of the lung, the uterus, and skeletal muscle blood vessels. β_2-receptors are found throughout the tracheal bronchial tree, but they are particularly concentrated in the small airways. When stimulated, β_2-receptors relax the smooth muscle in the lungs to cause bronchodilation. This action of the β_2-receptors on bronchial smooth muscle is the basis for many of the bronchoactive drugs. In addition, stimulation of the β_2-receptors in the blood vessels of the skeletal muscle causes them to dilate, increasing blood supply and sometimes causing tremor, a common side effect listed for many of the bronchodilators. In the uterus, stimulation of the β_2-receptors can stop contractions of premature labor. A summary of the sympathetic receptors and their effects is given in Table 5-1.

Clinical Pearl

Magnesium sulfate can be given intravenously to stop premature labor contractions, because it relaxes the uterine smooth muscle. It has also been shown to be an effective bronchodilator when administered intravenously as a 2-g dose over 20 minutes in asthma patients with a life-threatening exacerbation.

TABLE 5-1 Summary of the Sympathetic Nervous System Receptors, Their Locations, and Their Actions

Receptor	Location	Action
Alpha	Arteries and veins	Vasoconstriction
$Beta_1$	Heart	Increase in rate and force of contraction
$Beta_2$	Lungs, skeletal muscle, and uterus	Smooth muscle relaxation

Learning Hint

Drugs that mimic the effects of the sympathetic (adrenergic) system are called *sympathomimetic* or *adrenergic*. Drugs that mimic the parasympathetic (cholinergic) system are called *parasympathomimetics*. Conversely agents that block the effects of the sympathetic nervous system are called *sympatholytics* or *antiadrenergics*, and those that block the effects of the parasympathetic system are *parasympatholytics* or *anticholinergics*.

5.2e The Sympathetic Nervous System in the Lung

The sympathetic nervous system exerts its effects by both direct and indirect means. The presence of nerve fibers results in direct stimulation of the receptor site. These receptors are referred to as *neuronal receptors*. However, some receptors are not wired directly to the nervous system by nerve fibers. These receptors are stimulated indirectly by circulating catecholamines (NE and epinephrine) in the bloodstream. They are referred to as *hormonal receptors* because they respond to chemical mediators that are released into the bloodstream from the adrenal medulla. As the chemical mediators or hormones circulate through the bloodstream, they stimulate receptors throughout the body, not just the receptors associated with nerve fibers. Their stimulation results in the same action as if they were transmitted to the receptor by nerve fibers.

The arteries and submucosal glands of the lung are well innervated by sympathetic nerve fibers, whereas the bronchiolar smooth muscle essentially lacks these fibers and therefore responds to circulating hormones or medications. For example the α- and β_2-receptors of the bronchial smooth muscle are stimulated by the circulating hormones epinephrine and NE, which are produced within our bodies. Similarly, when we administer inhaled bronchodilators, the drug combines with the β_2-receptors in the lung, causing indirect or hormonal stimulation of the receptor rather than neuronal stimulation.

Epinephrine stimulates both α- and β-receptors equally, whereas norepinephrine acts mainly on the α-receptors. Recall, however, that in Chapter 1 we learned that "pure" reactions do not occur with any drug. Even though some drugs are *highly selective* for a particular receptor, there is always some potential for stimulation of other receptors as well. Table 5-2 summarizes these effects.

TABLE 5-2 Summary of the Major Effects of Sympathomimetics, Parasympatholytics, Sympatholytics, and Parasympathomimetics

Effects	Sympathomimetic	Parasympatholytic	Sympatholytic	Parasympathomimetic
Bronchial smooth muscle	Relaxes	Relaxes	Constricts	Constricts
Mucus secretion		Decreases		Increases
Heart rate	Increases	Increases	Decreases	Decreases
Blood pressure	Increases	Increases	Decreases	Decreases
Pupils	Dilate	Dilate	Constrict	Constrict
Blood flow to skeletal muscles	Increases	Increases	Decreases	Decreases
Salivation	Decreases	Decreases	Increases	Increases
Digestion	Decreases	Decreases	Increases	Increases
Blood glucose	Increases	Increases	Decreases	Decreases
Insulin	Decreases	Decreases	Increases	Increases

time for review

Note the similar actions of the sympathomimetic and parasympatholytic agents. The same effect results from very different actions on the autonomic nervous system. This is the reason for using more than one drug to treat bronchoconstriction. It is a concept that will be reinforced throughout this chapter. What do you think the relationship between sympatholytic and parasympathomimetic agents would be?

5.3 BRONCHODILATORS

Bronchodilators can be divided into three categories based on their mechanism of action:

- Sympathomimetics (β-adrenergics)
- Anticholinergics (parasympatholytics)
- Methylxanthines

The sympathomimetics cause bronchodilation directly by increasing **cyclic adenosine monophosphate** (cAMP), a substance that causes bronchial smooth muscle relaxation. Anticholinergics, also known as muscarinic antagonists, block the bronchoconstricting effects of the parasympathetic system by decreasing **cyclic guanosine monophosphate** (cGMP), a substance that causes bronchial smooth muscle constriction. Several mechanisms have been proposed for the bronchodilation action of methylxanthines, but none has been definitively established. Sympathomimetics and anticholinergics are most commonly administered as inhaled aerosols. Methylxanthines are administered orally or, very rarely, intravenously. Their different modes of action may lead to the use of combination drug therapy for optimal management of bronchospasm in some patients. Figure 5-6 shows the change in balance that leads to sympathomimetic bronchodilation.

CONTROVERSY

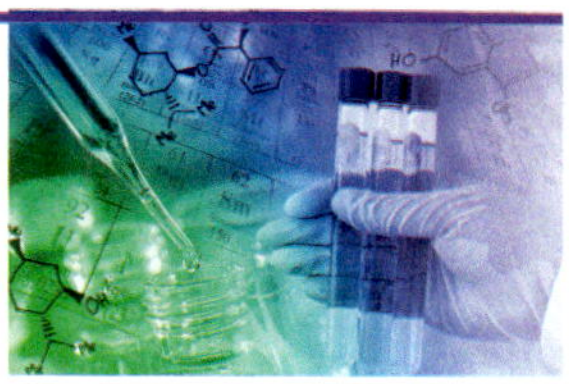

For quite some time methylxanthines were thought to bronchodilate by increasing levels of cAMP by inhibiting phosphodiesterase, the enzyme that deactivates cAMP. Currently there are several other theories to explain its mechanism of action. Furthermore methylxanthines may not actually produce bronchodilation at therapeutic doses, but they are weak bronchodilators at very high doses, which can increase the chance of adverse effects. They are called narrow therapeutic index medications because the toxic and therapeutic dosages are very close to each other. Due to this, theophylline, the only methylxanthine still in use, is used infrequently today to treat pulmonary diseases.

FIGURE 5-6 Sympathetic Stimulation Favoring Bronchodilation

Note that anything that enhances cAMP (sympathomimetics) or anything that decreases or lightens cGMP (anticholinergics) tips the scales toward bronchodilation.

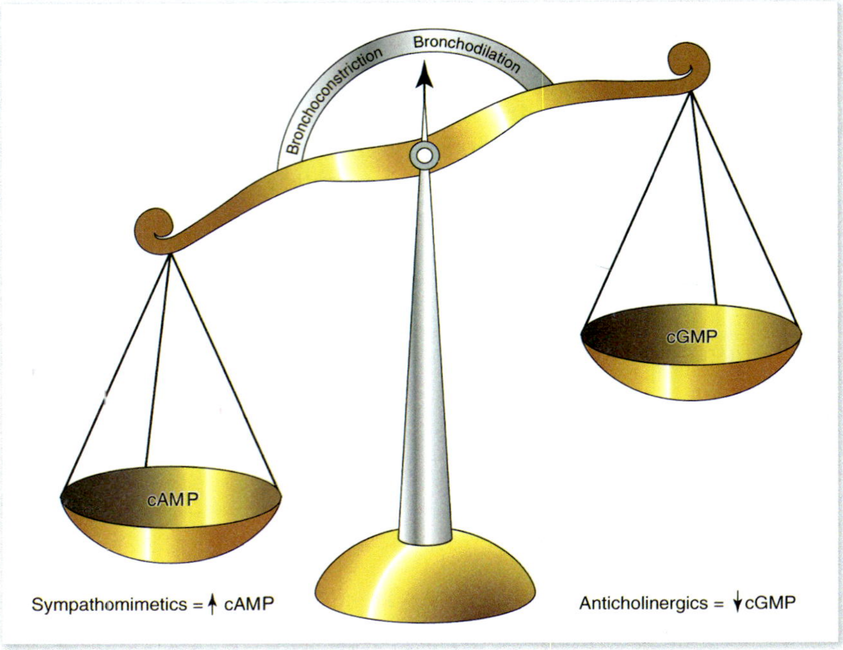

5.3a Sympathomimetic (Adrenergic) Bronchodilators

Stimulation of the sympathetic nervous system causes bronchodilation (β_2-effect), increase in heart rate/force of contraction (β_1), and vasoconstriction (α-effect) in the pulmonary system. Drugs that mimic these effects are called *sympathomimetic* or *adrenergic agonists*. Sympathomimetics have three potential effects, depending on the receptor or receptors that are stimulated:

- Alpha (α)-stimulation results in vasoconstriction, which reduces blood flow and thereby decreases swelling. In the upper airway, this can result in decongestion. For example, the active ingredient in many OTC nasal decongestants is phenylephrine, a potent α-receptor stimulant that temporarily relieves swelling in the nasal passages. α-Receptor-stimulating drugs can also be administered to the supraglottic region, where soft-tissue swelling can cause airway obstruction.
- β_1-Receptor stimulation results in increased heart rate and force of contraction. These drugs are discussed in later chapters concerning cardiovascular medications.
- β_2-Receptor stimulation results in bronchial smooth muscle relaxation, inhibition of inflammatory response, and increased mucociliary clearance.

5.3b Mechanism of Action

When a β_2-agonist binds to the β_2-receptor, it activates special stimulatory proteins (G proteins) that activate the membrane-bound enzyme adenyl cyclase. Adenyl cyclase, in turn, increases synthesis of cyclic adenosine 3′-5′-monophosphate (cAMP). cAMP causes relaxation of smooth muscle by inactivating an enzyme that initiates the interaction of actin and myosin. You may recall that actin and myosin are the proteins that work together to shorten or contract smooth muscle fibers. cAMP also decreases the amount of intracellular calcium, thus causing relaxation because calcium is needed for contraction.

cAMP also has anti-inflammatory properties related to its ability to inhibit mast cell chemical mediator release. This is discussed in depth in Chapter 7, but it is theorized that the prevention of the influx of calcium not only relaxes smooth muscle but also prevents the influx of calcium into mast cells. Calcium influx is believed to cause a powerful contraction and expulsion of the mast cells' chemical mediators, which leads to an inflammatory response.

cAMP is constantly broken down by another enzyme, phosphodiesterase. The cAMP becomes AMP, which is inactive, so it does not produce bronchodilation. In fact, when AMP is present in large quantities, it actually interferes with bronchodilation.

Learning Hint

Increased intracellular calcium = increased smooth muscle contraction; decreased intracellular calcium = decreased smooth muscle contraction.

5.4 DEVELOPMENT OF THE β-AGONISTS

Although natural substances have been used for their bronchodilating effects since ancient times, it was not until the 1900s that epinephrine was administered subcutaneously and later by aerosol for the treatment of bronchospasm. Since then various agents have been developed by altering the structure of the molecule. This has resulted in medications that are more potent and longer acting and that have fewer side effects. A perfect bronchodilator has yet to be developed, but a better understanding of pharmacokinetics has allowed many improvements. The first group of bronchodilators to be studied and developed were called catecholamines. The basic catecholamine molecule consists of a catechol nucleus and an amine side chain. The nucleus is made up of a benzene ring and two hydroxyl groups (see Figure 5-7).

FIGURE 5-7 Basic Catecholamine Molecule

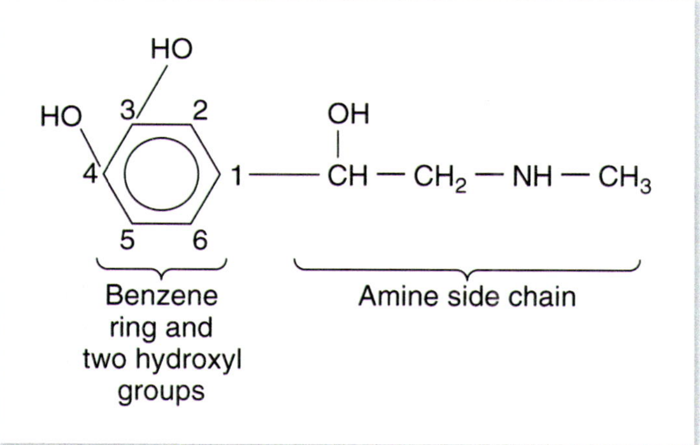

Drug researchers discovered that by making some changes to the structure of the benzene ring, they could make drugs that are much more resistant to degradation by enzymes, which enables them to stay active longer. β-Agonists also needed to be more β_2-specific so that the patients would have fewer cardiac side effects. Increasing the length of the side-chain portion of the molecule has, in fact, resulted in agents that are β_2-specific and therefore safer. (This is sometimes referred to as the *keyhole theory of specificity*.)

Changes to the benzene ring have resulted in three chemical classes of sympathomimetic **beta-agonists (β-agonists)**. These three classes are the catecholamines, resorcinols, and saligenins. For example catecholamines have hydroxyl molecules (OH) attached to their benzene ring at positions 3 and 4, whereas resorcinols have hydroxyl groups at 3 and 5. Please refer to the diagrams in Figure 5-8. You will also see some dramatic differences when you compare the side chain of epinephrine, a catecholamine, to that of salmeterol, a saligenin. The specific actions and examples of each class will be given.

FIGURE 5-8 Catecholamine, Resorcinol, and Saligenin Chemical Modifications

Note: Increasing length of amine side chain results in more β_2-specificity.

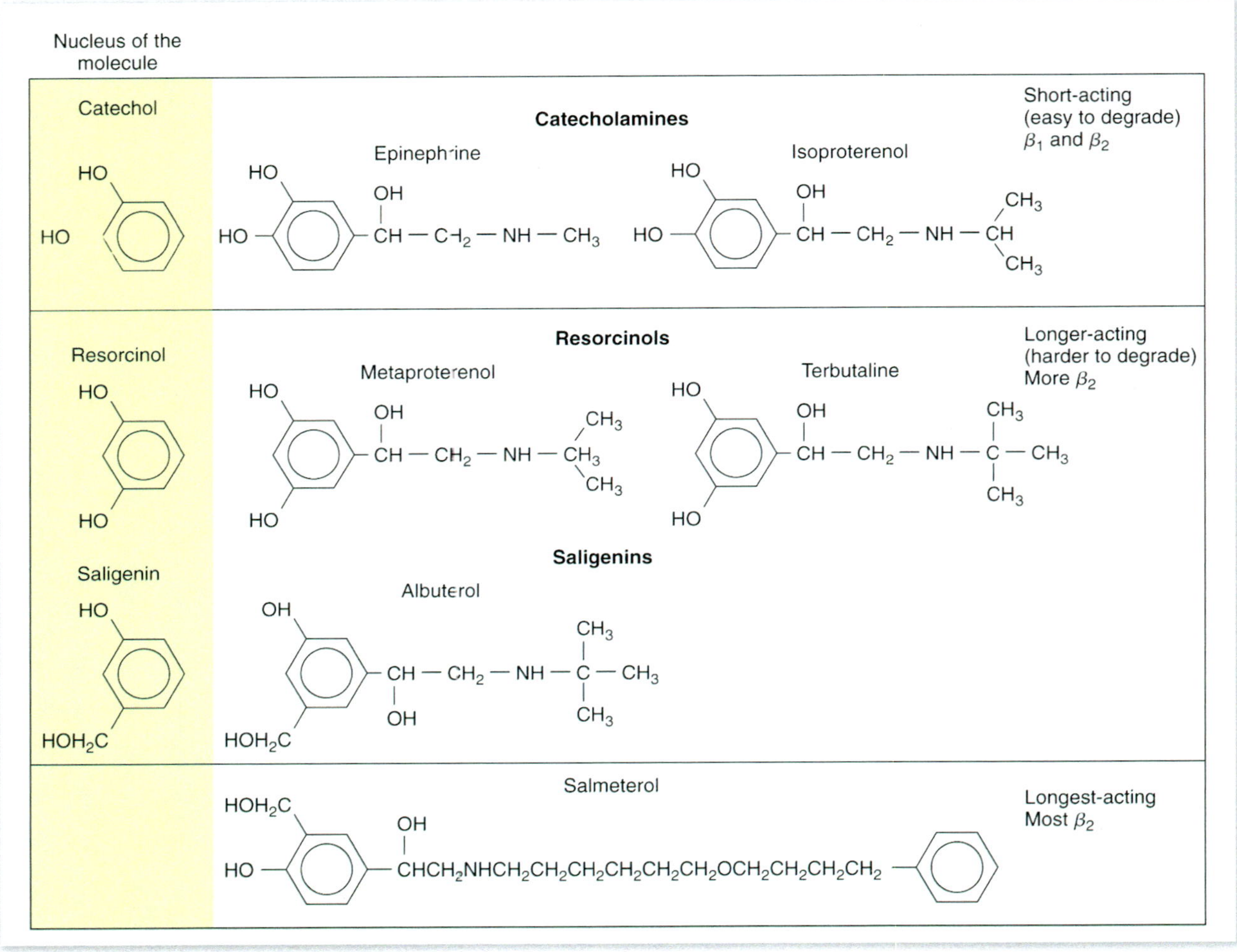

5.4a Catecholamines

Catecholamines are the oldest group of inhaled bronchodilators. All sympathetic bronchodilators are catecholamines or derivatives of catecholamines. Their basic molecular structure consists of a benzene ring and an amine side chain.

Catecholamines are effective and potent dilators. They have a rapid onset and reach their peak effect quickly. However, their duration of action is rather short (only about 0.5 to 3 hours), so they require frequent dosing. This does limit their usefulness in respiratory care because patients don't like having to take medication so frequently. The catecholamines are rapidly *deactivated* by the enzymes COMT (catechol-O-methyltransferase) and MAO (monoamine oxidase). COMT is found in the liver, kidneys, and throughout the body. None of the catecholamines can be given orally, because they are degraded in the GI tract where MAO is found.

Drugs in this class are no longer used as inhaled bronchodilators. Examples of catecholamines include epinephrine, norepinephrine, racemic epinephrine, dopamine, isoproterenol, isoetharine, and bitolterol. Only isoetharine and bitolterol were once used as inhaled bronchodilators, because they produced fewer cardiac side effects than other drugs in this class. The catecholamine racemic epinephrine is used to treat upper-airway swelling, because its primary effect is vasoconstriction, but it also acts as a relatively weak bronchodilator. The other catecholamines (including epinephrine) are used intravenously primarily for their effects on heart rate and blood pressure. Catecholamines may turn pink in color due to inactivation when exposed to heat, light, and air.

Clinical pearl

Administering catecholamines that have been rendered inactive by light or heat may cause a phenomenon known as beta-blockade. Here the drug still has affinity for the receptor site, but once bound does not activate the response and thus acts as an antagonist. If many of the β_2-receptors are "blocked," then even administering another active drug will have little or no effect.

Racemic Epinephrine

Racemic epinephrine is a synthetic form of epinephrine that has both α- and β-effects. It is used as a topical vasoconstrictor (α-effect) for treatment of airway edema associated with croup and laryngeal edema.

time for review

Why are catecholamines stored in dark containers?

5.4b Resorcinols

The catecholamines are not suitable for maintenance therapy of bronchospastic airways because of their short duration of action. Drug researchers sought to modify the catechol nucleus so that it would be resistant to breakdown by COMT and therefore be longer acting. The result was the development of metaproterenol (no longer available in dosage form for inhalation) and terbutaline (Brethine®, Brethaire®). Another advantage of the resorcinols is that they can be taken orally, because they also resist the action of enzymes in the GI tract and liver. Because of their longer duration, they were the first true maintenance drugs for treatment of reactive airway disease, although they could still be used for rescue therapy because of their rapid onset.

Metaproterenol

Metaproterenol is currently only available as a tablet or syrup. The inhaled forms have been removed from the market. The drug is slower to reach its peak effect (30 to 60 minutes), but its duration is 4 to 6 hours. Metaproterenol has a more bulky side chain, which makes it more β_2-specific than the catecholamines. It is considered to be β_2-selective, but metaproterenol has substantial cardiac side effects because of its structural similarity to isoproterenol. As just mentioned, it is no longer available in the United States for inhalation.

Terbutaline

Terbutaline is both β_2-specific and longer acting than catecholamines. Like metaproterenol, terbutaline is β_2-selective, but it has very few cardiac side effects. The onset of action is also 5 to 15 minutes from administration. It reaches its peak effect in about 30 to 60 minutes, and the duration is 4 to 6 hours. Terbutaline is no longer available as an MDI for use in the United States. Terbutaline is available in parenteral form and can be administered subcutaneously to treat bronchospasm or intravenously to stop premature labor by relaxing uterine smooth muscle.

time for review

What advantages do the resorcinols have over the catecholamines?

5.4c Saligenins

Saligenins are the most recently developed and most widely prescribed of all bronchodilators. They have largely replaced the catecholamine and resorcinol bronchodilators because modifications of the catechol nucleus have made this class the most β_2-specific. Like the resorcinols, they have the same rapid onset of action and a duration of 4 to 6 hours. Salmeterol (Serevent®) and formoterol (Foradil®) are long-acting β-agonists. Formoterol has a more rapid onset of action than salmeterol. Levalbuterol is the R isomer of albuterol (albuterol is a mixture of both the R and S isomers). It appears to have no clinically important advantage over albuterol. Pirbuterol (Maxair®) is structurally very similar, so it is also included with this group. The new kid on the block is indacaterol (Arcapta™ Neohaler™). It is a long-acting bronchodilator similar to salmeterol and formoterol. A table at the end of this section summarizes the therapeutic effects of β-agonists.

Albuterol (Proventil® HFA, Ventolin® HFA)

Albuterol is a frequently administered bronchodilator. It is very β_2-specific and has very few side effects because of its long side chain. The onset of action is 15 minutes. It reaches its peak effect in 30 to 60 minutes and has a duration of 4 to 6 hours. Albuterol is available as a syrup for children, oral tablets, extended-release tablets, nebulizer solution, MDI, and DPI (see Figure 5-9).

FIGURE 5-9 **Ventolin® HFA Metered-Dose Inhaler**

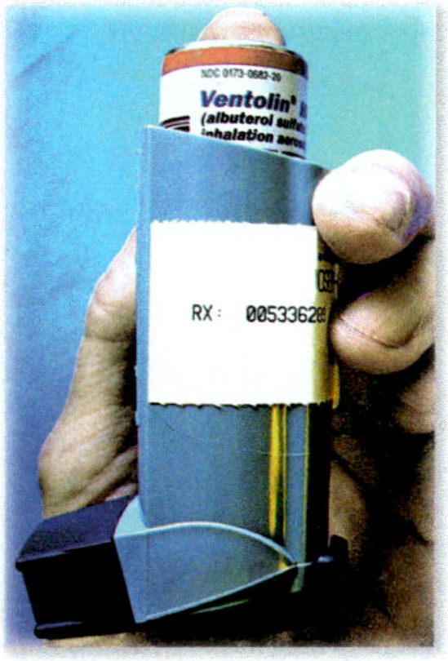

Pirbuterol

Pirbuterol is the result of a very slight modification to the nucleus, but it has the same side chain as albuterol. It is available orally, as a syrup for pediatric patients, and as an MDI with a breath-actuated inhaler device. Pirbuterol is said to be less potent by weight than albuterol and is similar to metaproterenol in both efficacy and toxicity. The side effects are the same as with other β_2-agonists.

BVT Lab

Visit www.BVTLab.com to explore the student resources available for this chapter.

Levalbuterol (Xopenex®)

Levalbuterol is the first drug in a new subclass of inhaled β-agonists. It is an R-isomer saligenin that appears to have little clinically significant advantage over albuterol. It is metabolized more slowly. Onset of action is about 15 minutes after administration. It takes 30 to 60 minutes for the drug to reach its peak effect, and it lasts for 3 to 8 hours. A 0.63-mg dose of levalbuterol is comparable to 1.25 mg of racemic albuterol in onset and action. A 1.25-mg dose of levalbuterol produced a greater increase in **forced expiratory volume in 1 second** (FEV_1) than a 2.5-mg dose of racemic albuterol. The duration is 8 hours, and side effects are similar to 2.5 mg of racemic albuterol. Beta-receptor-mediated toxicities are primarily dependent on the dose of the inhaled beta-agonist. Therefore levalbuterol does not appear to offer clinically significant advantages over albuterol.

Salmeterol (Serevent®)

Salmeterol is very *lipophilic*, unlike most β-agonists, which are *hydrophilic*. This means that, whereas other β-agonists approach the β-receptor directly from the extracellular space, salmeterol diffuses into the cell's bilayer phospholipid membrane and enters the receptor from a lateral approach. The long side-chain tail anchors itself into a hydrophobic region of the receptor, and the active saligenin head is left free to stimulate the active part of the β_2-receptor by engaging and disengaging itself. This action provides prolonged (12-hour) duration of action. Salmeterol's long action makes it ideal for maintenance (prevention of bronchospasm), but it cannot be used as a rescue treatment for acute bronchospasm because of its very slow onset (see Figure 5-10). Rescue medication such as albuterol should be given *in addition to* the patient's regularly scheduled dose of salmeterol for treatment of acute episodes.

FIGURE 5-10 Serevent® Diskus®

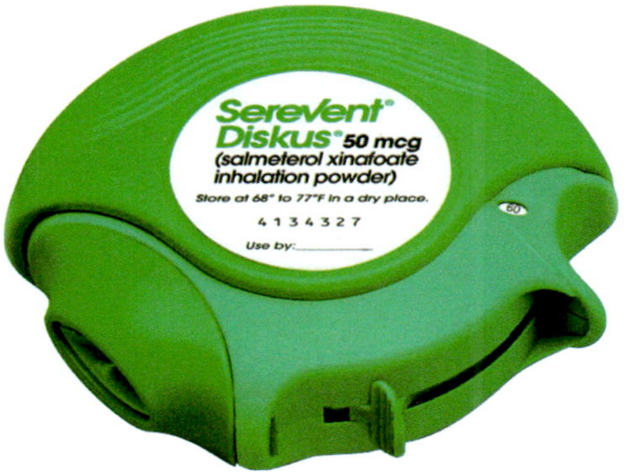

Formoterol (Perforomist®, Foradil®)

Formoterol is both a fast- and long-acting β_2-agonist. Like salmeterol, it is used as a maintenance drug in the treatment of asthma in adults and children 5 years or older. Formoterol is available as a DPI using the Aerolizer® inhaler or as a solution that can be nebulized. The dose is 12 mcg (1 capsule), or 20 mcg nebulized, every 12 hours. The onset of action is faster than that of salmeterol (2 to 3 min), and it decreases airway resistance more than salmeterol. Even though it has a rapid onset, it is not recommended as a rescue drug for acute asthma, because repeated administration of long-acting drugs produces an increased risk of toxicity as they accumulate in the body.

Arformoterol (Brovana®)

Arformoterol is a long-acting beta-agonist indicated for the treatment of COPD and is administered b.i.d. (once in the morning and once in the evening); the dosage is 15 mg by nebulized solution.

Olodaterol (Respimat® Soft Mist™ Inhaler)

Olodaterol is a once daily maintenance, long-acting beta-agonist for the treatment of COPD.

Indacaterol (Arcapta™ Neohaler™)

Indacaterol has a rapid 5-minute onset of action, but its peak effect and duration of action are 4 and 24 hours, respectively. Similar to formoterol and salmeterol, it is only used as a long-acting bronchodilator.

Summary of Therapeutic Effects of β-Agonists

	Pulmonary	Cardiovascular
Bronchodilation	Vasodilation	Inotropism/increased cardiac output
Anti-inflammatory	Increased mucociliary clearance	Decreased peripheral vascular resistance

5.4d Side Effects of β-Agonists

Most of the side effects of β-agonists are associated with the older drugs such as epinephrine and isoproterenol. Each new drug developed was made more β_2-selective by altering the chemical structure of the catecholamine molecule. However even the newer β_2-selective agents can cause some side effects.

The terms *tachyphylaxis* and *tolerance* are used to describe the desensitization of the β_2-receptor to β-adrenergic drugs. More specifically, tachyphylaxis refers to the decreased response to a drug that occurs shortly after administration. In the case of β-agonists this may occur within seconds of administration. This effect is transient, meaning that if the drug is stopped, the receptors rapidly return to their responsive state.

Tolerance is a decreased response to a drug that occurs with long-term use. After hours of exposure to β-agonists, there is an actual decrease in the number of β_2-receptors. This process is called **downregulation**. These receptors are not so easily restored, and new receptors must actually be synthesized. Infection and inflammatory mediators also decrease responsiveness to the medication. Administration of systemic corticosteroids can reverse desensitization of the β_2-receptors as a result of both tachyphylaxis and downregulation. However, inhaled corticosteroids do not appear to reverse these processes. The clinical importance of both tachyphylaxis and tolerance is a matter of ongoing debate.

CONTROVERSY

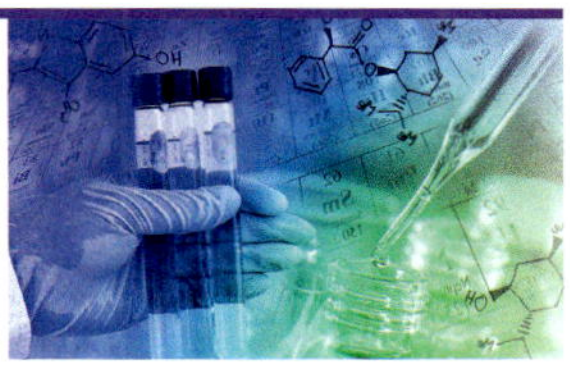

The **asthma paradox** is the unexpected increase in asthma deaths in recent years despite better understanding and treatment of the disease. The question of whether the use of β-agonists somehow increases the severity or risk of death from asthma has yet to be answered. Numerous studies have appeared on the effects of various adrenergic agonists in asthma, but they show conflicting results. Several theories attempt to explain the asthma paradox. Some of them implicate β-agonist usage, whereas others suggest that delays in seeking proper medical attention, increased exposure to allergens, or underusage of anti-inflammatory agents are possible causes.

In general, β-agonists are considered to be safe and effective, especially when delivered by inhalation. The guidelines based on Expert Panel Report 3 by the National Heart, Lung, and Blood Institute of the National Institutes of Health recognize that β-agonist therapy plays an important role in the management of asthma.

Summary of Side Effects of β-Agonists

Tachycardia	Nervousness
Arrhythmias/palpitations	Insomnia
Increased pulse and blood pressure	Dizziness
Hyperglycemia	Headache
Hypokalemia	Nausea
Tremor	

Table 5-3 lists and compares the sympathomimetic bronchodilators, including their brand names, routes and dosages, times of onset and peak action, durations, and receptor selectivities.

TABLE 5-3 Comparison of Some Typical Inhaled Sympathomimetics

Drug	Route	Dose	Frequency	Onset (min)	Peak (min)	Duration (hr)	Receptor
Catecholamines							
racemic epinephrine							
S2®	Neb	0.25–0.5 ml	q3–q6 hr	3–5	5–20	0.5–2	α, β
Resorcinols							
metaproterenol							
metaproterenol	PO; as a tablet or syrup	20 mg	t.i.d.			4–6	β_2, β_1
Saligenins							
albuterol							
Ventolin®	HFA	2 puffs	t.i.d.–q.i.d.	15	30–60	5–8	β_2, β_1
Proventil®	HFA	2 puffs	t.i.d.–q.i.d.	15	30–60	5–8	β_2, β_1
Proventil®	Neb	0.25–0.5 ml	t.i.d.–q.i.d.	15	30–60	5–8	β_2, β_1
indacaterol							
Arcapta™ Neohaler™		75 mcg	once daily	5	240		β_2
levalbuterol							
Xopenex®	Neb	0.31–3.78 mg	t.i.d.	15	30–60	3–8	β_2, β_1
Xopenex® HFA	MDI	2 puffs	q4–q6 hr	5–10	77	3–6	β_2, β_1
pirbuterol							
Maxair®	MDI	2 puffs	q4–q6 hr	5	30	5	β_2, β_1
salmeterol							
Serevent®	DPI (Diskus®)	2 puffs	q12 hr	20	3–5 hr	12	β_2
Formoterol							
Foradil®	DPI (Aerolizer®)	1 capsule	q12 hr	3–4	30–60	12	β_2
Perforomist®	Neb	20 mcg	q12 hr	3–4	30–60	12	β_2
arformoterol							
Brovana®	Neb	15 mcg	b.i.d. (morning and evening)	3–4	30–60	12	β_2

5.4e Classification by Duration of Action

In the clinical setting it is often more practical to classify sympathomimetics by the duration of their action rather than by their chemical classification. Bronchodilators are now classified as either short-acting beta-agonists (SABAs) or long-acting beta-agonists (LABAs), especially since the introduction of agents such as salmeterol that last up to 12 hours. Albuterol and levalbuterol are now classified as SABAs. Because of their relatively rapid onset of action, these all can be used as **rescue therapy.** They can provide rapid relief of symptoms, but they may need to be readministered rather frequently. Salmeterol is an example of a true long-acting bronchodilator or LABA, with a duration of 12 hours or more. It is most beneficial as **maintenance therapy**, because it takes a long time to start working, but it does last a long time. Table 5-4 compares these drugs.

TABLE 5-4 Classification of Sympathomimetics by Duration of Action

Short-acting (6–8 hr) SABAs	Long-acting (12–24 hr) LABAs
albuterol	salmeterol
Ventolin®	Serevent®
Proventil®	formoterol
levalbuterol	Foradil®
Xopenex®	Perforomist®
pirbuterol	indacaterol
Maxair® Autohaler®	Arcapta™ Neohaler™
	arformoterol
	Brovana®
	olodaterol
	Striverdi® Respimat®

PATIENT & FAMILY EDUCATION

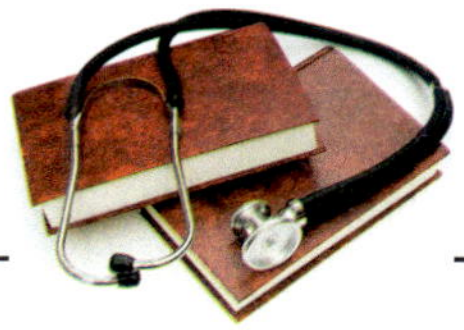

New Warning Labels

Ongoing FDA analyses of studies showing an increased risk of severe exacerbations of asthma symptoms resulting in hospitalizations and death have prompted the FDA to require a risk evaluation and mitigation strategy (REMS) and class-labeling changes for all LABAs. The REMS will require a revised medication guide written specifically for patients and a health-care professional education plan about the appropriate use of LABAs. When LABAs are felt to be clinically appropriate for an asthmatic patient, they should only be used with an asthma controller medication such as an inhaled corticosteroid. Combination products containing both a LABA and an inhaled corticosteroid are strongly encouraged to ensure compliance with both medications.

time for review

Contrast rescue versus maintenance bronchodilator therapy.

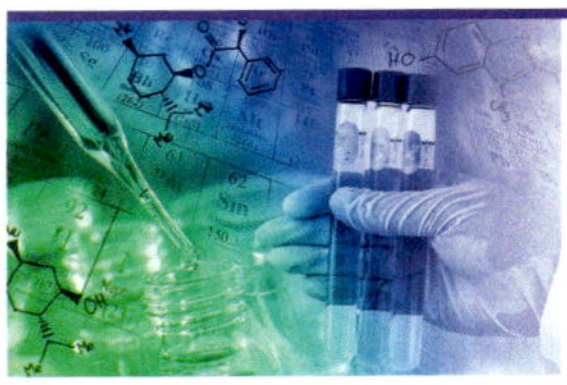

Controversy

MDIs used propellants based on chlorofluorocarbons (CFCs) from their inception. However, production of CFCs was ended in 1996 because of environmental and safety issues. CFCs were associated with toxicity when patients overused their MDIs, as well as damage to the Earth's ozone layer. A temporary exemption was granted for CFCs used for MDIs, but now all CFC propellants have been replaced with a safer hydrofluoroalkane (HFA) propellant or with DPIs that do not require propellant. DPIs are a safe alternative for patients who can use them, but not everyone can use them. They are especially problematic during emergency situations, when patients may not inhale deeply or quickly enough. Please refer to Chapter 4 for more on DPI usage. Changing MDIs from CFC to HFA propellants has required reformulating the drugs and redesigning the actuator in order to ensure dose equivalency between the two types.

As indicated in Table 5-3, most of the β-agonists are available for inhalation either by nebulization, MDI, or DPI. All but the catecholamines can be given orally (as tablets or syrups). Remember, catecholamines are deactivated in the stomach.

Life Span Considerations

For adult patients, any type of aerosol device is effective when used correctly. Patient preferences may play a role in device selection, along with cost, ability to demonstrate correct use of the inhaler device, and convenience.

For children 6 years and younger, MDI plus a spacer device should be used. In children ages 6–12 years, bronchodilators may be administered with either an MDI plus spacer or a breath-actuated or dry-powder inhaler. For steroid administration in this age group, an MDI plus spacer may be best to prevent oral thrush. Teenagers may use any of the three available options but may prefer dry powder inhalers in schools and on ski slopes, for example. The best device for a given patient is one he or she will use consistently and correctly.

Delivering the drug directly to the target organ (the lung) is obviously desirable in order to reduce side effects, but the efficacy of the inhalation route during acute attacks of airway obstruction has been questioned. Maximum aerosol deposition depends on the patient's ability to take a slow, deep breath followed by a breath-hold. Shortness of breath may compromise the patient's technique. Furthermore the reduction in diameter of the spastic airways may decrease deposition of aerosol particles in the bronchioles. In spite of this, several studies have failed to show any significant difference between inhaled and parenteral (intravenous or subcutaneous) administration of β-agonists. No reason has been identified to avoid the inhalation route during severe acute episodes of bronchospasm. In fact the *Guidelines for the Diagnosis and Management of Asthma* of the National Heart, Lung, and Blood Institute recognize the benefit of frequent (every 20 minutes) and continuous nebulization of selective β_2-agonists such as terbutaline and albuterol during severe acute asthma attacks.

Although it is recognized as sometimes being necessary, this aggressive dosing is not standard therapy. There is a risk of arrhythmias (**premature ventricular contractions** or PVCs), hypokalemia, hyperglycemia, and significant tremor. Patients must be closely supervised and monitored with a cardiac monitor. In most instances, this requires the patient to be in an intensive care unit or emergency department. In spite of this, frequent and continuous nebulization with albuterol or levalbuterol can be both safe and effective.

5.5 ANTICHOLINERGIC (PARASYMPATHOLYTIC) BRONCHODILATORS

Another class of bronchodilators is the anticholinergic agents. Their mechanism of action is entirely different from that of the sympathomimetics. Remember that the parasympathetic nervous system plays an opposing role to that of the sympathetic system. Stimulation of the parasympathetic nervous system increases bronchoconstriction and mucus production. Administration of an anticholinergic can block the effects of the parasympathetic system and thus cause bronchodilation.

The prototypical anticholinergic agent is atropine. It is an alkaloid found in several plants, including *Atropa belladonna* (the nightshade plant) and *Datura stramonium* (jimsonweed). Ingredients in these plants have probably been used for thousands of years for their effects on the CNS. As early as the seventeenth century, the fumes from burning *Datura stramonium* were inhaled for cough and shortness of breath. In the 1980s, interest in anticholinergic agents as adjuncts to β-adrenergics was renewed. This renewed interest was due largely to a better understanding of the role of the parasympathetic nervous system in bronchospasm and also to the introduction of ipratropium bromide, an atropine derivative with fewer side effects. Ipratropium bromide (Atrovent®) is the most commonly used anticholinergic bronchodilator today.

5.5a Mechanism of Action

In contrast to the sympathetic nervous system, the lungs are innervated directly by the vagus nerve, which is a major nerve of the parasympathetic nervous system. Nerve fibers reach the airway epithelium, submucosal glands, smooth muscle, and probably mast cells. The muscarinic receptors are present in the airways from the trachea to the bronchioles; however, they are concentrated in the large airways.

When a parasympathetic nerve fiber is stimulated, ACh is the neurotransmitter that stimulates a muscarinic receptor in the bronchial smooth muscle. Once stimulated, the inactive enzyme guanosine triphosphate (GTP) is converted to its active form, cGMP. However cGMP causes constriction of the bronchial smooth muscle (see Figure 5-11). Stimulation of parasympathetic nerves in the lung also causes other parasympathetic responses, such as slowing of the heart rate and increased secretions.

FIGURE 5-11 Parasympathetic Stimulation Favoring Bronchoconstriction

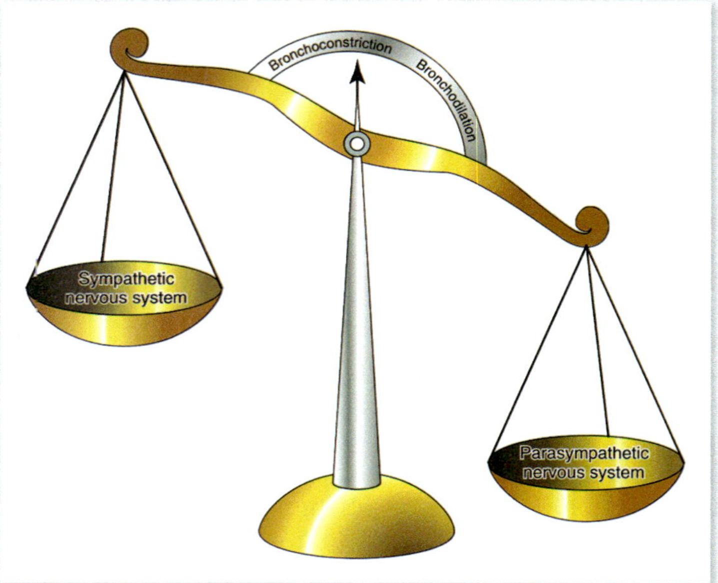

Parasympatholytic (anticholinergic) agents block ACh at the muscarinic receptor site in the airways (see Figure 5-12). Effects of parasympatholytics include drying of pulmonary secretions, increased heart rate, and bronchodilation. Notice that these are opposite (*-lytic*) effects to those of parasympathetic stimulation. The degree of bronchodilation that can be achieved with an anticholinergic bronchodilator is dependent on the degree of bronchial tone already present due to the parasympathetic system. In healthy individuals, there is minimal airway dilation following the administration of an anticholinergic agent, because there is only a basal level of parasympathetic tone to be blocked. However, in certain disease states, the parasympathetic activity is increased, and significant bronchodilation can be achieved with administration of an anticholinergic agent.

FIGURE 5-12 Diagram of Parasympathetic Neurotransmission Blockage (Parasympatholytic) Leading to Bronchodilation

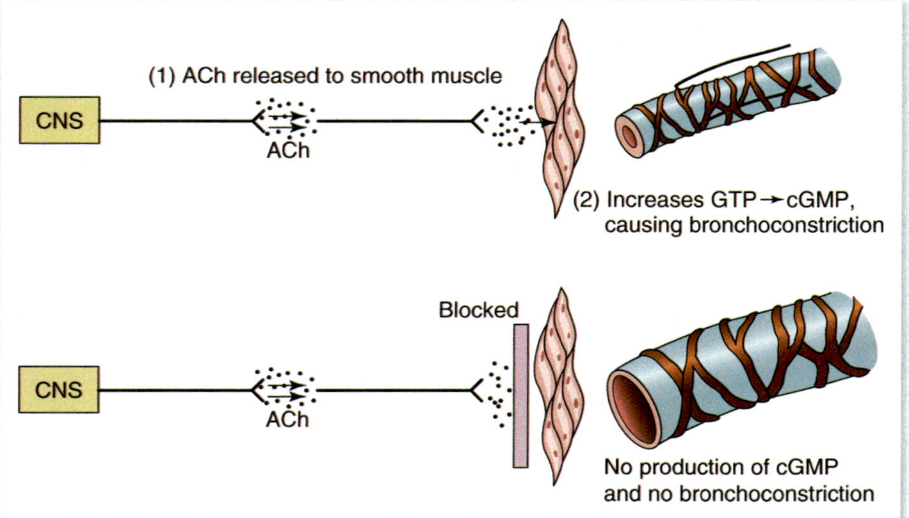

For example a portion of the bronchospasm seen in COPD patients is caused by vagally mediated innervation of airway smooth muscle. In other words the bronchospasm is due to overstimulation of the parasympathetic nervous system, and this problem should respond to an anticholinergic agent. Inhalation of irritants such as cigarette smoke, cold air, high inspiratory flow rates, noxious fumes, and histamine release cause a nerve impulse to be sent from the airway to the CNS, then from the CNS back to the airways by way of the parasympathetic nervous system, which constricts the airway smooth muscle and increases mucus secretion and cough. This parasympathetic reflex bronchoconstriction can be blocked very effectively by an anticholinergic agent. Anticholinergics such as ipratropium or tiotropium are indicated in the routine management of COPD. They are also used in conjunction with short-acting β_2-agonists in the emergency treatment of severe asthma.

5.5b Atropine Sulfate

Atropine sulfate is the prototypical parasympatholytic and does relax airway smooth muscle. However it is not commonly used as a bronchodilator because of its many side effects. It inhibits mucus production and reduces mucociliary clearance. Since atropine is lipophilic and can cross biologic barriers easily, CNS effects and other adverse effects can occur even at small doses. Restlessness, irritability, drowsiness, fatigue, and mild excitement have been reported. At higher doses, disorientation, hallucinations, coma, and acute psychotic reactions can occur. Relaxation of the muscles that control the lens of the eye causes blurred vision. Vagal blockade increases heart rate. The GI effects of atropine include dryness of the mouth (due to blockade of salivary gland secretion) and decreased motility in the gut. Clinically, atropine is primarily a cardiac drug and will be discussed in Chapter 15.

Clinical pearl

The inhibition of mucus production and impaired mucociliary clearance can cause thick retained airway secretions, which obstruct the airways and can lead to collapse of the lung.

time for review

Why is atropine contraindicated in cystic fibrosis patients who have thick tenacious secretions?

5.5c Ipratropium Bromide (Atrovent®)

Ipratropium bromide (Atrovent® HFA) is available as a solution for nebulization, MDI, and as a nasal spray pump (see Figure 5-13). It is also available with albuterol (a sympathomimetic) in a single MDI canister (Combivent® Respimat®) or as a solution (DuoNeb®) for patients who have demonstrated a response to both classes of drugs. The onset of bronchodilation begins within minutes but then increases more gradually to its peak effect in 1 to 2 hours. The duration of bronchodilation is about the same as that of a β-agonist in asthmatics, but it acts for 1 to 2 hours longer than a β-agonist in COPD patients. Since it has a quick onset, it is considered a short-acting muscarinic antagonist or SAMA. It has little or no effect on mucociliary clearance from the lung, even though it does decrease hypersecretion of mucus in the nose. This is one of the main reasons why it is

Clinical pearl

Anticholinergics are also indicated for allergic and nonallergic rhinitis, because they block muscarinic receptors in the mucus-producing glands in the nose to help the "runny nose."

preferred over atropine. Since it is hydrophilic and cannot cross biologic barriers easily, it has little or no effect on heart rate, blood pressure, or the GI tract, but there are rare cases of dry mouth, headache, blurred vision, cough, nausea, and nervousness (see Table 5-5). Patients with prostatic hyperplasia, urinary retention, and glaucoma should be monitored for possible systemic side effects.

FIGURE 5-13 Atrovent® HFA

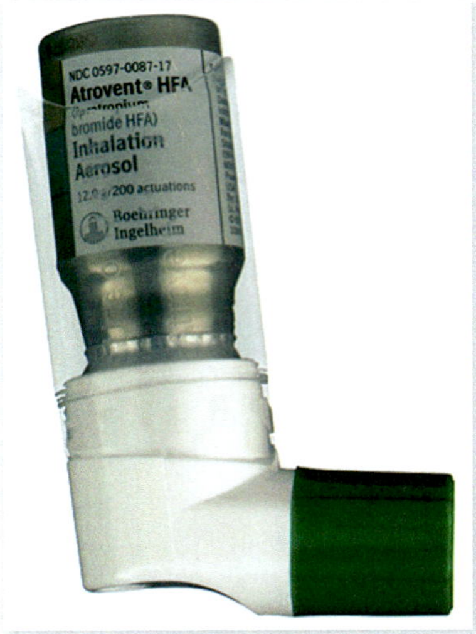

TABLE 5-5 Common Parasympatholytics

Drug and Trade Names	Dosage	Frequency	Onset (min)	Peak (hr)	Duration (hr)
SAMAs					
ipratropium bromide					
Solution for nebulization	500 mcg/unit dose	t.i.d., q.i.d.	1–5	0.25	4–8
Atrovent® HFA MDI	2 puffs	q.i.d.	15	1–2	4–6
ipratropium bromide and albuterol					
Combivent® Respimat®	2 puffs	q.i.d.	15	2	6–8
DuoNeb®	3 ml	q.i.d.	5	0.8	4–5
LAMAs					
tiotropium bromide					
Spiriva®	1 inhalation/day	once daily	30	3	>24
aclidinium					
Tudorza® Pressair®	1 inhalation	twice daily	10	3	12

5.5d Tiotropium Bromide (Spiriva®)

Tiotropium bromide (Spiriva®) is a long-acting muscarinic antagonist (LAMA) bronchodilator (see Figure 5-14). It is indicated for long-term, once-daily maintenance treatment for COPD. The onset of action is 30 minutes. Peak effect is reached within 3 hours, and 90% of the peak effect on FEV_1 is maintained for over 24 hours. Tiotropium is not indicated as a rescue drug for acute symptoms of shortness of breath. It is available as a DPI, referred to as a HandiHaler®, and as a spray for oral inhalation. This product is called Spiriva® Respimat®. The HandiHaler® device comes with a packet of 30 "blisters." Each blister contains one 18-mcg capsule of tiotropium. Spiriva® Respimat® is supplied in a carton containing a drug-filled cartridge and an inhaler device. The safety profile of tiotropium is the same as for ipratropium, and serious side effects are relatively uncommon. Dry mouth is the most common adverse reaction. Other side effects are consistent with anticholinergic effects, such as urinary retention, constipation, increased heart rate, blurred vision, and glaucoma.

Aclidinium (Tudorza® Pressair®)

Aclidinium (Tudorza® Pressair®) is a long-acting anticholinergic bronchodilator. It is indicated for the long-term, twice-daily, maintenance treatment of COPD. The onset of action is minutes. Peak concentrations in plasma are reached in 10 minutes. Several trials comparing aclidinium to placebo showed a statistically significant increase in FEV_1 in favor of aclidinium over placebo. Aclidinium is not indicated as a rescue drug for acute symptoms of shortness of breath. It is available as a DPI. The brand name medication is called Tudorza® Pressair® and is a multi-dose, dry-powder inhaler that delivers 400 mcg of aclidinium per actuation. The safety profile of aclidinium is similar to tiotropium and ipratropium. Serious side effects are relatively uncommon. Dry mouth is the most common adverse reaction. Other side effects are consistent with anticholinergic effects, such as urinary retention, constipation, increased heart rate, blurred vision, and glaucoma.

FIGURE 5-14 **Spiriva® HandiHaler®**

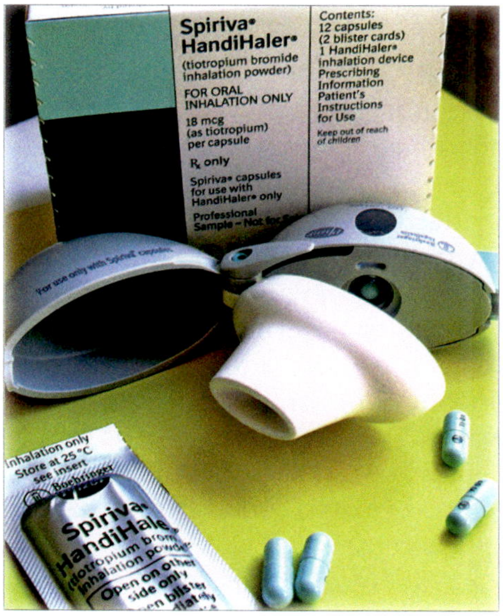

Clinical pearl

Care must be taken to protect patients from getting anticholinergic drugs into their eyes. In patients with narrow-angle glaucoma (which is common and often not diagnosed in elderly patients), anticholinergics can increase intraocular pressure. Using MDIs with holding chambers can help reduce the risk, as can instructing patients to keep nebulizers in their mouth, using breath-actuated nebulizers when possible, and being very careful with placement when mask treatments are necessary.

Clinical pearl

Anticholinergic (also known as antimuscarinic) bronchodilators have a different side effect profile than β_2-adrenergic bronchodilators, and no tolerance to bronchodilation has been observed with their use. Combination therapy using an anticholinergic (ipratropium) and a short-acting β_2-agonist (albuterol) results in greater bronchodilation with fewer side effects than either drug alone. In December of 2013, the FDA approved Anoro™ Ellipta® (Figure 5-15), which is a combination prescription medication containing two long-acting bronchodilators. It contains umeclidinium bromide, a LAMA, and vilanterol, a LABA. Anoro™ is approved only for use in COPD and is *not* used to treat asthma, as LABAs such as vilanterol can increase the risk of death in asthma patients.

FIGURE 5-15 Anora™ Ellipta™

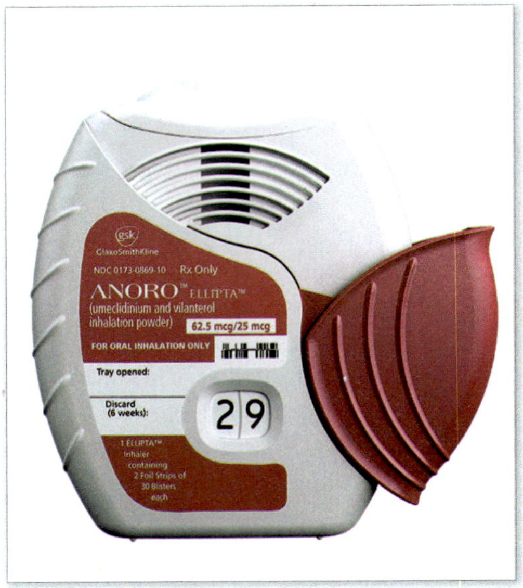

Copyright: GlaxoSmithKline. Used with permission.

5.5e Monitoring Outcomes of Inhaled Bronchodilator Therapy

Patients should be assessed before, during, and after treatment in order to get an accurate assessment of the effectiveness of the medication(s). The clinician should obtain baseline data such as heart rate, respiratory rate, breath sounds, and oxygen saturation by pulse oximeter. Measuring arterial blood gases may also be indicated if acid–base status is in question. The practitioner should inquire about the patient's perceived level of **dyspnea** (subjective) and observe the patient's breathing pattern and use of accessory muscles. Measurement of **peak expiratory flow rate** (PEFR) or FEV_1 should be performed before and after the treatment. These can be sensitive indicators of airway obstruction and actually quantify airway obstruction and posttreatment improvement. However, both PEFR and FEV_1 are effort-dependent. These are valuable only if the patient gives a maximum effort. Patients in acute bronchospasm may be unable to perform the forced exhalation required, because it can cause coughing and increase bronchospasm.

Signs of a positive bronchodilator response include improved appearance, reduced dyspnea, decreased use of accessory muscles, improved vital signs, increased sputum production, decreased wheezing coupled with increased intensity of breath sounds, increase in FEV_1 or PEFR, and improved oxygenation.

Side effects are relatively uncommon with the newer β_2-selective sympathomimetics. Side effects are even less common when the drug is given by inhalation, compared with oral and intravenous administration. However, although adverse reactions may be uncommon, some patients are more sensitive than others, and problems are possible. The most common side effect is muscle tremor due to stimulation of β_2-receptors in the skeletal muscles. There are also some β-receptors in the heart and blood vessels, so increased heart rate and vasodilation are possible. It is generally accepted that an increase in heart rate of greater than 20% of the baseline heart rate (or 20 beats/minute) is significant. If either tremor or increase in heart rate develops, the treatment should be stopped and the patient monitored until the effects subside; the physician should also be notified. The entire event should be documented in the patient's medical record.

Often, when the clinician changes the route of administration (e.g., from oral to inhaled), the selection of a more β_2-selective agent or a smaller dose may alleviate unwanted effects from bronchodilator therapy.

Patient & Family Education

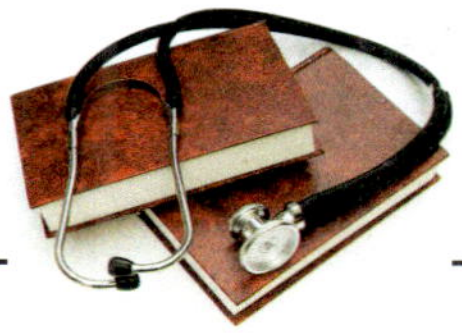

Inhaler Education Is Critical

Research consistently supports that adults and children, alike, misunderstand instructions concerning aerosol device use. Of patients with asthma or COPD, 1 in 3 misused his or her inhaler. In patients with prior instruction, the error rate was 23.1% compared to an error rate of 52.6% in patients without previous instruction. To ensure proper use, require both adults and children to demonstrate how their aerosol device should be used.

time for review

List the positive clinical responses to bronchodilator therapy.

5.6 METHYLXANTHINES

Theophylline and its salt, aminophylline, are the primary xanthines used clinically. However there are also a few other well-recognized members of the xanthine group (or *methylxanthines*, as they are sometimes called). These include theobromine and caffeine. All of these substances can be found naturally in certain plants. For example caffeine is found in coffee beans and cola. Tea leaves contain both caffeine and theophylline. Caffeine and theobromine are found in cocoa. Various parts of these plants have been used for their stimulant effects on the CNS for centuries. Xanthines are administered orally or intravenously, and there are many different brand names. Even though they are not administered by aerosol, it is important for the clinician to understand the role they may play in bronchodilation.

5.6a Mechanism of Action

The traditional explanation of the xanthines' mode of action is that they produce bronchodilation by inhibiting phosphodiesterase, which is the enzyme that deactivates cAMP. This indirectly increases bronchodilation by increasing cAMP. Although this is true, at the dosages commonly used in humans, theophylline is a relatively poor inhibitor of phosphodiesterase and therefore a weak bronchodilator. Several other theories of how xanthines work have been investigated, but at this time there is no definite explanation for how they work. In fact it is possible that there are multiple mechanisms behind their actions.

5.6b Nonbronchodilating Effects of Theophylline

Even though theophylline is a weak bronchodilator, it has several other effects that produce clinical improvement. For example theophylline has been shown to increase the strength and endurance of muscle contraction, including that of the diaphragm. This may help prevent respiratory failure by increasing the patient's **ventilatory drive**, the strength of the stimulus to breathe. Experiments performed in animals have shown theophylline's ability to decrease inflammation and immune cell function, which results in a decrease in the late phase increase in airway obstruction that occurs in asthma. The diuretic effect of xanthines is well known to those who drink caffeinated beverages such as coffee, tea, and cola.

Theophylline has a slow onset and long duration of action and is well tolerated by many patients. However, patients should be monitored closely, because there is wide variability in its therapeutic effect. This variability in response is most likely due to its being metabolized at different rates by different people. In addition a variety of other medications interact with theophylline, increasing side effects and serum drug levels. Toxicity can result, and patients with liver disease and congestive heart failure (CHF) must also be carefully monitored. The therapeutic range for theophylline is narrow (5 to 15 mcg/ml). Side effects increase when blood concentrations are close to 20 mcg/ml, and toxic levels can exist (more than 20 mcg/ml). Serum levels should be monitored as appropriate.

Side effects involve the CNS, cardiovascular effects, and the GI tract. CNS side effects include dizziness, headache, restlessness, irritability, insomnia, and seizures. Cardiovascular side effects include diuresis, palpitations, tachycardia, arrhythmias, and hypertension. GI side effects include nausea, vomiting, diarrhea, epigastric pain, and anorexia. Common brand names for theophylline include:

- Theo-24®
- Theochron®
- Elixophyllin®

Clinical pearl

Methylxanthines may be prescribed as maintenance therapy for COPD, and this will be discussed in the "putting it all together" section of this book (Chapter 13). Caffeine is used in the treatment of apnea of prematurity because of its stimulation of the CNS.

For patients with chronic asthma, theophylline is a potentially useful, inexpensive medication when symptoms are not controlled by usual doses of inhaled glucocorticoids. For patients with chronic COPD, theophylline may be useful as a third-line agent to improve functional impairment, but individual response is variable and the dose must be carefully individualized to maximize benefit and minimize toxicity. For either disease, theophylline may be a useful oral alternative in patients who are poorly adherent to inhaled medications.

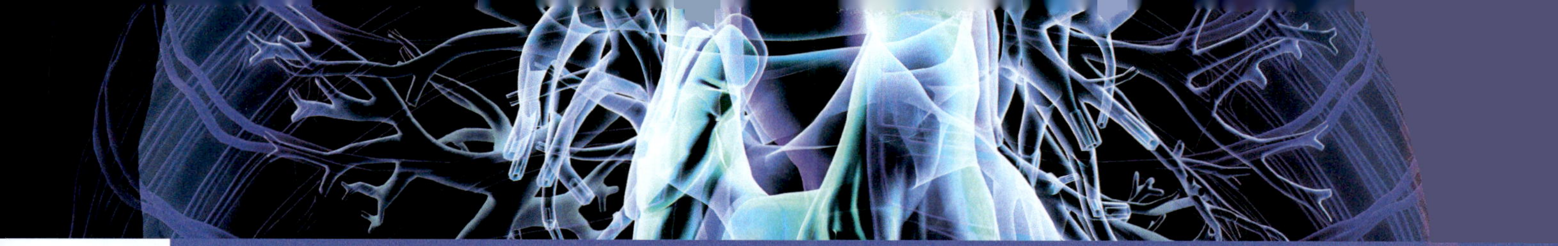

Summary

To obtain the best possible results from inhaled bronchodilators, the health-care practitioner responsible for administering these medications must be familiar with the three mechanisms of bronchoconstriction (bronchospasm, airway edema, and mucus plugging) as well as the numerous agents for treatment, their doses, route of administration, and potential for side effects.

Bronchodilation can be achieved via three classes of medications: β-adrenergic agents, anticholinergic agents, and methylxanthines. The β-adrenergic agents work by stimulating the sympathetic effects of bronchodilation in the lungs. Ideal agents are β_2-specific, to avoid unwanted cardiac (β_1) side effects. Anticholinergic agents work by blocking the parasympathetic response of bronchoconstriction and thus cause bronchodilation.

Although the methylxanthines, especially theophylline and aminophylline, are traditionally classed as bronchodilators, they are actually poor bronchodilators at therapeutic levels. Their real benefit as a maintenance drug in COPD may be due to increased ventilatory drive or by strengthening the contraction of the diaphragm, thereby increasing airflow and improving ventilation. In asthma, they decrease airway inflammation. Because they have a long duration of action, they may be used to control symptoms through the night. However, their benefits should always be weighed against their numerous side effects, especially because long-acting sympathomimetics are now available.

REVIEW QUESTIONS

1. You are called to the emergency department to assess a 14-year-old girl. She is short of breath and complains of tightness in her chest. She has a history of asthma. Upon assessment, you note that her respirations are 31/min and her heart rate is 110. On auscultation, you note a prolonged expiratory wheeze. Which of the following medications would you recommend, and why?
   (a) ipratropium bromide
   (b) albuterol
   (c) salmeterol
   (d) caffeine

2. Which of the following are advantages of ipratropium bromide over atropine for treatment of bronchospasm?
   (a) fewer cardiac side effects
   (b) no effect on mucus clearance from the lung
   (c) more rapid onset of action
   (d) all of the above

3. Which of the following would you recommend for an asthmatic patient who complains of waking up in the early morning hours with shortness of breath?
   (a) albuterol
   (b) epinephrine
   (c) ipratropium bromide
   (d) salmeterol

4. How should a patient who is receiving theophylline be monitored to determine the appropriate dose?
   (a) Measure peak expiratory flow rate (PEFR) before and after administration of the medication.
   (b) Measure FEV_1 before and after the administration of the medication.
   (c) Measure serum blood levels of the medication and ask the patient about side effects.
   (d) Auscultate breath sounds after administration of the medication.

5. A patient with asthma has failed to improve after treatment with 0.5 ml nebulized albuterol. Which of the following would be most appropriate?
   (a) ipratropium bromide (Atrovent®)
   (b) salmeterol (Serevent®)
   (c) isoproterenol (Isuprel®)
   (d) levalbuterol (Xopenex®)

6. Explain why you chose the drug you did for the patient in Review Question 5.

7. During an albuterol treatment, the patient complains of feeling "shaky." You note that the patient's heart rate has increased from 90 to 128 beats/minute. Which of the following would you recommend?
   I. Stop the treatment.
   II. Notify the patient's nurse and physician.
   III. Stay with the patient and continue to monitor him.
   IV. Tell the patient that the treatment is almost done and encourage him to finish.

   (a) I only
   (b) IV only
   (c) II and IV
   (d) I, II, and III

8. Which of the following medications are available as a DPI?
   I. isoetharine
   II. levalbuterol
   III. Serevent®
   IV. tiotropium

   (a) I and II
   (b) III only
   (c) III and IV
   (d) I, II, III, and IV

9. Which of the following drugs would be most useful in treating an acute asthma attack?
   I. salmeterol (Serevent®)
   II. albuterol (Proventil®)
   III. ipratropium (Atrovent®)
   IV. levalbuterol (Xopenex®)

   (a) I only
   (b) I, II, and III
   (c) II, III, and IV
   (d) III and IV

10. A COPD patient takes albuterol by MDI and ipratropium by MDI four times per day. His physician would like to change him to long-acting medications. Which of the following would you recommend?
   I. DuoNeb®
   II. Serevent®
   III. Combivent®
   IV. Spiriva®

   (a) I only
   (b) II and IV
   (c) III only
   (d) IV only

11. Which of the following can be used to monitor the effectiveness of bronchodilator therapy?
    (a) PEFR
    (b) FEV_1
    (c) use of accessory muscles
    (d) all of the above

12. A patient with COPD experiences increased bronchospasm after using her albuterol inhaler. Her doctor feels that it may be due to the propellant in her MDI. What do you suggest?

13. Explain why a bronchodilator may not be helpful in treating a child with croup.

CASE STUDY 1

A 66-year-old male

A 66-year-old male with a history of COPD is admitted to the emergency department with shortness of breath. He is not currently taking any medication for his breathing. The patient states that he usually gets short of breath only upon exertion, but he developed a "cold" several days ago that made his breathing worse. He has been placed on oxygen. The doctor wants him to have breathing treatments. What medication, dose, and route of administration would you suggest?

(a) How should the effectiveness of the treatments be monitored?

(b) After several days of breathing treatments and antibiotics, the patient is ready for discharge, but he still becomes short of breath during the night. What maintenance medication(s) do you suggest?

CASE STUDY 2

A 9-year-old boy

A 9-year-old boy presents with a complaint of chest tightness, cough, and shortness of breath. This usually occurs during periods of exertion, but he has also woken up several times during the night with similar symptoms. His general health has been good and his physical exam, including breath sounds, is normal at this time. What possible diagnosis should be explored?

(a) How should this boy be assessed for airflow obstruction?

(b) What medication, dose, and route of administration would you suggest?

(c) How should he monitor his response to his medication?

Case Studies Continue

CASE STUDY 3

A patient with COPD

A patient with COPD Is currently taking albuterol by MDI four times a day. The patient states that her inhaler does not seem to work as well as it used to. She still gets short of breath and it is sometimes hard to wait for the next dose. She is not taking any other medications at this time. Which of the following would you recommend?

(a) Continue albuterol as ordered.

(b) Give albuterol by nebulizer.

(c) Discontinue albuterol and give Serevent®.

(d) Continue albuterol and add tiotropium once a day.

Explain your answer.

The physician asks if you think the patient would do better with levalbuterol (Xopenex®). What do you think?

If levalbuterol is ordered, should another drug be used with it? Why or why not?

Chapter 6

Mucokinetics and Surfactants

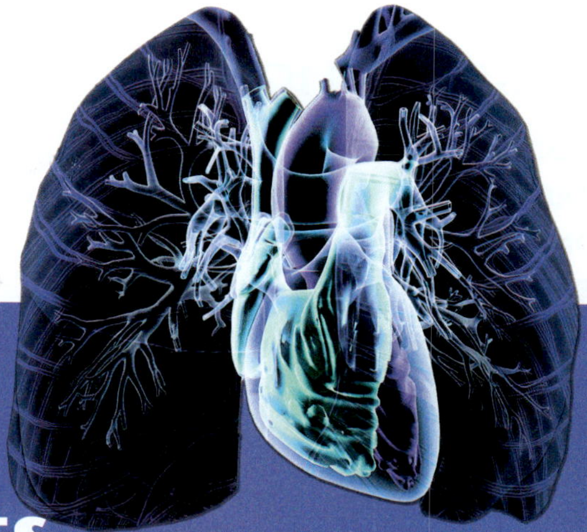

OBJECTIVES

Upon completion of this chapter you will be able to

- Define key terms related to mucokinetic and surfactant agents.
- Describe the production, function, and clearance of mucus in the healthy lung.
- State the indications for bland aerosols and mucolytic agents.
- Compare and contrast the mechanisms of action of bland aerosols and mucolytic agents.
- Describe how surface tension relates to oxygenation and the work of breathing.
- Describe the role of surfactants in the lungs and surfactant replacement agents.
- Describe the mechanisms of action of expectorants and antitussive agents.

KEY TERMS

aliquot
bronchial gland
bronchorrhea
endogenous surfactant
exogenous surfactant
expectorant
goblet cell
hydrophilic
hypertonic
hypotonic
isotonic
maintenance therapy
rhinorrhea
stomatitis
surface tension
surfactant
viscoelastic

ABBREVIATIONS

ACCP	American College of Chest Physicians
ARDS	acute respiratory distress syndrome
DNase	deoxyribonuclease
FVC	forced vital capacity
NaCl	sodium chloride, or salt
PDA	patent ductus arteriosis
PEP	positive expiratory pressure
RDS	respiratory distress syndrome of newborns
SP	surface proteins

This chapter encompasses a rather diverse group of drugs with widely varying effects. We will need to review the physiology of mucus production, mucus function, and the effects that various disease states have on them. We will look at the role of *bland* (unmedicated) aerosols and mucolytics and the importance of bronchial hygiene techniques in the management of retained secretions. The consequences of retained secretions can be very serious and include infections, airway obstruction, and collapse (atelectasis). It is therefore important to understand the pharmacologic aids available to you to assist in good bronchial hygiene.

Finally we will take a closer look at the lower respiratory tract, where surfactants play a critical role in maintaining the integrity of the alveolar surface. This integrity is vital to the role of adequate gas exchange and therefore must be maintained. This chapter will provide the reader with a basis for understanding current and future roles for surfactant replacement therapy.

6.1 THE MUCOCILIARY SYSTEM

6.1a Anatomy and Physiology

The three layers of the airway are the mucosa, submucosa, and adventitia (see Figure 6-1). The mucosa (inner layer of the airway) is made up of different types of specialized epithelial cells, which rest on a basement membrane. Most numerous are the pseudostratified ciliated columnar epithelia, but there are also secretory cells such as goblet cells, serous cells, and clara cells. The goblet cells produce a relatively small amount of mucus, which is secreted into the airway. The serous cells produce less-viscous mucus, which makes up the sol layer of the mucus—we'll get to that in a minute. The role of the clara cells is not completely clear, but they are known to have a high degree of metabolic activity and to contain a lot of enzymes. The bronchial glands are found in the submucosal layer. They produce most of the mucus found in the airways. Together, the **goblet cells** and **bronchial glands** produce about 100 ml of mucus each day. Most of the mucus is reabsorbed, but about 10 ml reaches the pharynx each day, where it is usually swallowed.

Learning Hint

The terms *mucous, mucus,* and *mucosa* are often confused. Mucus is a secretion of the mucous membranes or mucosa. For example the respiratory mucosa or mucous membranes secrete the substance mucus, which protects the airways.

FIGURE 6-1 Illustration of the Three Layers of the Airway and a Micrograph of the Respiratory Epithelium

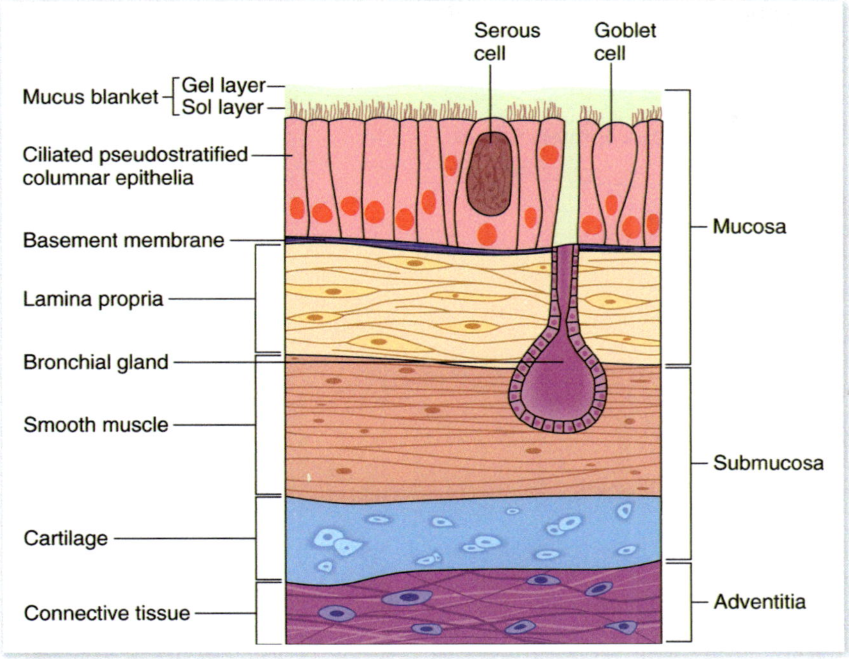

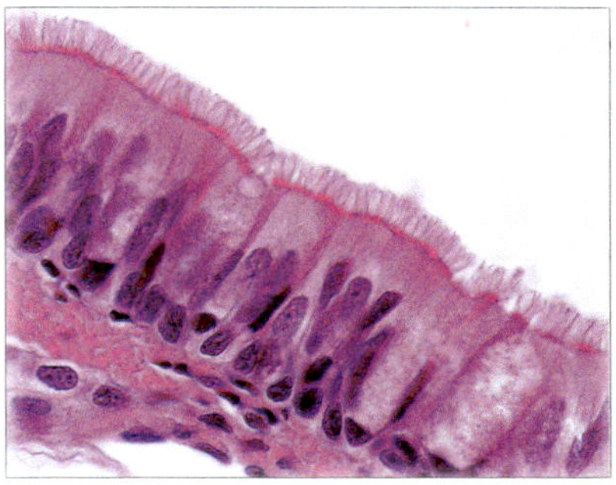

Source: Shutterstock

The mucociliary system, or mucociliary escalator as it is sometimes called, consists of the mucosal blanket that lines the airways from the naso- and oropharynx to the terminal bronchi. It also includes the cilia, which propel the mucus up the airway. Cilia are tiny hairlike projections that arise from the surface of the mucosal cells. There are about 200 cilia per cell, and they are about 6 microns in length. The cilia beat about 1,000 times per minute in a coordinated fashion to propel the mucus toward the upper airway. In healthy lungs, the mucus moves forward at a speed of about 2 cm/min.

The mucociliary system is an important part of the pulmonary defense system. It protects the lungs from inhaled debris, and it contains enzymes that give it antimicrobial properties that help prevent infection. Mucus helps to warm and humidify inspired gases, and it prevents excessive loss of heat and moisture from the airways. It is important to note that no cilia or mucus are found in the lower airways from the respiratory bronchioles to the alveoli.

Learning Hint

Exposure to irritants such as cigarette smoke increases the size and number of the bronchial glands, which accounts for the excessive mucus production and cough that many smokers have.

6.1b Structure and Composition of Mucus

The layer of mucus (or *mucosal blanket*) that covers the surface of the airways is about 5 to 10 microns thick and is made up of two distinct layers, the gel layer and the sol layer. The gel layer floats on top of the sol layer and is about 1 to 2 microns thick; as its name implies, it is rather gelatinous. It is sticky and works a lot like flypaper to trap inhaled particles and bacteria. The sol layer is deeper (about 4 to 8 microns thick) and has a more watery consistency, which enables the cilia to beat freely. The beating of the cilia within the sol layer helps propel the gel layer toward the larynx.

The mucus molecule itself is very large and complex. It is about 95% water, so it is imperative that there is a sufficient amount of water available in the body to produce normal mucus. Once mucus has formed, it does not absorb

Learning Hint

The consistency of the mucus plays an important part in mucus clearance. If mucus is too thick, it becomes very difficult for the cilia to move the mucus (think of trying to row a boat through pudding). Mucus that is too thin is not easily managed either. If your garage is flooded, would you use a rake to move the water to the floor drain?

Learning Hint

The structure of the mucus molecule has been compared to a round bottle brush, and the molecules tend to form long, flexible strands that are **hydrophilic**, meaning they attract water like a sponge. A general concept of the molecular structure will be helpful in understanding how some of the mucolytic agents work.

water readily. The remaining 5% of mucus composition comprises long, flexible strands of protein and lipid molecules that form polypeptide chains, with many carbohydrate side chains attached. The side chains are cross-connected with disulfide, physical, ionic, and hydrogen bonds (see Figure 6-2).

FIGURE 6-2 The Mucus Structure

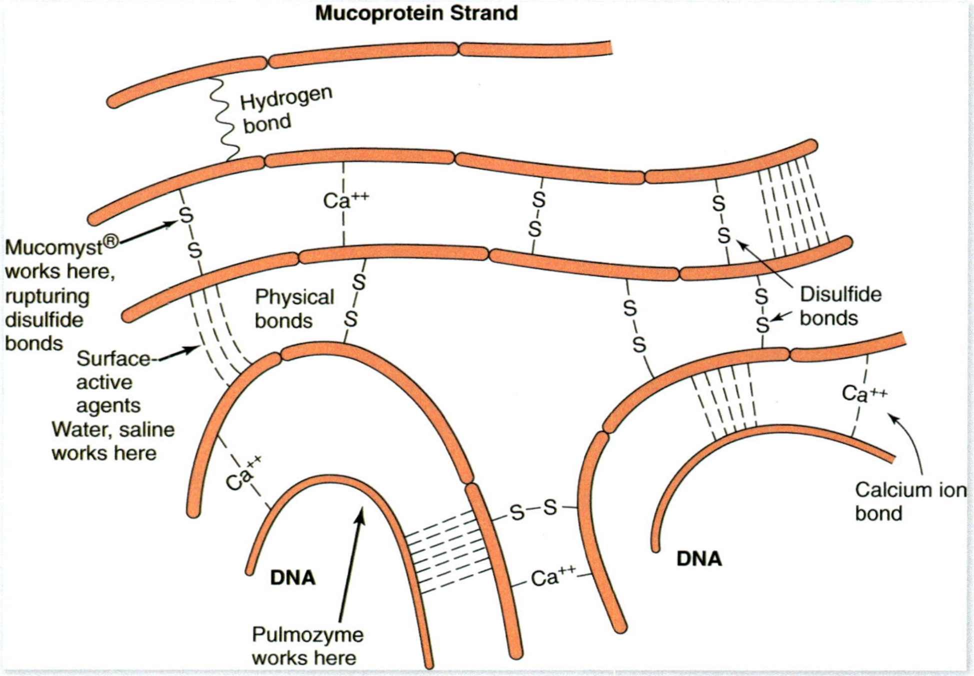

See Table 6-1 for a summary of the functions of mucus in the healthy lung.

TABLE 6-1 Mucus Function in the Healthy Lung

Preventing water from moving into and out of the epithelia
Shielding epithelia from direct contact with toxic materials, irritants, and microorganisms
Preventing infection by the action of antimicrobial enzymes
Lubrication of the airway

Proper function of the mucociliary system is critical to the maintenance of a healthy pulmonary system. The volume, consistency, and structure of mucus produced can be altered in various disease states, including primary pulmonary disease and systemic dehydration. Mucus production increases when the respiratory tract is irritated and during increased parasympathetic stimulation. In certain disease states (such as cystic fibrosis, pneumonia, and chronic bronchitis), mucus production increases significantly. The airways can produce more than twice the normal amount of mucus. Simultaneously, mucus clearance can also be impaired, resulting in an overwhelming accumulation of mucus in the lungs. See Table 6-2 for a more complete listing of disease states that increase the volume and/or thickness of mucus.

TABLE 6-2 **Diseases That Increase the Volume or Thickness of Mucus**

Chronic bronchitis
Asthma
Cystic fibrosis
Acute bronchitis
Pneumonia

The frequency with which the cilia beat is also adversely affected by disease state, environmental conditions, and chemicals. Many factors can slow or stop the beating action of the cilia, which decreases the rate of mucus clearance from the lung. Thick mucus, dry gas, smoke (including cigarette smoke), noxious gases, infection, positive-pressure ventilation, foreign bodies (including endotracheal tubes), high concentrations of oxygen, and certain drugs such as atropine are all known to slow the beating of the cilia. Table 6-3 identifies factors that impair the function of the cilia.

TABLE 6-3 **Factors That Impair Ciliary Activity**

Endotracheal tubes
Extremes of temperature
High concentrations of oxygen
Dust, fumes, and smoke
Dehydration
Thick mucus
Infections

Either increased mucus production or impaired mucus clearance can result in a pulmonary system that is completely overwhelmed with thick, retained secretions that obstruct the airways. Although the mechanisms controlling mucus composition and production are not completely understood, the pharmacologic approach to secretion management generally falls into one of the following broad categories:

- Those that increase the depth of the sol layer (water or saline solution and expectorants)
- Those that alter the consistency of the gel layer (mucolytics)
- Those that improve ciliary activity (sympathomimetic bronchodilators and corticosteroids)

A variety of pharmacologic agents and bland aerosols alter the structure of mucus. Mechanical techniques such as deep breathing, assisted coughing, and suctioning can be applied to aid in the removal of secretions. Respiratory care practitioners are frequently called on to assist with mobilization of retained secretions by applying various combinations of humidity, bland and medicated aerosols, and mechanical techniques.

Of course the purpose of this chapter is to focus on the pharmacologic approaches for the control of mucus. This includes bland aerosols, which increase mucus clearance, mucus production, and productive coughing. Mucus-controlling drugs (mucolytics) achieve their effect by changing the molecular structure of the

BVT Lab

Flashcards are available for this chapter at www.BVTLab.com.

mucus gel so that the cilia can work more efficiently. The pharmacologic basis for the mucus-controlling agents that are currently available will be reviewed in this chapter. Because mucus is composed largely of water, the importance of maintaining adequate systemic hydration has been emphasized as a very important aspect of maintaining proper consistency and clearance of mucus. See Table 6-4 for factors that lead to dehydration and thereby thicken mucus.

TABLE 6-4 Factors That Lead to Dehydration and Thick Mucus

Increased respiratory rate
Increased depth of breathing
Systemic fluid loss
Infections

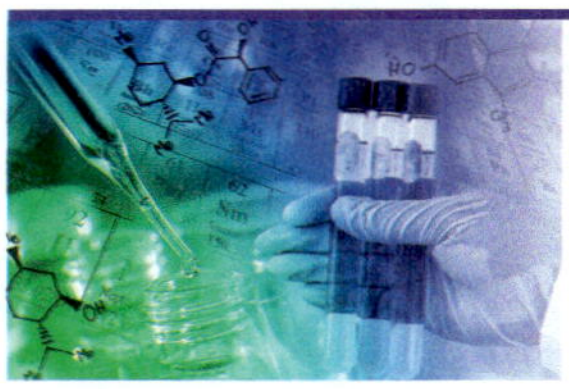

CONTROVERSY

The Importance of Proper Hydration

While proper hydration is stressed in mucus clearance, good empirical evidence doesn't fully exist that supports this belief. While an older study, one small study in 1987 found no difference in sputum volume, elasticity, respiratory symptoms, or ease of expectoration among stable COPD patients who were fully hydrated, were dehydrated, or had a normal fluid intake (Shim et al., 1987).

PATIENT & FAMILY EDUCATION

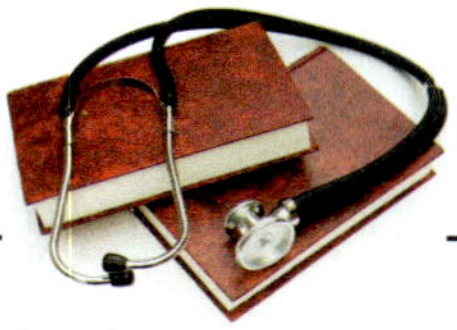

It is important to emphasize to both patients and their families that COPD is an irreversible, chronic lung disease that generally worsens with time. The most important strategy to decrease mucus production in smokers is to stop smoking. Currently there are no medications, including the ones discussed in this chapter, that are capable of reversing the damage done to the lungs.

6.2 BLAND AEROSOLS

6.2a Definitions

Bland aerosols do not affect the mucus molecule directly; instead they dilute the mucus by altering its water content. They are also referred to as wetting agents. Bland aerosols include the following agents:

- Water
- Normal saline
- Hypotonic saline
- Hypertonic saline

Historically, treatment of thick, retained secretions has been aimed at thinning thick mucus by adding water or saline to the respiratory tract by inhalation. Once it has formed, the gel layer of the mucus is somewhat resistant to the addition and removal of water. However it is critical to have an adequate amount of water available as mucus is being formed so that the mucus will have normal **viscoelastic** properties (the ability to change from thick to thin and back).

Bland aerosols may not be as effective as once thought at thinning thick mucus by topical hydration or mixing; instead, their benefit may be due to a different mechanism. All bland aerosols are somewhat irritating to the airway (although they are not all equally irritating) and may have varying benefits; in some cases they may produce harm, depending on the patient's underlying disease. Irritation tends to increase the production of thinner mucus, possibly by stimulating the goblet cells' and bronchial glands' production of mucus. Mucus clearance is increased by restoring the sol layer and stimulating cough, and this effect can be clinically useful.

6.2b Delivery Methods

Several methods are available for delivering water and saline to the lung. One method is the use of humidification devices, which work by bringing dry gas into contact with water, where the gas passes over or bubbles through the water. The water molecules evaporate and therefore increase the humidity of the gas. Another method of delivering water to the airway is the use of nebulizers. Nebulizers produce aerosols, which are small droplets of solution suspended in a gas. When the aerosol is inhaled, water particles are deposited in the airway. The final method is to instill the liquid directly into the respiratory tract. We will discuss each of these techniques briefly.

Humidifiers

Simple humidifiers are used mainly for oxygen delivery (see Figure 6-3). The amount of humidity that they add to the gas is highly variable and depends on how long the gas is in contact with the water, the surface area available between the gas and the water, and the temperature of the gas. The type of humidifier commonly used in conjunction with oxygen therapy is intended to minimize the drying effects of oxygen, not to serve as therapy for thick secretions. Heating inspired gas greatly increases the amount of water vapor that the gas can carry. Systems that deliver heated, humidified gas are most often used with mechanical ventilators. In-depth knowledge of how to deliver and monitor gas that is heated to body temperature and 100% relative humidity is an important aspect of ventilator management.

FIGURE 6-3 A Simple Humidifier

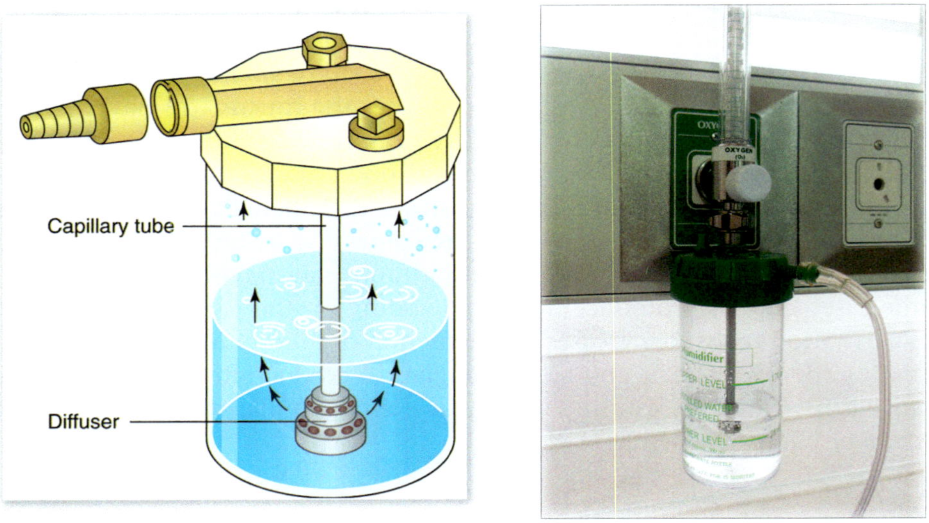

Source: Shutterstock

Aerosols

The most common method of administering water and saline solutions to the respiratory tract is by aerosol. Small-volume (handheld) nebulizers, large-volume nebulizers, and ultrasonic nebulizers have all been used. Small-volume nebulizers typically contain 3 to 5 ml of aerosol, of which only about 1 ml is actually deposited in the lung. For this reason small-volume nebulizers are used for medication delivery, as discussed in Chapter 4, and sputum induction, when stimulating the cough is the goal of the therapy.

Large-volume and ultrasonic nebulizers are capable of delivering significant volumes of aerosol to the lungs (see Figure 6-4). Although they are clinically very useful, ultrasonic nebulizers have been shown to cause runny, watery secretions in infants. Secretions of this consistency also impair the function of the mucociliary system. This condition has been, again, compared to trying to rake water.

Direct Instillation

Direct instillation of fluid (usually normal saline) into the respiratory tract is sometimes performed on patients with artificial airways, during bronchoscopy, and on rare occasions through a transtracheal catheter. Fluid injected into the upper airway is very irritating and causes a strong cough.

The once-common practice of *routinely* instilling saline into the airway during suctioning is now discouraged. It was once thought to improve mucus clearance by thinning thick secretions, but it is now understood that the saline does very little to thin thick secretions, and only about 20% of the instilled fluid is recovered during suctioning. Current evidence suggests that instilling saline down the endotracheal tube dislodges large numbers of bacteria from the inside of the patient's endotracheal tube into the lungs, which may increase the risk of pneumonia for the patient. The main benefit of saline instillation appears to be that it does stimulate a vigorous cough. This practice should be reserved for situations where patients do not cough adequately during suctioning. Saline is routinely instilled during bronchoscopy, when the patient's airway is anesthetized and coughing is minimal. More of the instilled solution can be recovered by suctioning through the bronchoscope.

Learning Hint

Have you ever experienced hard coughing or choking while you were drinking a fluid that accidentally entered your airway? That experience is similar to what patients experience when solutions are instilled into their airways.

FIGURE 6-4 A Nebulizer

A large-volume nebulizer, which can be connected via large bore tubing to a face mask, face tent, or tracheostomy mask to deliver aerosolized humidification

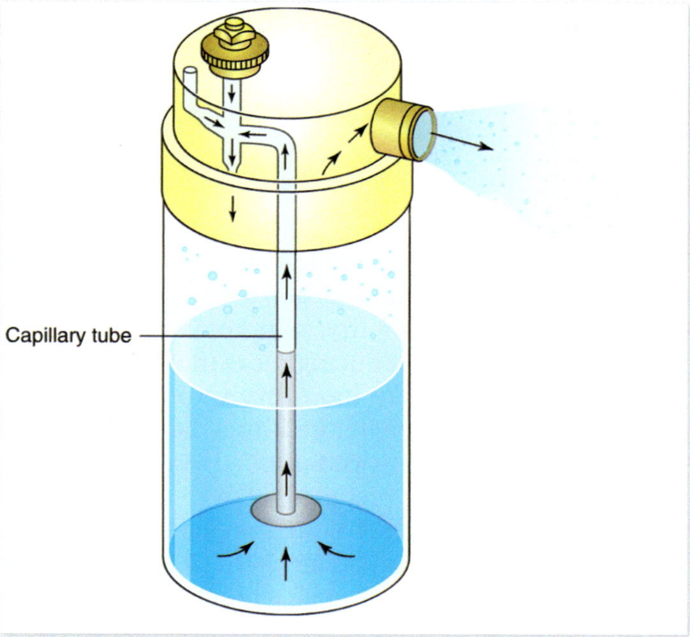

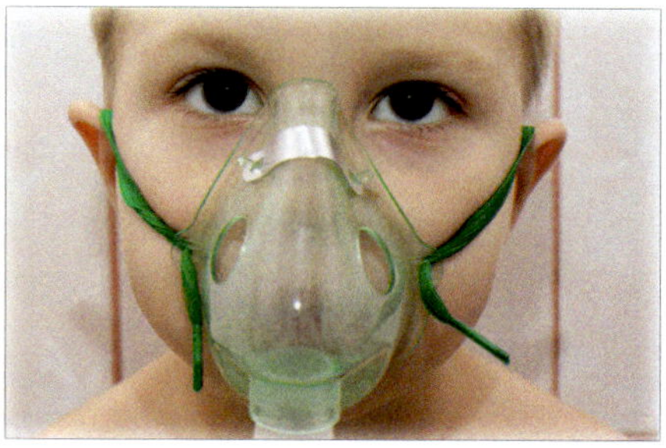

Source: (*Shutterstock*)

6.2c Bland Solutions

Sterile and Distilled Water

Sterile water is free of microorganisms, but it may also contain additives to make it bacteriostatic. Distilled water is both sterile and pure (it has no additives, and all other constituents, such as naturally occurring minerals, are removed). Although any solution intended for inhalation must be sterile, water does not need to be distilled. In fact distilled water tends to be a bit more irritating than sterile water. Sterile water is commonly used as the diluent for other aerosolized medications, in humidifiers, in large-volume nebulizers, and in croup tents.

A cool mist of sterile water may have a soothing (humectant) effect on inflamed upper airways, as in croup, but there is little evidence that a significant amount of water deposits in the lower airways. It is also theorized that, because sterile water is hypotonic, it is more readily absorbed by mucus, and it may thin mucus more effectively than saline—but again, there is little objective evidence that either water or saline mixes well with mucus.

Devices that produce very dense aerosols tend to be more irritating to the airways. Dense aerosols are more likely to cause cough and even bronchospasm in susceptible individuals (such as asthmatics). However, the irritation and cough make these aerosols useful for sputum induction. It is a good idea to monitor the breath sounds of patients receiving aerosol treatments for sputum induction, because wheezing may indicate bronchospasm.

BVT Lab

Visit www.BVTLab.com to explore the student resources available for this chapter.

Normal Saline

Normal saline (0.9% sodium chloride) is physiologically normal. Because it is **isotonic** with body fluids (meaning that it has the same tonicity as other body fluids), it is less irritating and not as likely to cause bronchospasm as water. However, the administration of either normal or hypertonic saline to patients with COPD can cause a significant decline in lung function and should not be routinely recommended. It is frequently used as a diluent for other aerosolized medications, such as bronchodilators.

Hypertonic Saline

Hypertonic saline is any solution that contains more than 0.9% sodium chloride (NaCl). The most commonly available solutions contain 5% and 10% NaCl. These solutions are very irritating and are used only for sputum induction, particularly when the patient has a dry, nonproductive cough. Remember, the airway responds to irritation by producing more mucus.

Hypertonic saline solutions are more likely to cause bronchospasm than any of the other bland aerosols. Therefore it may be necessary to pretreat some patients with a bronchodilator. It is certainly advisable to monitor the patient throughout the treatment and be prepared to stop the treatment or administer a bronchodilator if necessary. As mentioned previously, hypertonic saline may cause a decrease in lung function in patients with COPD; however, it is beneficial in patients with cystic fibrosis because it aids in improving mucus clearance and subsequently lung function.

Hypotonic Saline

Saline is also available in a solution of 0.45%, or half-normal saline. Commercially available solutions for ultrasonic nebulizers are usually 0.45% strength. **Hypotonic** saline is less irritating than either sterile water or hypertonic saline. In addition to ultrasonic nebulizers, it can be used in any large-volume nebulizer or as the diluent for nebulized medications. Table 6-5 lists the common concentrations of saline.

TABLE 6-5 Common Concentrations of Saline

Percentage Solution	Solution Type
0.45%	Half-normal
0.9%	Normal
5%	Hypertonic
10%	Hypertonic

time for review

Why might hypertonic saline be better than sterile water or normal saline for sputum induction for a patient who has a dry, nonproductive cough?

6.3 MUCOLYTICS

6.3a Definition

When there is infection and/or dehydration of the pulmonary system, the gel layer of the mucus becomes thickened. Waste products of inflammation such as white blood cells (leukocytes), DNA, and other cellular debris add to the thickening of the mucus. Thick mucus cannot be mobilized by the action of the cilia, and when the cilia cannot keep the gel and sol layers in motion, the layers combine and a vicious cycle of thickening mucus ensues. In this situation humidity, mucolytic agents, and expectorants, or combinations of these agents, may be needed.

Mucolytics are drugs that control mucus by their direct action of altering the structure of the mucus molecule. In essence they facilitate expectoration of mucus by liquefying it. Mucolytics break down the complex molecular strands to thin the thick mucus. Two mucolytic agents are currently approved by the FDA for administration by aerosol to treat abnormal pulmonary secretions. They are acetylcysteine (Mucomyst®) and dornase alfa (Pulmozyme®). Investigation continues in this area, and new agents may be forthcoming.

Clinical pearl

Pioneer folk medicine recommended dissolving baking soda (sodium bicarbonate) in boiling water and breathing in the vapors to treat colds. Sodium bicarbonate is a weak base, and mucus becomes less adhesive in an alkaline environment. Increasing the pH of the mucus weakens the bonds of the polysaccharide chains. Alkalinization also activates proteases that are found in purulent sputum to help digest the excess protein molecules. There is also evidence that it potentiates the effects of acetylcysteine. However it has not been proven to improve mucus clearance, so its use cannot be recommended.

Acetylcysteine (Mucomyst®, Mucosol®)

Acetylcysteine is used to treat thick, viscous secretions, such as may be seen in cystic fibrosis, chronic bronchitis, tuberculosis, and acute tracheobronchitis. It acts by disrupting the disulfide bonds in the mucus. The long mucopolysaccharide strands are cross-connected with numerous bridges, including disulfide bonds. The long strands become a matted network of complex molecules. Breaking the disulfide bonds releases the mucopolysaccharide strands. The structure of the gel layer is broken down, and the viscosity and elasticity of the mucus is therefore reduced (see Figure 6-5). Since nebulized acetylcysteine can cause acute bronchospasm, it should be given after treatment with an inhaled beta-agonist, if it is used at all. Good bronchial hygiene therapies such as chest percussion, postural drainage, cough training, and positive expiratory pressure (PEP) therapy should be considered the first-line treatment. Oscillatory therapy combined with PEP therapy increases airway vibrations and facilitates secretion mobilization.

Dose and Administration Acetylcysteine can be given by aerosol or by direct instillation to the tracheobronchial tree. It is supplied in 10% and 20% solution strengths, and the dosages are as follows:

20% solution: 3 to 5 ml t.i.d. or q.i.d.
10% solution: 6 to 10 ml t.i.d. or q.i.d.

For instillation, 1 to 2 ml of either strength can be used.

FIGURE 6-5 Mucolytic Effects of Acetylcysteine (Mucomyst®)

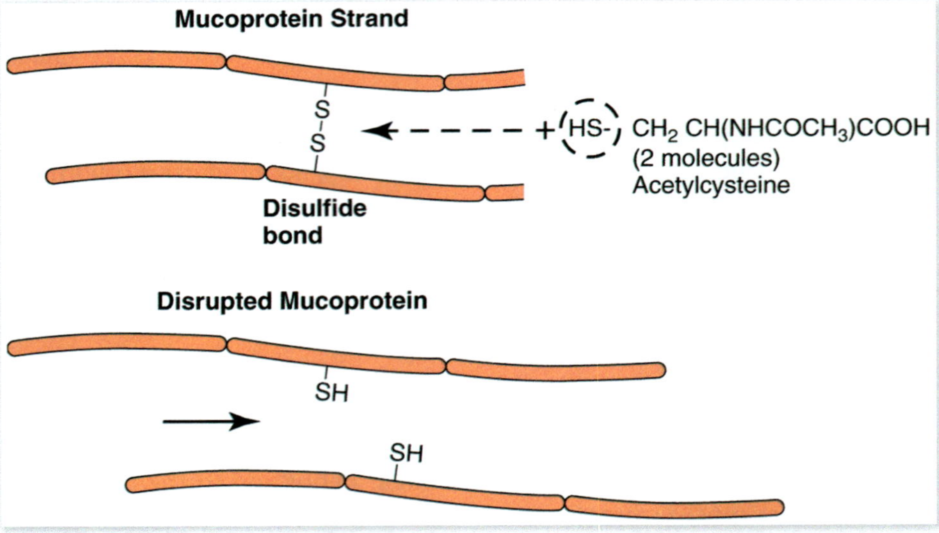

Clinical pearl

When the 10% solution is used, the volume of the dose is 6 to 10 ml, which exceeds the optimal fill volume of most small-volume nebulizers. The dose will have to be divided, and the treatment time will therefore be very long.

Adverse Reactions Acetylcysteine is often poorly tolerated by patients because of its sulfurous odor and because its low pH (2.2) may cause bronchospasm, which may occur when the drug is administered by nebulization. Acetylcysteine is most likely to cause bronchospasm in patients with reactive airway disease, but bronchospasm can also occur in patients without any primary pulmonary disease. The 10% strength of acetylcysteine is less likely to cause bronchospasm than the 20% solution.

When acetylcysteine is to be nebulized, most clinicians opt to use the 20% solution in combination with a short-acting bronchodilator administered beforehand to prevent bronchospasm. It is better to administer the bronchodilator before the acetylcysteine, because even albuterol takes 15 minutes to onset of action and reaches its peak effect in 30 to 60 minutes.

Other complications of acetylcysteine include nausea, **rhinorrhea**, **bronchorrhea**, and **stomatitis**. *Rhinorrhea* and *stomatitis* are secondary consequences of irritation of mucous membranes. Excessive thin and watery secretions result. *Bronchorrhea* is the term used to describe excess thin, watery secretions in the airways. Rhinorrhea is what you would commonly call a runny nose.

Once a larger mucus molecule is broken down, it must be cleared, or mucus plugging can result. Deep breathing and coughing are essential to clear the mucus from the airways. Mucus plugging can occur in patients with ineffective cough or artificial airways. It is advisable to monitor patients carefully for changes in breath sounds or signs of respiratory distress. Suction equipment should be available for patients who cannot cough effectively.

Although it is flavorless, some patients object to the disagreeable odor caused by the release of hydrogen sulfide. Nausea and vomiting have been attributed to the smell. Acetylcysteine is corrosive to metal and irritating to mucous membranes, so patients should rinse their mouths and nebulizers (if they have metal parts) after treatments.

Other Uses Acetylcysteine is a potent antioxidant that is also used as an antidote in acetaminophen (Tylenol®) overdose. In this situation, acetylcysteine (Acetadote® is the brand name for the IV form) may be given orally or intravenously. If given orally, it may be mixed in cola or some other soft drink or, orange juice, or given by nasogastric tube. The package insert is a good reference for complete information on dosing, but we recommend calling a poison control center.

Clinical pearl

The hydrogen sulfide smell of acetylcysteine has been compared to that of rotten eggs, but it is actually flavorless. If the patient is to drink it, mixing it with cola makes it more palatable and reduces the risk of the patient vomiting.

Dornase Alfa (Pulmozyme®)

Dornase alfa is a clone of the natural human enzyme that digests extracellular DNA. Dornase alfa is a solution of recombinant human deoxyribonuclease (DNase). It received FDA approval in 1994.

Pulmonary secretions in cystic fibrosis are extremely thick and sticky because of abnormal chloride exchange mechanisms, which increase sodium and water absorption from the airway. This thickens airway mucus, impairs mucus clearance, and leads to infection. Because of their chronic pulmonary infections, cystic fibrosis patients have large numbers of neutrophils that congregate in the airways. As the neutrophils break down, a lot of their DNA is also left in the airways. This results in further thickening of the mucus.

Dornase alfa is indicated as **maintenance therapy** in the management of the viscous pulmonary secretions seen in cystic fibrosis. It is a proteolytic enzyme that breaks down the DNA material, decreasing the viscosity of the mucus and restoring its ability to flow. The change in sputum viscosity is dose-dependent—with higher doses producing thinner mucus.

Dose and Administration Dornase alfa is available in single-dose ampules containing 2.5 mg of drug in 2.5 ml of solution, administered once a day. Further analysis has suggested that patients older than 21 years of age with a forced vital capacity (FVC) greater than 85% of predicted may benefit from twice-a-day treatment. Dornase alfa should not be diluted or mixed with other medications. The solution should be refrigerated and protected from light. Medication that has been at room temperature for more than 24 hours or appears discolored should be discarded. The manufacturer recommends that dornase alfa should be nebulized only with the Hudson "T" Up-Draft II® disposable nebulizer, Marquest Acorn II® and Pulmo-Aide® compressor, PARI LC (reusable) Jet Plus® with PARI PRONEB® compressor, or the SideStream® Durable jet nebulizer with the MOBILAIRE™ or Porta-neb compressor, because these are the only ones that it has been tested with.

Clinical pearl

Under normal circumstances, the amount of sodium that the patient absorbs from the saline used as diluent for breathing treatments is so insignificant that it is not even considered. However in some patients, such as infants and adults who are on sodium-restricted diets, reducing sodium intake may be very critical. If breathing treatments are being given very frequently, it may be advisable to consider using sterile water as the diluent in order to avoid increasing the patient's sodium intake.

Adverse Effects Dornase alfa has been shown to be safe and well tolerated. Side effects are minimal but include voice alteration, pharyngitis, laryngitis, rash, chest pain, and conjunctivitis. It is contraindicated in patients with hypersensitivity to dornase alfa or to Chinese hamster ovary cell products (from which it is derived).

6.3b Expectorants

Expectorants increase the production and expectoration of mucus by increasing the amount of fluid in the respiratory tract and stimulating cough. They are one of the main ingredients in many OTC cough and cold medications. Expectorants are thought to work either by increasing vagal gastric reflex stimulation (parasympathomimetic) or by absorption into the respiratory glands to stimulate mucus production directly. Hypertonic saline, which was discussed earlier in this chapter, is also considered to be an expectorant. Guaifenesin is one of the most commonly used expectorants. Other examples include terpin hydrate, ammonium chloride, and potassium iodide (see Table 6-6).

TABLE 6-6 Mucolytics and Expectorants

Drug	Trade Name	Adult Dosage
acetylcysteine	Mucomyst®	1–10 ml of 10%, or 2–20 ml of 20%, nebulized 3–4 times daily
dornase alfa	Pulmozyme®	2.5 mg daily via jet nebulizer
guaifenesin	Robitussin®	200–400 mg PO every 4 hours
potassium iodide	SSKI®	300–600 mg (0.3–0.6 ml), diluted in 240 ml fluid, PO 3–4 times daily

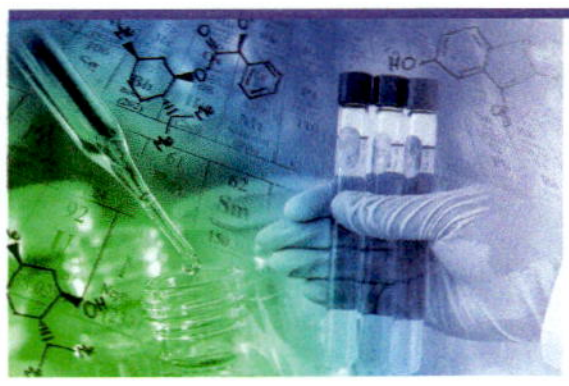

CONTROVERSY

There is some controversy about the effectiveness and use of expectorants. One problem is the difficulty of obtaining objective data to assess their effectiveness. The simplest and most frequently recommended method for preserving mucus clearance is still to drink plenty of water and other liquids that do not cause diuresis. Tea and alcohol should be avoided because of their diuretic effects. While maintaining hydration is frequently recommended, as previously discussed, there is little objective evidence that this strategy works to improve clinically important outcomes in diseases such as COPD.

6.3c Antitussives/Cough Suppressants

Stimulation of vagal sensory endings in the larynx, bronchi, or even the stomach can cause a cough. The cough that results from irritation of these nerve endings may not be contributing to clearance of the airways, as it may be dry and nonproductive. More coughing leads to more irritation of the nerve endings, and so on. It may be necessary to suppress this type of dry, hacking, nonproductive cough. Cough suppressants depress the cough center, which is thought to be located in the medulla. There are both narcotic and nonnarcotic preparations to choose from. Codeine is one of the common narcotic cough suppressants, and dextromethorphan is a nonnarcotic cough suppressant.

Cough suppressants should never be given to patients with thick retained secretions. They need to cough to clear them. You can also find combinations of drugs in OTC cold preparations, such as an antitussive and an expectorant. The rationale is that a frequent, dry, hacking cough is better replaced by a less frequent but more productive cough. However, the practice of combining an expectorant to stimulate mucus production with an antihistamine to dry secretions in OTC medications is questionable. The American College of Chest Physicians (ACCP) published evidenced-based clinical practice guidelines on cough suppressant therapy and concluded that antitussives can be useful in patients with chronic bronchitis but have little efficacy for cough due to upper-airway infection. Suppressant therapy is most effective when used for short-term decrease in coughing.

6.3d Conclusion

The mucociliary system preserves and protects the lungs from disease and dehydration. The normal structure and function of the mucociliary system should be maintained. When possible, avoid factors that contribute to excess mucus production, such as smoking, pollution, and allergens. When the integrity of the mucociliary system is compromised, therapy should be geared toward increasing mucus clearance and maintaining adequate hydration. This may be achieved through a variety of mechanisms, including:

- Administration of bronchodilators
- Adequate systemic hydration
- Deep breathing and coughing
- Postural drainage
- Mucolytics
- Expectorants

6.4 SURFACE-ACTIVE AGENTS

6.4a Alveolar Physiology and Surfactant Synthesis

Throughout Chapter 5 and so far in Chapter 6, we have been discussing the anatomy and physiology of the conducting airways. We have also explored many of the pharmacologic agents that act on the airways themselves and the mucus they contain. Now we turn our attention to the area of the lungs beyond the terminal bronchioles, where gas exchange takes place. This is known as the *respiratory zone* of the lungs, and it includes the respiratory bronchioles, alveolar ducts, alveoli, and pulmonary capillaries (see Figure 6-6).

FIGURE 6-6 The Respiratory Zones of the Lung

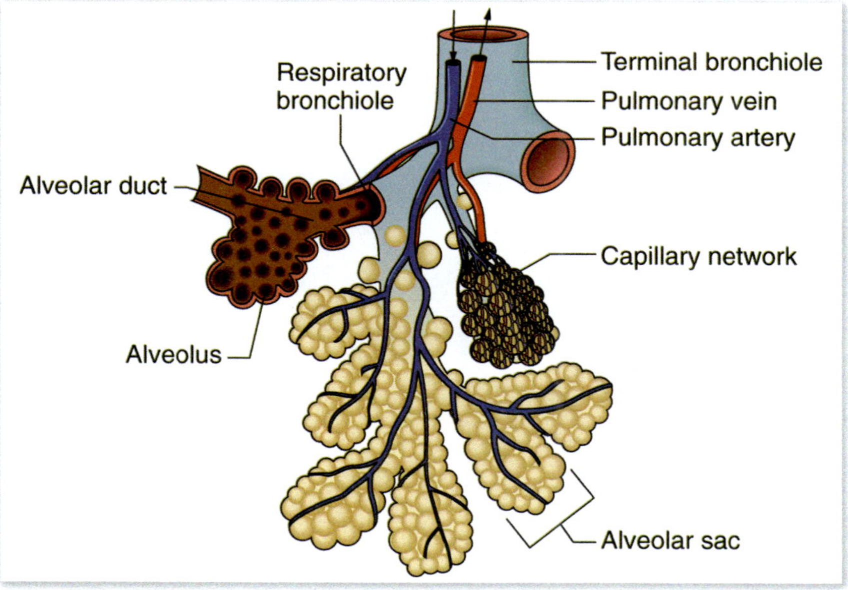

The walls of the respiratory bronchioles are made up of very thin, flattened squamous cells and a thin layer of connective tissue. They lack the smooth muscle and mucus-producing cells of the conducting airways. Alveolar ducts branch from the respiratory bronchioles, and the walls of the alveolar ducts are made up entirely of alveoli. Each alveolar duct ends in a cluster of alveoli, which together are called an alveolar sac. Each alveolar sac opens into about 10 to 16 alveoli.

The alveoli are made up of type I and type II pneumocytes. The type I pneumocytes are large, very thin, flat cells with tight junctions between them. Type I pneumocytes make up about 93% of the total alveolar surface area. They are ideally suited to allow for the diffusion of gases.

Type II pneumocytes are small, cuboidal cells found mainly in the corners between type I pneumocytes (see Figure 6-7). The type II pneumocytes manufacture a complex substance called **surfactant**. Surfactant consists of 80% phospholipids, 10% neutral lipids (cholesterol), and 10% surface proteins (SPs). The phospholipids are phosphatidylcholine, phosphatidylglycerol, phosphatidylinositol, and phosphatidylethanolamine. The surface proteins are SP-A, SP-B, SP-C, and SP-D. The theorized role of each of these proteins is listed in Table 6-7. Surface proteins B and C (SP-B and SP-C) appear to be critical to maintaining normal surfactant function, whereas SP-A and SP-D are not (see Table 6-7).

FIGURE 6-7 Structure of an Alveolus

Alveolar structure and cell types: Type I: squamous pneumocyte for diffusion; Type II: granular pneumocyte for surfactant production and cellular repair; Type III: alveolar macrophage for immune function

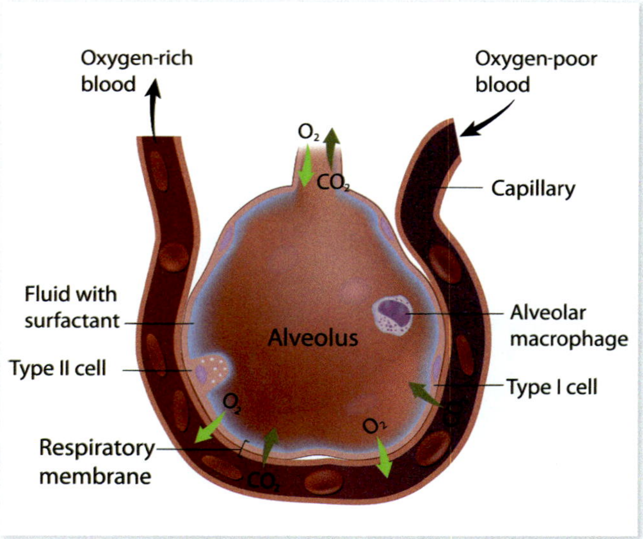

Source: Shutterstock

TABLE 6-7 Surfactant Proteins

Protein	Function
SP-A	Has host-defense properties; activates macrophage function; facilitates phagocytosis of pathogens
SP-B	Critical to surface tension–lowering property of surfactant
SP-C	Facilitates surfactant spreadability
SP-D	Functions as host-defense mechanism by binding to pathogens

Learning Hint

Try blowing up several balloons of different sizes. Note that some balloons require much more effort to blow up than others. This is because they have a higher surface tension. The balloon that is easiest to blow up has the lowest surface tension.

6.4b Surfactant Function

Surfactant is critical to maintaining the condition of the alveolar surface so that gas exchange can occur. Clinically, surfactant performs the following three functions:

- Prevents alveolar collapse
- Enables the lung to expand easily
- Prevents leakage of fluid from the alveolar capillary membranes

To understand the importance of surfactant, we must first understand surface tension. The surface of a liquid acts as if there were an elastic skin constantly pulling in, attempting to contract the liquid into the smallest surface area. This force is called **surface tension**. It is created by uneven forces of attraction on the molecules at the surface of the liquid. The molecules under the surface have equal forces of attraction all around them. The molecules at the surface are in contact with air (this is called the *gas–liquid interface*); there is no attraction between the surface molecules and air, so the surface molecules are pulled inward and down, creating the force called surface tension (see Figure 6-8). It is this surface tension that makes liquid contract into a small sphere, such as the water drops that "bead" on a freshly waxed car. Without surface tension, the water drop would spread out into a large puddle.

FIGURE 6-8 Surface Tension

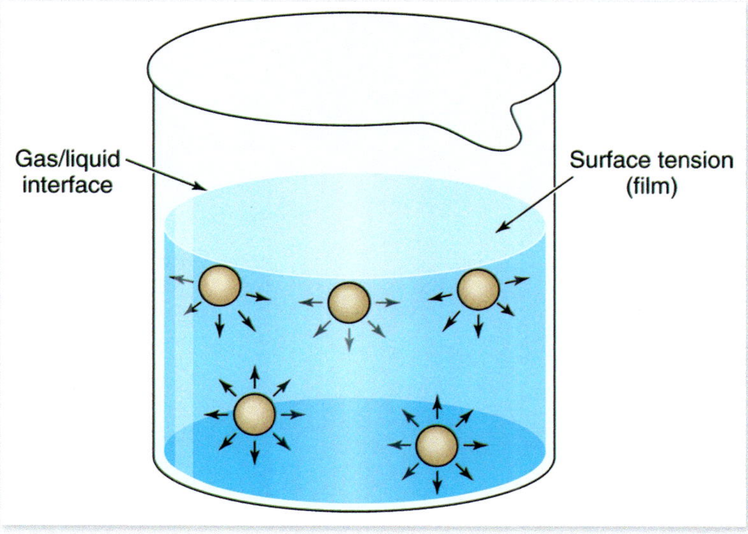

The surface of alveoli also has a layer of fluid, comprised largely of water. The greater the surface tension of the fluid, the smaller the sphere becomes; in turn, the smaller the sphere becomes, the greater the surface tension gets. By the law of LaPlace, the alveoli will eventually decrease to their critical volume. Below this volume, the force of the surface tension will cause the alveoli to collapse, resulting in atelectasis. Once alveoli collapse, the pressure required to reopen them is much greater than the pressure required to inflate an alveolus that is just above its critical volume. This pressure is called the critical pressure.

Surfactant is secreted by the type II pneumocytes and stored in vesicles called lamellar bodies. The lamellar bodies unravel in the alveoli, and the surfactant forms a thin film called a monolayer on the inner surface of the alveoli. The air–liquid interface is replaced with an air–lipid interface, which has a much lower surface tension. In this way the alveoli are stabilized above their critical volumes and do not collapse. Lower surface tension allows the alveoli to expand into a larger sphere, which provides a larger surface area for greater gas diffusion. The lower surface tension also makes it easier to inflate the alveoli, which results in a lower work of breathing.

time for review

How can the law of LaPlace be used to explain why a balloon can be very difficult to blow air into initially, but once started, blowing becomes easier?

The action of surfactant and its effect on surface tension is a very dynamic process. Surface tension varies with alveolar volume. On inspiration, the alveolar volume increases, spreading the surfactant molecules farther apart, and surface tension increases. This helps to prevent alveolar overdistension. On exhalation, the surfactant molecules are tightly packed, decreasing surface tension and preventing collapse (see Figure 6-9).

FIGURE 6-9 The Effects of Surfactant on Alveolar Surface Tension

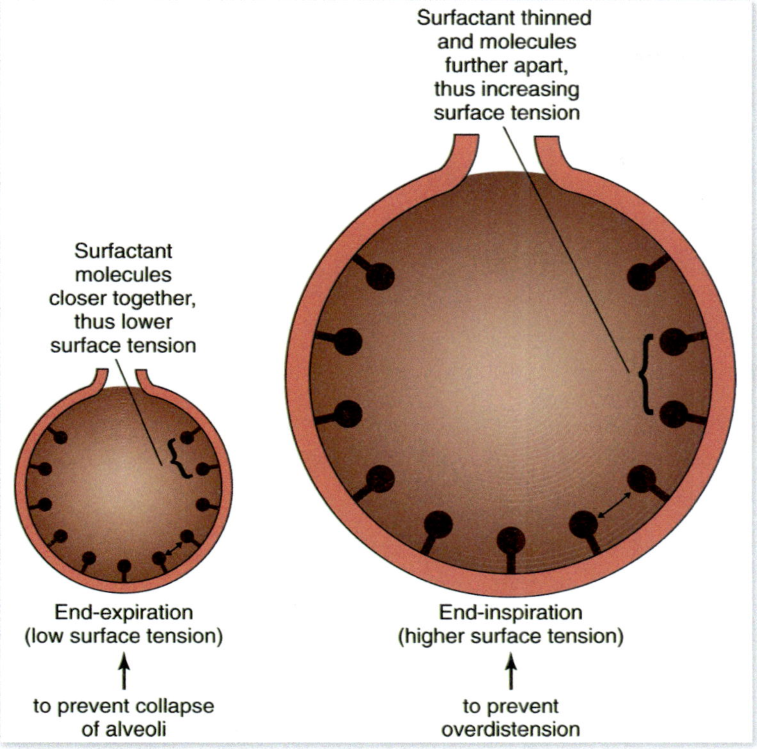

Surfactant has a relatively short half-life and must be continuously replaced at the alveolar surface. During exhalation, old surfactant is squeezed out of the monolayer, and new surfactant is added on inspiration. Under normal circumstances most of the surfactant (90%–95%) is taken back up and recycled by the type II pneumocytes.

Because inflation and deflation are important in maintaining a healthy monolayer and low surface tension in the alveoli, you can see that lung collapse or atelectasis disrupts surfactant production. Hypoxia can also damage the type II pneumocytes and interrupt surfactant production, and repeated collapse and reopening of alveoli cause a lot of lung damage, inflammation, and leaking of protein-rich fluid into the alveoli. This also disrupts surfactant function.

time for review

Infants born prematurely may not have mature type II pneumocytes. What complications might ensue?

6.4c Indications for Surfactant Replacement Therapy

The major indication for surfactant replacement therapy is to prevent or treat respiratory distress syndrome (RDS) in infants. RDS is a disease associated mainly with prematurity (less than 34 weeks' gestation) and low birth weight. The type II pneumocytes in these infants are not mature enough to produce surfactant. An inadequate amount of surfactant leads to alveolar collapse, hypoxemia, and increased work of breathing for the infant.

Surfactants have been used anecdotally and successfully to treat several other conditions, including:

- Meconium aspiration syndrome
- Full-term infants with RDS
- Pulmonary hemorrhage
- Congenital diaphragmatic hernia
- Severe pneumonia
- Any condition in which there is loss of surfactant and low lung volume

In these cases, the type II pneumocytes may have been damaged by perinatal asphyxia, or the surfactant may be deactivated by aspiration.

6.4d Types of Exogenous Surfactants

The surfactant that is produced naturally in lung tissue is called **endogenous surfactant**. **Exogenous surfactants** are produced outside the body and administered as a therapy. Two types of exogenous surfactants are currently available: natural/modified and synthetic. Synthetic surfactants are mixtures of synthetic components that are produced in the laboratory. This means that the drug is free of infection and foreign proteins, which is an advantage, but it may not perform as well as natural surfactant because of the organic chemicals that are substituted for the natural proteins.

Natural surfactant is obtained from animals by alveolar wash. The surfactant is then extracted from the liquid by centrifugation or simple filtration. The surfactant is modified by adding and removing certain components to improve its function in the lung, reduce protein contamination, and ensure sterility. This preparation consumes a lot of time, which adds to the cost of the drug. There is also a concern over the possibility of viral infection and immunologic reaction to foreign proteins. However, the advantage of natural surfactants is that they contain the phospholipids and proteins (SP-B and SP-C) necessary for absorption and spreading of the phospholipids.

Both natural and synthetic surfactants have been shown to be effective, but natural surfactants act more quickly and are associated with lower mortality, less barotrauma, and lower oxygen requirements. There were no significant differences in head-to-head trials of various natural surfactants.

6.4e Therapeutic Approaches

There are two therapeutic approaches to surfactant administration. In very premature infants (less than 30 weeks' gestation) there is a high probability that RDS will occur, so surfactant is given as soon as possible (usually within minutes) after birth. This is referred to as prophylactic treatment. Theoretically this strategy may prevent lung injury, but it is also associated with unnecessary treatment of some babies. Clinical trials suggest that prophylactic treatment compared to rescue treatment decreases morbidity and death in infants who are less than 30 weeks gestational age when they are delivered.

Rescue treatment is indicated for infants who demonstrate serious signs and symptoms of RDS. The advantage of rescue treatment is that only babies that really need it receive treatment, and there is more time to ensure good tube placement prior to administration of the surfactant. The down side of this approach is that it may allow for the progression of lung injury.

6.4f Representative Drugs

Calfactant (Infasurf®)

Calfactant is a natural surfactant.

Dose and Administration Calfactant is supplied as a refrigerated suspension that does not have to be warmed to room temperature before use. The dose is 3 ml/kg of body weight administered intratracheally every 12 hours. Three doses is the maximum.

Beractant (Survanta®)

Beractant is a natural/modified surfactant comprised of natural bovine (cow) lung extract modified with three other additives.

Dose and Administration The dose is 4 ml/kg of birth weight administered by direct tracheal instillation. The dose can be repeated in 6 hours for up to 4 doses if required on the basis of clinical judgment.

Poractant Alfa (Curosurf®)

Poractant alfa is a natural porcine surfactant that must be kept refrigerated prior to use.

Dose and Administration The initial dose is 2.5 ml/kg birth weight. This may be followed by up to two additional doses of 1.25 ml/kg birth weight at 12-hour intervals.

Lucinactant (Surfaxin®)

Lucinactant is a synthetic surfactant that also requires refrigeration prior to use. As discussed above, natural surfactants are favored over synthetic surfactants such as lucinactant due to improved clinical outcomes with natural surfactants.

Dose and Administration 5.8 ml/kg birth weight should be administered through the endotracheal tube up to a total of four doses within the first 48 hours of life.

6.4g General Techniques of Surfactant Administration

All forms of surfactant are administered intratracheally. This requires placement of an endotracheal tube. The tube must be positioned properly above the carina to ensure even distribution to both lungs. The baby should be suctioned before administration of surfactant to remove any secretions that would interfere with medication delivery. Specific brands may call for modifications to the general guidelines for surfactant administration.

The surfactant should be allowed to come to room temperature. The calculated dose is drawn into a syringe. The intubated baby is placed on his or her side. The dose is divided into four **aliquots**, or equally divided portions; two aliquots are administered with the baby turned to the right side and two aliquots are administered with the baby turned to the left side. This procedure is intended to distribute the surfactant as widely as possible throughout the lung. However there is no real evidence to support this practice. There are three methods for instilling surfactant into the endotracheal tube:

Sideport Adapter

The solution is instilled down the baby's endotracheal tube through the sideport of a special adapter on the endotracheal tube. This technique allows the medication to be instilled while the infant is attached to the ventilator. However reflux of the solution may occur (see Figure 6-10a).

Catheter

The baby is briefly disconnected from the ventilator while a 5-French catheter is placed directly in the endotracheal tube to instill the surfactant. The catheter is withdrawn and the infant is returned to the ventilator after each instillation.

Double-Lumen Endotracheal Tube

This endotracheal tube has a catheter embedded into the wall of the tube to provide distal instillation like a catheter, while the baby remains attached to the ventilator as with the sideport adapter (see Figure 6-10b).

6.4h Adverse Reactions

Babies must be monitored closely following surfactant administration because there may be rapid improvements in lung compliance. As the lung compliance increases, tidal volumes may increase significantly. Ventilator pressure will need to be decreased to prevent alveolar damage or rupture. Oxygen levels in the baby's blood may also increase rapidly, so the oxygen concentration will also need to be decreased. Monitoring may include breath sounds, chest radiographs, chest movement or tidal volume changes, arterial blood gases, and oxygen saturation measurements. The hazards can be divided into those that occur during administration and those that occur after administration.

Clinical pearl

The transient decrease in oxygen is due to the initial diffusion barrier of the drug. This is very transient and should not be significant, especially with proper preoxygenation. The bradycardia and/or hypotension may be secondary to hypoxemia or may be a result of vagal stimulation.

During Administration:

- Reflux of solution
- Transient decrease in oxygenation
- Bradycardia and/or hypotension

After Administration:

- Hyperoxygenation
- Hyperventilation (decrease in $PaCO_2$)
- Patent ductus arteriosis (PDA)

FIGURE 6-10 Surfactant Administration Techniques: (a) Sideport Adapter; (b) Double-Lumen Endotracheal Tube

Note: The baby is pictured on his/her back, but should be turned side-to-side during administration.

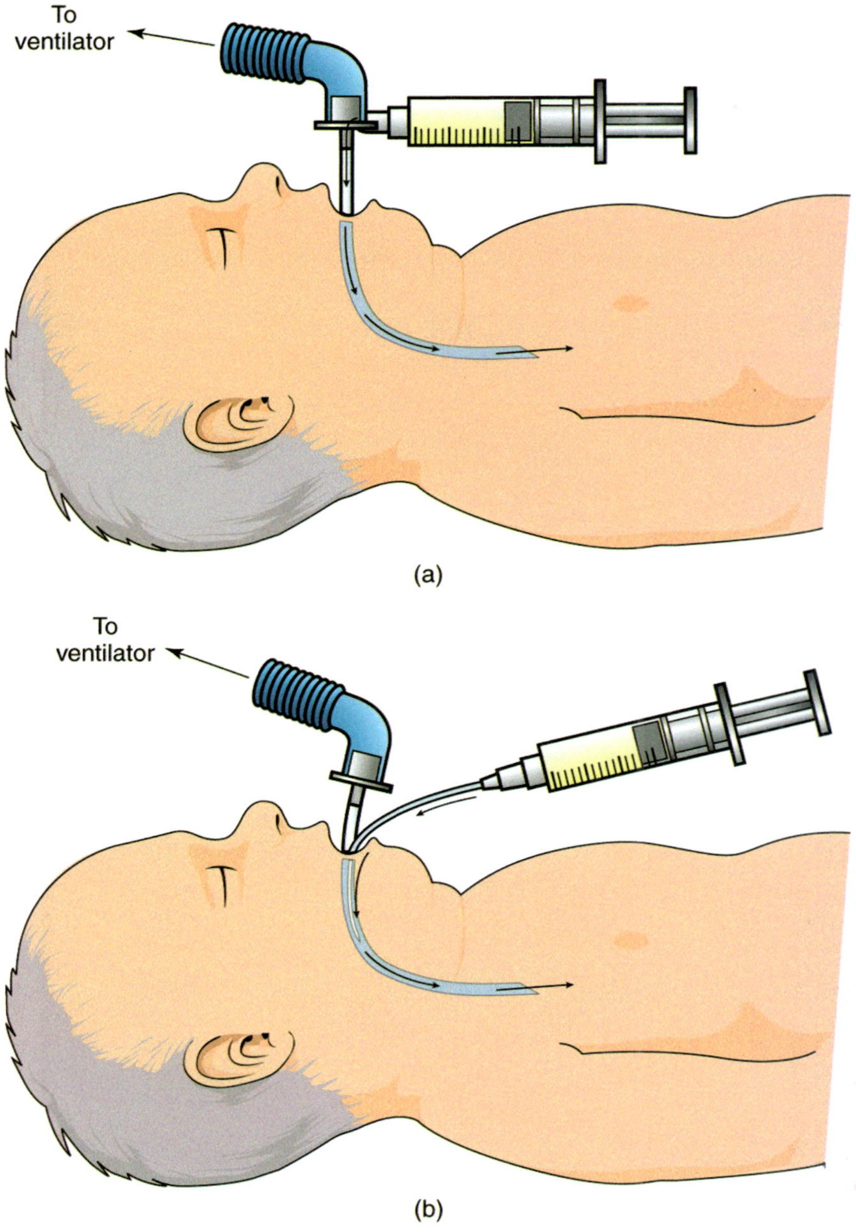

Uncommon Side Effects:

- Apnea
- Pulmonary hemorrhage

6.4i Surfactant Administration in Adult Patients

So far surfactant has not been proven to be successful in treatment of adults and children with acute RDS (ARDS). Only a few studies of adults with ARDS have been done, and the results have been conflicting. There are differences in the pathophysiology of ARDS. In RDS of the newborn, the problem is a primary surfactant production deficiency, whereas in ARDS, the surfactant deficiency is secondary to lung injury and inflammatory response. This may account for the different responses to surfactant replacement therapy. Beractant, poractant alfa, and calfactant are available in the United States, and several other surfactants are available throughout the world. See Table 6-8 for the commercially available surfactants.

TABLE 6-8 Commercially Available Surfactants in the United States

Generic Name	Trade Name	Type	Dose
beractant	Survanta®	Natural/modified	4 ml/kg
calfactant	Infasurf®	Natural/modified	3 ml/kg
poractant alfa	Curosurf®	Natural/modified	2.5 ml/kg
lucinactant	Surfaxin®	Synthetic	5.8 ml/kg

LIFE SPAN CONSIDERATIONS

Respiratory distress syndrome (RDS) in children is nearly always found in infants born prematurely. Acute respiratory distress syndrome (ARDS) can be found in both children and adults and is generally due to a severe illness that affects the lungs by damaging the alveoli. Unfortunately the similarity of these terms can cause confusion for health-care professionals *but* not for readers of this text.

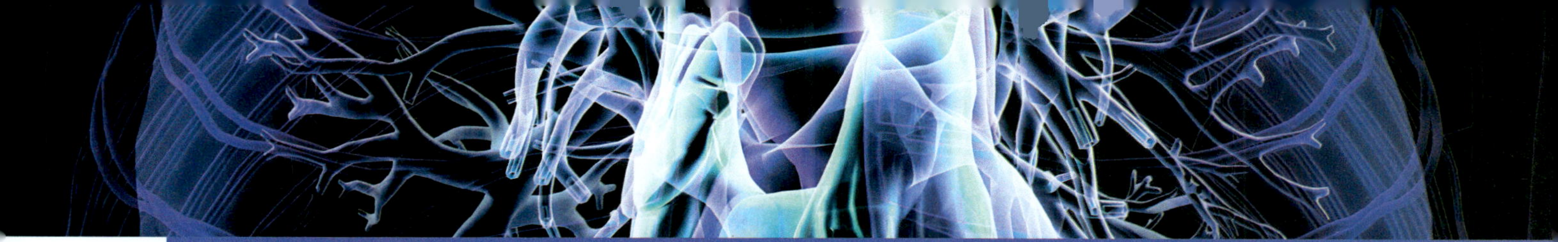

Summary

Proper function of the mucociliary system is critical to maintain proper pulmonary hygiene. Bland aerosols can deliver high levels of humidity to assist proper function. In addition mucolytic drugs can be administered to thin mucus to facilitate expectoration of thickened secretions that occur in many pulmonary disease conditions. Expectorants and antitussive agents can also assist in helping to treat pulmonary irritation and secretion problems.

Proper functioning of surfactant at the alveolar level is needed to maintain proper surface tension to prevent both collapse and overdistension of the alveoli. Exogenous surfactant replacement therapy can prevent or treat premature or low-birth-weight infants with respiratory distress syndrome (RDS).

REVIEW QUESTIONS

1. What layer(s) make up the mucosal blanket that covers the airways?
   (a) sol
   (b) gel
   (c) (a) and (b)
   (d) none of the above

2. Bland aerosols are aerosols that
   (a) have no taste
   (b) are boring
   (c) are colored
   (d) are nonmedicated

3. A patient with a dry, nonproductive cough who requires a sputum induction for tuberculosis testing may benefit most from what solution?
   (a) hypertonic
   (b) hypotonic
   (c) sterile water
   (d) isotonic

4. The drug dornase alfa (Pulmozyme®)
   I. is indicated for maintenance therapy for secretions in cystic fibrosis patients
   II. ruptures disulfide bonds in sputum
   III. should not be mixed with other medications
   IV. should be refrigerated and protected from light

   (a) I, II, and III
   (b) I, III, and IV
   (c) I and IV
   (d) IV only

5. During surfactant replacement administration, the patient should be monitored for what hazards or conditions?
   I. improved lung compliance
   II. transient decrease in oxygenation
   III. reflux of solution
   IV. bradycardia

   (a) I, II, III, and IV
   (b) I and II
   (c) I and III
   (d) II, III, and IV

6. State four functions of mucus in maintaining a healthy pulmonary system.

7. What is the typical dose range for acetylcysteine, and how can it be delivered?

8. Which of the following would be best to prevent bronchospasm in a patient who is ordered nebulized acetylcysteine?
   (a) Administer 2 puffs of salmeterol before the acetylcysteine.
   (b) Add 2.5 mg of albuterol to the acetylcysteine.
   (c) Administer 2.5 mg of albuterol after the acetylcysteine.
   (d) Pretreat the patient with 2.5 mg of albuterol by nebulizer 20 minutes prior to the acetylcysteine.

9. You are preparing to administer beractant to an 800-g male with RDS. Which of the following is the appropriate dose?
   (a) 4 ml
   (b) 3.2 ml
   (c) 5 ml
   (d) 2 ml

10. Critical functions of surfactant in the lung are that it
    I. improves oxygenation
    II. prevents alveolar collapse (atelectasis)
    III. reduces the risk of intrapulmonary hemorrhage
    IV. decreases the work of breathing

    (a) I only
    (b) I and II
    (c) I, II, and IV
    (d) I, II, III, and IV

11. What is the primary indication for surfactant replacement therapy?
    (a) pneumonia
    (b) meconium aspiration
    (c) respiratory distress syndrome (RDS)
    (d) pulmonary hemorrhage

12. How is surfactant administered?
    (a) by MDI
    (b) by instilling the solution directly into the endotracheal tube
    (c) by aerosol
    (d) intravenously

13. Calfactant is ordered for a baby weighing 1.5 kg. What dose should be given?
    (a) 4.5 ml
    (b) 6.0 ml
    (c) 3.75 ml
    (d) 7.5 ml

Case Study 1

A COPD patient

A COPD patient is admitted with pneumonia. He is not able to produce his usual amount of sputum. The patient states that when he does cough up sputum, it is very thick and yellow. Upon auscultation, you note that he has expiratory rhonchi bilaterally and crackles over the right middle and lower lobes. He is already receiving aerosol treatments with albuterol and ipratropium bromide. He is also on antibiotics.

(a) What other medication may help to reduce the viscosity of this patient's sputum?

(b) What other therapies and recommendations do you have for this patient?

(c) What would you tell this patient concerning systemic hydration?

Case Study 2

A baby boy

A baby boy is born at 29 weeks' gestation. He weighs 2 kg. He is admitted to the neonatal intensive care unit with respiratory distress, nasal flaring, and grunting. His oxygen requirement has increased to 70%.

(a) What pathologic process should be suspected?

(b) What medication is indicated, and when and how should it be given?

(c) Would this be considered prophylactic or rescue therapy?

(d) What patient parameters should be monitored before and after medication administration?

Chapter **7**

Anti-Inflammatory and Antiasthmatic Agents

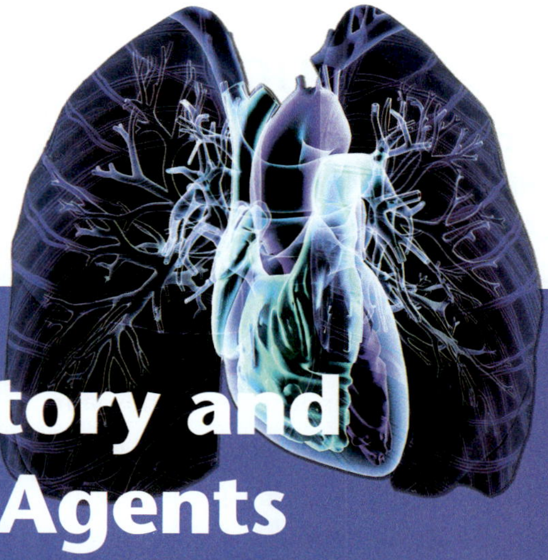

OBJECTIVES

Upon completion of this chapter you will be able to

- Describe the inflammatory process as it relates to airway disease.
- List the chemical mediators involved in allergic reactions.
- Discuss the physiology of corticosteroids.
- Define *hypothalamic pituitary adrenal axis, suppression,* and *steroid dependency.*
- Be able to describe the pharmacotherapy of oral, parenteral, and inhalational corticosteroids.
- Be able to differentiate the anti-inflammatory and antiasthmatic classes of medications available to treat asthma according to their mechanism of action and clinical use.

KEY TERMS

antigen
bronchial hyperresponsiveness
chemical mediators
corticosteroid
exercise-induced bronchospasm
glucocorticoid
histamine
leukotriene
mineralocorticoid
prostaglandin

ABBREVIATIONS

ACTH	adrenocorticotropic hormone
BHR	bronchial hyperresponsiveness
CAM	cellular adhesion molecule
CBC	complete blood count
CRF	corticotropin-releasing factor
EAR	early asthmatic reaction
EIB	exercise-induced bronchospasm
FEV_1	forced expiratory volume in 1 second
FVC	forced vital capacity
H_2	histamine 2
HPA	hypothalamic pituitary adrenal axis
ICS	inhaled corticosteroid
IgE	immunoglobulin E
LAR	late asthmatic reaction
MRI	mediator-release inhibitor
PEF	peak expiratory flow
PG	prostaglandin
PGE_1	prostaglandin E_1
PGE_2	prostaglandin E_2
$PGF_{2\alpha}$	prostaglandin $F_{2\alpha}$

Learning Hint

Remember from Chapter 5 that bronchospasm is the contraction of the smooth muscle layer *within* the airway and is treated by a fast-acting bronchodilator. The inflammatory process produces pressure and swelling *around* the airway, which compresses or constricts the airway. Just relaxing the smooth muscle layer with a bronchodilator will not solve the problem; the inflammation and associated swelling must be relieved. That is where anti-inflammatory medications come into play.

In Chapter 5 we learned about the role of bronchodilators to treat bronchospasm within the smooth muscle layer of the airway. Bronchospasm can be the result of an immediate reaction to an airway irritant, but the story doesn't end there. What about the subsequent airway inflammation that can result from bronchospasm, disease processes such as asthma or chronic bronchitis, or mechanical lung trauma? In this chapter we focus on the anti-inflammatory and antiasthmatic classes of medications, which are frequently used in association with bronchodilators to treat and/or lessen the subsequent pulmonary inflammation. To distinguish the roles of these classes of drugs, it is first important to review how the airway can be affected by inflammation and what the various pathways are that lead to the inflammatory response.

Lung inflammation can result from diseases, infections, inhalation of toxic substances, or trauma. The resulting mucosal edema, bronchoconstriction, and increased mucus production can be life threatening because of increases in airway resistance from swelling and decreasing ventilation leading to poor gas exchange.

Inflammation occurs in response to a stimulus that causes release of chemical mediators that travel to the site of injury. Several different pathways containing chemical mediators lead to inflammation in the lungs. Different drugs discussed in this chapter work on different mediator pathways. This is the rationale for using combinations of drugs: to attack the specific pathway(s) leading to the inflammatory response in each particular situation.

7.1 THE INFLAMMATORY PROCESS

7.1a The Immune Response

The major function of the body's natural defense mechanism—the immune system—is to neutralize, destroy, and eliminate foreign materials called **antigens**. It accomplishes this through the ability of white blood cells (leukocytes) to produce specific antibodies to combat foreign invasion. Antigens stimulate both the immune and inflammatory processes. Table 7-1 lists some of these common antigens.

TABLE 7-1 Common Antigens

Dust mites	Smoke
Animal dander	Sulfites
Mold	Viruses
Pollen	Bacteria

BVT Lab

Flashcards are available for this chapter at www.BVTLab.com.

The *immune system* has two functional units: *humoral* (circulating) *immunity* and *cell-mediated immunity.* Either or both units can respond to an antigen and activate the white blood cells known as lymphocytes, as well as macrophages. Humoral immune response involves activation of *B lymphocytes,* while cell-mediated immunity involves production of *T lymphocytes.*

B lymphocytes produce antigen-specific antibodies called *immunoglobulins* that act to remove or destroy the antigen. We currently know of five major classes of immunoglobulins that are found naturally in the body or are produced by B lymphocytes in response to foreign objects. See Table 7-2 for a list of the classes of immunoglobulins. T lymphocytes remove or destroy antigens directly or may act indirectly with help from macrophages and neutrophils.

TABLE 7-2 Immunoglobulins

Type	Characteristics
IgG	Most common; 80% of total immunoglobulins in plasma; protects against childhood diseases
IgM	10% of total immunoglobulins; numbers increase in chronic infections
IgE	Hypersensitivity reactions, allergic rhinitis, allergic asthma; bound to mast cells
IgA	Mucous membranes in respiratory tract; salivary and bronchial secretions; transfer immunity to the child
IgD	Role unknown; may be B cell maturation

7.1b Mast Cell Chemical Mediator Release

The most common immune system–produced antibody involved in allergic asthma and rhinitis (runny/stuffy nose) is immunoglobulin E (IgE). Once IgE becomes exposed to an antigen, it fixes itself to the surface of a mast cell membrane. Mast cells can be found throughout the body, but for our discussion we will focus on those found in the respiratory tract. In essence, once the antigen attaches to the mast cell, the mast cell becomes "sensitized" and awaits reexposure of the antigen, much like a police officer waiting to leap out and grab a known perpetrator that he's seen before. Upon reexposure, an antigen–antibody reaction occurs, which consists of a cascade of **chemical mediators** spilling out from the ruptured mast cell (degranulation). Mediators released include histamine, heparin, and other chemical factors.

Within the airway, these chemicals can immediately lead to bronchospasms. Eventually, these chemicals and others produced as a result of the cleanup of the mast cell rupture (arachidonic acid metabolism producing leukotrienes and prostaglandins) cause *inflammation;* the inflammatory reaction causes further airway smooth muscle contraction, mucosal edema, cellular infiltration, and mucus secretions with plugging. See Figure 7-1, which represents the initial mechanism that leads to mast cell rupture or degranulation.

Clinical pearl

Mast cells are found throughout the body. If the sensitized mast cell ruptures (degranulates) in the airway, bronchoconstriction may result. If sensitized mast cells in the eyes are exposed to an antigen, the eyes may water, become red, and swell. Likewise mast cell degranulation in the nasal passages can lead to rhinitis and upper-airway congestion.

FIGURE 7-1 Mast Cell Rupture or Degranulation in the Airways

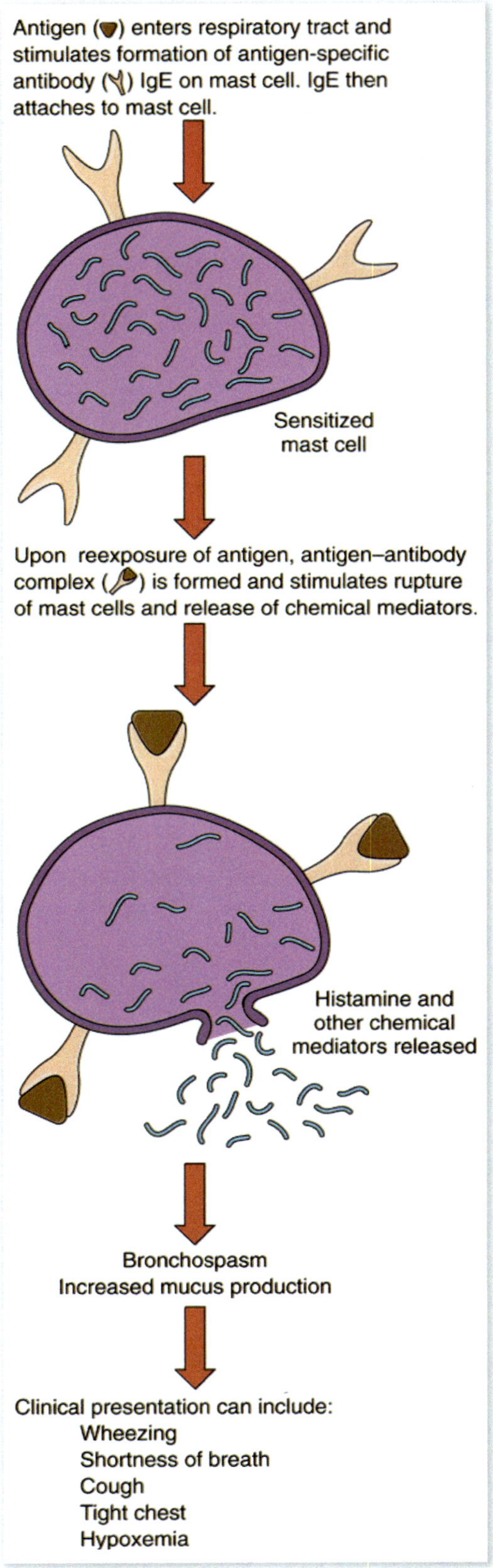

7.1c Types of Asthma

Because asthma represents a disease of chronic inflammation, it can be used to illustrate the inflammatory response. Keep in mind that the inflammatory response is a needed body response; it is only *hyperactivation* of this response that can cause serious consequences.

There are two main types of asthma: allergic asthma and nonallergic asthma. Most people have the allergic kind, caused by an external antigen such as pollen, dust, smoke, or pets. This is the kind that can lend itself to treatment with *immunotherapy,* commonly known as allergy shots, if we know the exact antigen that triggers the immune and inflammatory response. Allergy shots work because an allergic individual exposed to small doses of an antigen or allergen produces antibodies that are specific to that antigen. The antibodies are then sensitized and can recognize and fight the antigen when it returns. Although allergy shots may sound like the most logical treatment possible, they are usually used only if drug therapy is not effective for allergies. This is because immunotherapy treatment can be lengthy, with symptom relief not occurring until after at least 6 months of therapy. Also there is always a risk of anaphylaxis in patients with severe asthma who receive allergy shots; some believe this is because too many mast cells become sensitized and the subsequent chemical mediator release can then be too great.

Nonallergic asthma is precipitated by infection, cold air, exercise, or stress, with no specific antigen being identified. No immune response is involved, but mast cells still degranulate, which then can result in an acute asthma attack. Lessening the frequency and severity of the attacks from either nonallergic or allergic asthma is accomplished by prophylactic antiasthmatic agents, which stabilize or desensitize mast cells, thus preventing their rupture and chemical mediator release. This is why these agents are also known as *mast cell stabilizers.* These agents are discussed later in this chapter.

Clinical pearl

Allergic asthma is sometimes also called *atopic* or *extrinsic asthma,* because it is known to be stimulated by a specific antigen source. Nonallergic asthma is also referred to as *intrinsic* or *nonatopic asthma.*

7.1d Phases of the Inflammatory Response

Regardless of the type of asthma, the inflammatory response related to an asthmatic attack and mast cell degranulation can have two distinct phases: early and late. The *early-phase response* of any inflammatory reaction consists of local vasodilation and increased vascular permeability, redness, and wheal (local, usually itchy, swelling or welt) formation. The immediate inflammatory response in asthma results in bronchial contraction, with wheezing, cough, dyspnea, and hypoxemia resulting from mast cell degranulation and the subsequent release of histamine and other chemical mediator substances. Please see Figure 7-1 again, which illustrates the early phase of the inflammatory response.

Bronchodilators almost always reverse bronchospasm in the early phase; however, in more difficult cases of asthma, the episode launches a series of steps leading to a slow inflammatory process that develops 6–8 hours later. This is termed the *late-phase response* and is very difficult to resolve. The late-phase reaction can be serious, and treatment is aimed at stopping inflammatory progression before it occurs at this stage. White blood cells, including lymphocytes, and other chemical mediators contribute to the late-phase inflammation. White blood cells infiltrate the asthmatic airways, as evidenced by an increase in eosinophils and neutrophils. Sloughing of airway cells and growth of goblet cells result in hypersecretion of mucus and mucosal swelling. Increased vascular permeability then occurs, causing further mucus secretion and mucosal swelling, which results in mucus plugging. In essence a "traffic jam" of cellular debris and secretions piles up.

Learning Hint

On the complete blood count (CBC), the presence of increased eosinophils hints at the presence of an active allergic response.

In addition, the destruction of the phospholipid mast cell membrane and its subsequent breakdown by phospholipase produces the fatty acid arachidonic acid. Arachidonic acid then produces two pathways that contribute to the late-phase response. The lipoxygenase pathways consist mainly of **leukotriene** release, and the cyclo-oxygenase pathway primarily releases **prostaglandins**, all adding to the late-phase responses of submucosal edema, mucus production, and hyperreactive airways. See Figure 7-2, which shows the early- and late-phase inflammatory responses.

FIGURE 7-2 The Early- and Late-Phase Inflammatory Response in the Airways

Note: Increased neutrophils, monocytes, and eosinophils migrating to inflamed airways also contribute to late-phase response.

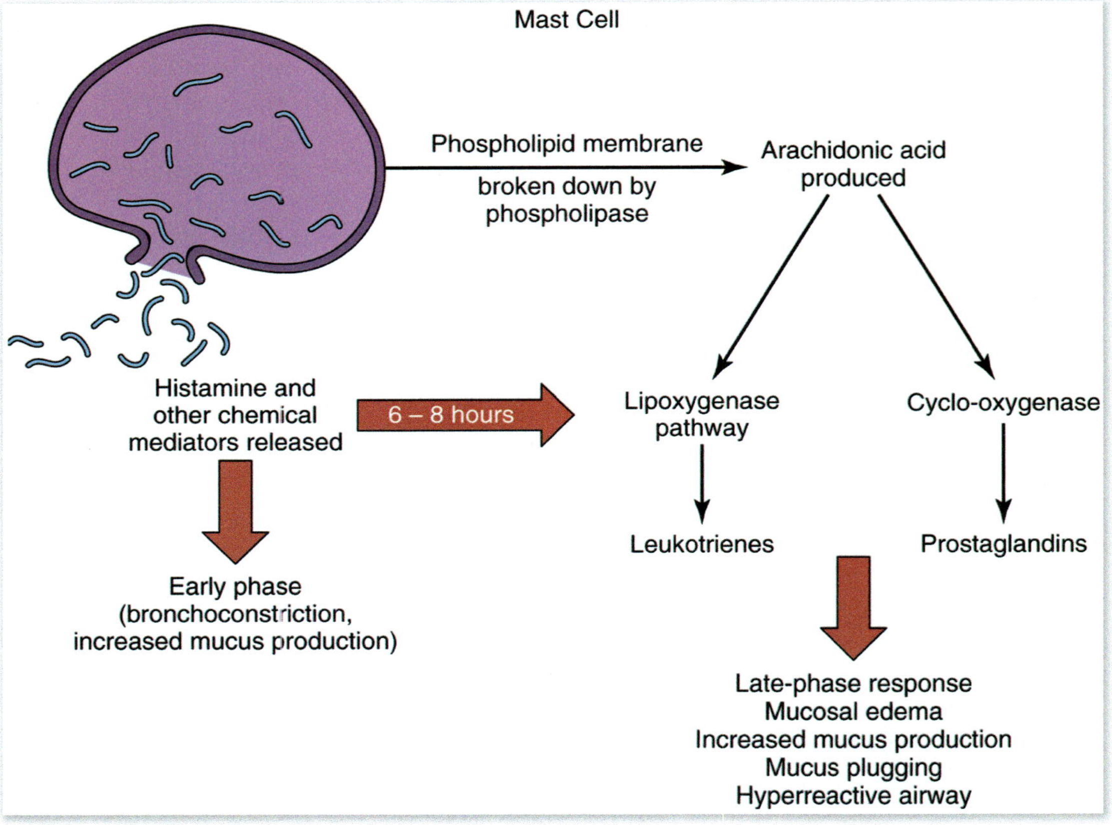

time for review

Contrast early- and late-phase responses; why do you think this is important for drug therapy?

Looking at Figure 7-2, logic tells us that the optimal blockage of the inflammatory response would be to stabilize the mast cell membrane and not allow it to begin the cascade of mediator release leading to both the early- and late-phase responses. This is the mechanism of action of the prophylactic antiasthmatics discussed later in this chapter. In addition this chapter discusses other categories of drugs that block specific inflammatory pathways, such as the leukotriene inhibitors, antihistamines, and prostaglandin inhibitors. For now we will focus on the drug category **corticosteroids**, which have a broad spectrum of activity and work on several of the different mediator pathways in both the early- and late-phase inflammatory responses.

Clinical pearl

Other drugs currently being researched for their ability to inhibit airway inflammatory response include monoclonal antibodies to specific cytokines as well as cellular adhesion molecules (CAM-1). These drugs work by preventing proteins in the immune system from becoming activated, which is also an underlying cause of allergic asthma symptoms. The drug omalizumab (Xolair®) binds to IgE and prevents IgE from binding to cells and triggering an allergic reaction. This drug is given subcutaneously.

7.2 CORTICOSTEROIDS

7.2a Corticosteroid Physiology

Corticosteroids can block both the initial immune response and the subsequent inflammatory process and are therefore a mainstay of treatment for allergic asthma. Before we can talk about corticosteroids and how they work, though, we must review corticosteroid physiology.

Body functions are controlled by the nervous system and the endocrine system working together in an integrated fashion. The endocrine system produces hormones, which are chemical substances secreted into the bloodstream that then circulate and exert physiologic effects on body cells and tissues. The adrenal glands contain two endocrine organs: the adrenal medulla and the adrenal cortex. The adrenal medulla secretes the hormones catecholamines, norepinephrine, and epinephrine and is functionally related to the sympathetic component (fight-or-flight) of the autonomic nervous system, as discussed in Chapter 3. In this chapter we focus on the adrenal cortex. Its role is secretion of steroid substances called adrenocortical hormones, or corticosteroids.

Corticosteroids are classified into **mineralocorticoids** and **glucocorticoids.** Depending on the chemical structure of the corticosteroid hormone, drugs differ in their mineralocorticoid and glucocorticoid activities. Mineralocorticoids are corticosteroids with salt-retaining activity that are important for electrolyte balance and fluid volume. Aldosterone (produced by the adrenal gland) and fludrocortisone (synthetic) are examples of mineralocorticoids. Aldosterone and fludrocortisone cause increased sodium and water reabsorption by the kidney into the bloodstream, which decreases urine production and thereby causes volume expansion within the bloodstream.

Clinical pearl

Spironolactone (Aldactone®) is a diuretic that works as an aldosterone antagonist.

Glucocorticoids affect carbohydrate, protein, and fat metabolism and are useful pharmacologically for anti-inflammatory activity and their ability to suppress immunologic activity. Synthetic corticosteroids have been developed to optimize anti-inflammatory activity (to be more glucocorticoid-like) and to minimize mineralocorticoid activity. Although the two classifications seem distinct, glucocorticoids also tend to have some mineralocorticoid activity (see Table 7-3).

TABLE 7-3 Glucocorticoid and Mineralocorticoid Activity of Oral Corticosteroids

Corticosteroid	Glucocorticoid Strength	Mineralocorticoid Strength
hydrocortisone	1	1
cortisone	0.8	0.8
prednisone	2.5–3.5	0.8
prednisolone	3–4	0.8
methylprednisolone	4–5	0–0.8
dexamethasone	20–40	0

time for review

Immunosuppression using high doses of corticosteroids may be beneficial after organ transplantation, but this has implications for precautions you should take when treating transplant patients. Can you think of what precautions you should take and why?

Other corticosteroids that are not as pertinent to cardiorespiratory pharmacotherapy, and therefore are not discussed here, are sex hormones, which have androgenic, estrogenic, or progestenic activity. Some of these types of corticosteroids have been used by weightlifters or as sexual hormone–replacement therapy. The term *steroid* is frequently used instead of *corticosteroid* in these contexts. All steroids except the sex hormones are essential for survival. (One could, of course, argue that the sex hormones are also essential—for the survival of the species.)

Corticosteroids are used to treat many diseases, such as rheumatoid arthritis, cancers, and pulmonary diseases. In respiratory disease, they are used to treat acute and chronic asthma, although their use in COPD is controversial, as discussed in Chapter 13. Administration routes used are inhalation, oral, and parenteral.

Treatment with corticosteroids is usually short term and adjunctive, but it can also be long term. Corticosteroids make some patients feel euphoric, and patients frequently want to be on steroids. Unfortunately therapeutic pharmacologic use can alter the balance of natural steroid production. This will be discussed shortly, as it relates to steroid dependence and adrenal suppression.

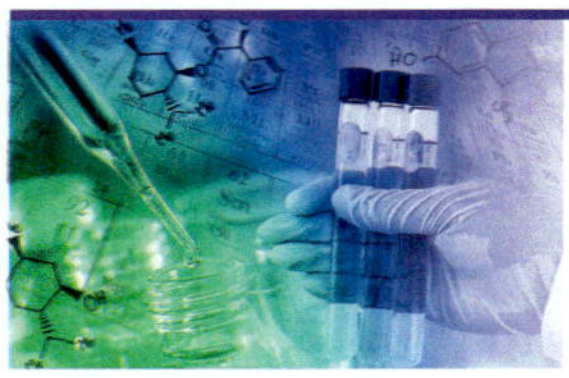

CONTROVERSY

Corticosteroids may provide significant benefits, but they also carry the risk of several side effects. The implications of their clinical use must be understood and jointly agreed to by both the patient and the health-care provider.

Clinical pearl

Corticosteroids are secreted daily by the adrenal cortex at the rate of about 10 to 30 mg/day. This release does not occur steadily but occurs in response to surgery, stress, infection, and emotion on a 24-hour diurnal rhythm cycle. Serum concentrations peak at about 8:00 a.m. Night-shift workers have very different patterns or diurnal rhythms, and dosing time of exogenous pharmacologic steroids may have to be reversed in their case.

The main internally produced or endogenous glucocorticoid is hydrocortisone. It is important to understand the production and control of the body's endogenous corticosteroids and the hypothalamic pituitary adrenal axis. Only then can the concept of adrenal suppression and steroid dependence be understood.

7.2b Hypothalamic Pituitary Adrenal Axis

The hypothalamic pituitary adrenal axis (HPA) controls corticosteroid release in the body. It is responsible for the normal diurnal variation in blood levels of steroids. For example, when we get up in the morning, the body must ready itself to face the day; hormone production begins and then peaks and troughs throughout the day according to our metabolic needs. One of the factors that influence corticosteroid release in the body is stress. In stressful situations corticosteroids work to decrease the effects of stress. They do this by raising blood glucose levels so that vital tissues, such as the brain and heart, get the glucose needed in stressful situations.

When the hypothalamus is stimulated, it sends impulses that cause corticotropin-releasing factor (CRF) to be released in the anterior pituitary gland. The anterior pituitary gland, under the influence of CRF, then causes adrenocorticotropic hormone (ACTH) to be released into the bloodstream. ACTH then circulates within the bloodstream to the adrenal cortex, where it stimulates the secretion of corticosteroids. This is under normal biofeedback mechanism control, by which high levels of corticosteroids in the bloodstream inhibit further release of CRF and ACTH (see Figure 7-3).

FIGURE 7-3 **HPA Mechanism for Release and Regulation of Corticosteroids**

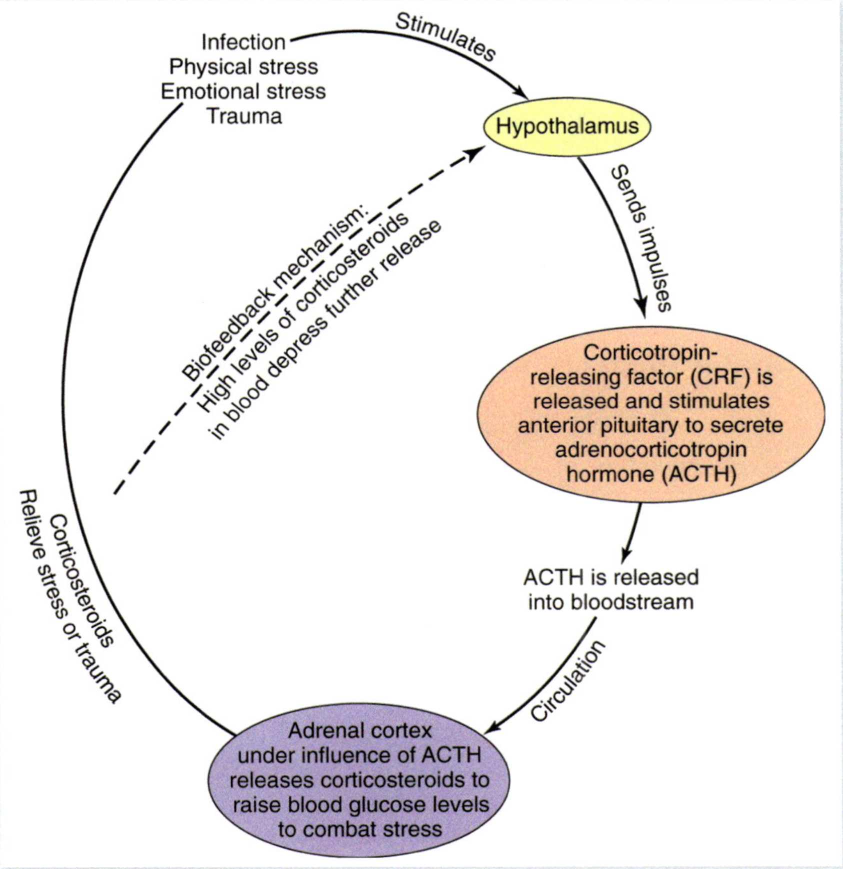

If exogenous pharmacologic corticosteroid drugs are used to treat diseases, adrenal or HPA suppression can occur, causing the adrenal glands to atrophy because they no longer have to work to produce these hormones. The body cannot tell the difference between corticosteroids it has produced itself and those that have been administered pharmacologically. The body just knows it has a higher level of hormones and tells itself to turn off its own production. It then becomes dependent on the administered pharmacologic corticosteroids. This means that short-term (up to 3 weeks even at high doses) pharmacologic exogenously administered corticosteroids can simply be stopped without a taper; but patients who have taken corticosteroids for longer periods must be tapered off slowly (generally a 10%–20% reduction every 1 to 2 weeks), to give the body time to pick up production and regain internal regulation.

7.2c Corticosteroid Mechanism of Action

Clinical pearl

It is well documented that corticosteroids, when used in conjunction with β_2-agonists, improve pulmonary functions such as forced vital capacity (FVC), forced expiratory volume (FEV_1), and peak expiratory flow rates (PEFs).

Corticosteroids have a variety of mechanisms of action, all related to blocking or diminishing the late-phase asthma responses by blocking the arachidonic acid cascade of metabolites (leukotrienes and prostaglandins). In addition corticosteroids remove circulatory lymphocytes, monocytes, eosinophils, and basophils by moving them to lymph, bone marrow, and the spleen. Fewer cells then reach the site of inflammation, and therefore there is less congestion. Corticosteroids also inhibit macrophage and leukocyte processing of antigens, so the ability of cells to respond to antigens is decreased, thus suppressing the immune response.

Corticosteroids also decrease the production of eosinophils, basophils, and monocytes. They have shown an additional beneficial effect, enhancing the responsiveness of the β_2-receptors by increasing the responsiveness of adenyl cyclase in airway smooth muscle to catecholamines or β-agonists (see Chapter 5). Corticosteroids do not have a direct relaxing effect on bronchial muscle but do facilitate the effect of β-agonists, thereby enhancing the desired bronchodilation effects of β_2-adrenergic drugs given for the hyperreactive airways. Taking all these factors into account, corticosteroids clinically reduce airway inflammation, decrease airway obstruction, improve oxygenation, and increase the response to β-agonists (see Table 7-4).

TABLE 7-4 Effects of Corticosteroids on Inflammation

Block arachidonic acid metabolites (leukotrienes and prostaglandins)
Decrease monocytes, eosinophils, and basophils
Decrease lymphocytes and macrophages
Inhibit late-phase inflammation
Increase β_2-receptors and responsiveness

The effects of corticosteroids are often time-dependent. Although the cellular and biochemical effects of corticosteroids are immediate, clinical response takes longer. Increased responsiveness to β-agonists occurs within 2 hours, and β-receptor density increases within 4 hours. Seasonal **bronchial hyperresponsiveness** (BHR) requires at least a week of therapy to reverse. **Exercise-induced bronchospasm** (EIB) sensitivity decreases after 4 weeks of therapy.

7.2d Corticosteroid Use in Airway Remodeling

Corticosteroids prevent or suppress airway inflammation, which results in reduction of bronchial hyperresponsiveness and prevention and reduction of airway remodeling. Airway remodeling is important because it is a change in the composition of the airway wall that occurs in some asthmatics over time. Think of a ball being thrown against the same spot on a wall. The first couple of times it may not leave a mark, but after repeated throws it will change the surface of the wall. The structural changes in the airway result from long-standing airway inflammation. One of the consequences is persistent airway obstruction that may not be responsive to treatment. Considering airway remodeling, use of corticosteroids as an early anti-inflammatory intervention makes sense.

BVT Lab

Visit www.BVTLab.com to explore the student resources available for this chapter.

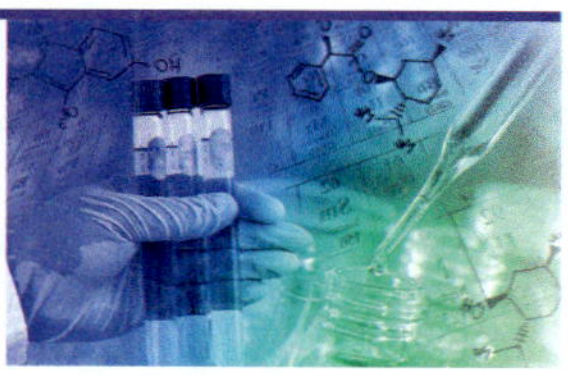

CONTROVERSY

Should drug therapy of asthma be disease-modifying and a primary prevention strategy, or should it simply produce symptom control?

7.2e Adverse Effects of Corticosteroids

Side effects of steroids can be considered as short term or long term, depending on the duration of use and route of administration (systemic or topical). The most common side effects of short-term use include appetite stimulation, stomach irritation, headache, and mood changes. The mood changes may be a sense of well-being or a steroid psychosis. Steroids can exacerbate acne and can cause hypokalemia, hyperglycemia, and leukocytosis. The hyperglycemia causes what is called steroid diabetes. Once the steroids are discontinued, these side effects usually go away.

Long-term side effects include osteoporosis or bone changes that could lead to fractures; immunosuppression, which can lead to increased risk of infection; and myopathy of skeletal muscles. See Table 7-5 for side effects of corticosteroids.

TABLE 7-5 Side Effects of Corticosteroids

Category	Side Effect
Immunologic	Immunosuppression Increased susceptibility to infections
Cardiovascular	Edema Hypertension
CNS	Euphoria Insomnia
Dermatologic	Thin skin Impaired wound healing Bruising Altered fat distribution
Endocrinologic	Diabetes Cushingoid state
Metabolic	Electrolyte imbalance Negative nitrogen balance
Musculoskeletal	Muscle weakness Osteoporosis Growth suppression
Ophthalmic	Glaucoma

Life Span Considerations

Controversy exists about the extent of effect that corticosteroids have on children's growth as a result of steroid-induced changes in bone growth and epiphyseal (growth-plate) maturation. Several studies actually show improved growth rates for children switched from oral steroids to inhaled steroids. This result could be due to better control of the asthma and less need for oral systemic steroids. The most recent data concerning the use of inhaled corticosteroids in children suggest no apparent affect on final adult height.

7.2f Oral and Parenteral Corticosteroid Administration

Sometimes oral steroids are given as pulse or burst doses—for example, 40 mg of prednisone per day orally for 3 days. At other times they are given on every-other-day regimens at 2 to 3 times the daily dose. Whatever the regimen, the lowest possible dose of steroid should be used to accomplish the therapeutic goal.

Corticosteroids often take days, not hours, to heal damaged airways. Although it is common to use parenteral administration, research results are ambivalent as to whether this route is faster-acting than oral administration. Objective improvement takes a minimum of 6 to 12 hours, and maximum improvement may take longer than a week. Objective measures such as pulmonary function tests may show improvement 12 hours after administration. In the emergency room, corticosteroids are warranted for patients with a poor response to β-agonists over 1 to 2 hours. Because of the delayed onset, many clinicians initiate early corticosteroid use to lessen or prevent the late-phase inflammatory response.

Hydrocortisone (Cortef®) and methylprednisolone (Solu-Medrol®) are most commonly given by injection. Methylprednisolone's advantage is less fluid retention in patients with heart disease, because of fewer mineralocorticoid effects (again, see Table 7-3). After hospitalized patients improve in 48 to 72 hours, the IV dose is tapered to an oral dose and the duration of treatment is based on clinical response. If the patient had been steroid-dependent before hospitalization, tapering the dose to what it was before hospitalization is the goal.

7.2g Inhaled Corticosteroids

The aerosol corticosteroids are chemically altered to minimize systemic toxicity and are available in metered-dose inhalers (MDIs), dry-powder inhalers (DPIs), and nebulizer solutions. A small portion of all aerosol steroids is deposited in the mouth and pharynx and then swallowed. The portion that is swallowed is absorbed into the bloodstream and metabolized by the liver. Inhalational or topical corticosteroids have advantages over oral or parenteral administration in terms of lessened systemic adverse effects. Typical side effects from aerosol administration include oropharyngeal fungal infections, with the most common being thrush (*Candida* yeast infection) (see Figure 7-4). Some patients may have changes in their voices and/or hoarseness (dysphonia) as a result of inhaled steroids. The incidence of dysphonia is usually not reduced with the use of a spacer but may be lowered with dry-powder inhalers. However, the minimization of systemic side effects via the inhalational route makes it ideal for treating airway inflammation. See Table 7-6, which provides a summary of advantages of aerosol and oral routes.

Clinical pearl

Thrush (candidiasis) is treatable with liquid antifungal antimicrobials that are swished in the mouth and swallowed. Using a spacer to reduce oropharyngeal deposition and rinsing the mouth with water or a mouthwash after taking a steroid MDI minimizes the occurrence of opportunistic fungal infections.

FIGURE 7-4 Oral Thrush Due to Inhaled Steroids

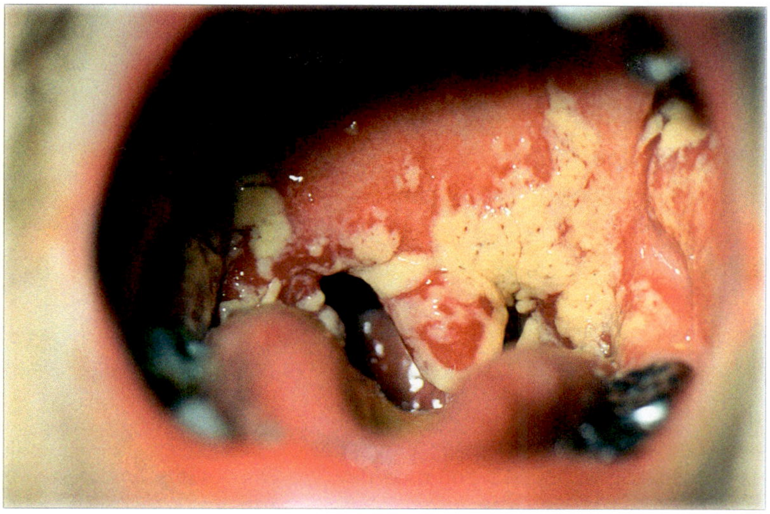

Source: Wikimedia Commons

TABLE 7-6 Comparison of Oral and Aerosol Corticosteroids

Characteristic of the Drug	Oral	Aerosol
HPA suppression	Yes	No*
Cushing's syndrome	Yes	No**
Steroid dependence	High risk	Low risk
Local therapeutic effects	No	Yes
Risk to growth development in children	Yes	No
Ease of use	Yes	No
Cost	Inexpensive	Expensive
Local airway reaction	No	Yes

*HPA suppression has been reported but the risk is small with recommended doses.
**Case reports of Cushing's syndrome have been reported. The risk is increased when high inhaled corticosteroid (ICS) doses are used with drugs that inhibit the metabolism of the ICS.

There is little advantage of one aerosol steroid over another when they are used at similar doses. Doses are usually classified as low, medium, or high. See Table 7-7 for comparative adult inhaled corticosteroid doses. Most inhaled steroids can be given twice daily. Doses should be adjusted to provide control with minimal side effects. Inhaled steroids have a different time course of response than oral steroids. Inhaled steroids produce symptom improvement in the first 1 to 2 weeks of therapy, with maximum improvement in 4 to 8 weeks. FEV_1 and PEF may take 3 to 6 weeks for maximum improvement. The BHR improvement can take 1 to 3 months and continue over 1 year.

Clinical pearl

The most important way to determine the right dose of an inhaled corticosteroid (ICS) for a patient is to carefully monitor the patient's response to therapy using clinical parameters, always attempting to find the lowest effective dose.

Table 7-7 Comparative Adult Inhaled Daily Corticosteroid Doses (divided doses twice daily)

Drug	Low Dose	Medium Dose	High Dose
beclomethasone dipproprionate HFA (Qvar®), 40 or 80 mcg/dose	80–160 mcg/day	>160–320 mcg/day	>320 mcg
budesonide DPI (Pulmicort®) 90 or 180 mcg/dose	180–600 mcg/day	>600–1,200 mcg/day	>1,200 mcg/day
ciclesonide HFA (Alvesco®) 80 or 160 mcg/dose	80–160 mcg/day	>160–320 mcg/day	>320 mcg/day
flunisolide (Aerospan®) 80 mcg/dose	320 mcg/day	>320–640 mcg/day	>640 mcg/day
fluticasone HFA (Flovent®) (MDI) 44, 110, 220 mcg/dose (DPI) 50, 100, 250 mcg/dose	88–264 mcg/day 100–300 mcg/day	>264–440 mcg/day >300–500 mcg/day	>440 mcg/day >500 mcg/day
mometasone furoate (Asmanex®) (DPI) 110 or 220 mcg/dose	110–220 mcg/day	>220–440 mcg/day	>440 mcg/day

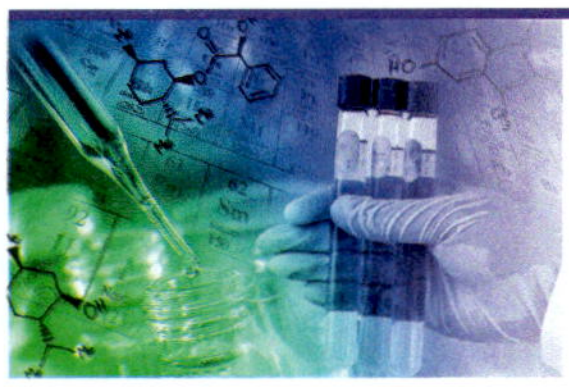

Controversy

There is no doubt that inhaled corticosteroids have less systemic adverse effects than their oral or parenteral cousins. A patient's risk of systemic adverse effects may depend on the delivery system, cumulative dose, and the absorption of the drug from the lung or the gastrointestinal tract when the drug is swallowed. Patients should have regular eye exams and bone health should be maintained by regular exercise and adequate calcium and vitamin D intake. Bone density testing to detect osteoporosis should be obtained in patients on high-dose inhaled corticosteroids.

Learning Hint

Corticosteroid inhalational products are not equivalent per puff or per microgram. Comparative doses are estimated and rely on clinician judgment.

7.2h Benefits of Daily Corticosteroid Use

Corticosteroids are the most potent anti-inflammatory agents for asthma and are most effective inhalationally for long-term control of persistent asthma (more specifics on this in Chapter 13). They not only effect improvement in bronchial hyperresponsiveness over time but also prevent and reverse airway remodeling. This has led to thoughts that the drugs may improve long-term outcomes from asthma. Once corticosteroids are discontinued, however, the lung function returns to pretreatment values over the course of a month or two. Because less drug is usually better in the long run, studies have looked at and determined that step-down dosing from oral corticosteroids to inhaled corticosteroids can be effective. There are many benefits of daily inhaled use. Table 7-8 lists these benefits.

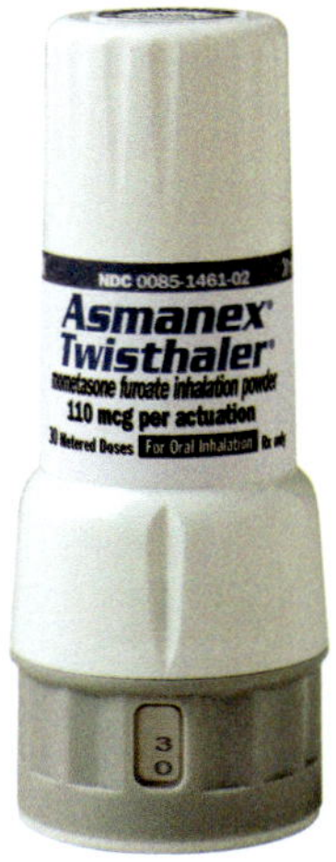

Source: Merck Archives; Merck, Sharpt & Dohme Corp., 2015

Table 7-8 Benefits of Daily Use of Inhaled Corticosteroids

Fewer symptoms
Fewer severe exacerbations
Reduced use of quick-relief β_2-agents
Reduction in airway remodeling
Improved lung function
Reduced airway inflammation

A combination of a long-acting bronchodilator salmeterol (Serevent®) and the corticosteroid fluticasone (Flovent®) is used in a DPI device called the Advair® Diskus® (Figure 7-5). In November 2005 the U.S. Food and Drug Administration (FDA) issued a public health advisory about potentially fatal effects of the salmeterol component. Although this drug has been shown to reduce the number of asthma episodes, in a small number of cases it was also shown to increase the chance of severe asthma episodes and death. In addition therapy with long-acting beta-agonists (LABAs) alone has been shown to be inferior to inhaled corticosteroids alone.

FIGURE 7-5 Advair® Drug Advertisement and Inhaler Device

The combination drug Advair® contains the bronchodilator drug salmeterol and the corticosteroid anti-inflammatory drug fluticasone. Notice the background magazine advertisement that points out that asthma has two main causes: airway constriction and inflammation. A combination drug such as Advair® treats both at the same time to prevent acute attacks.

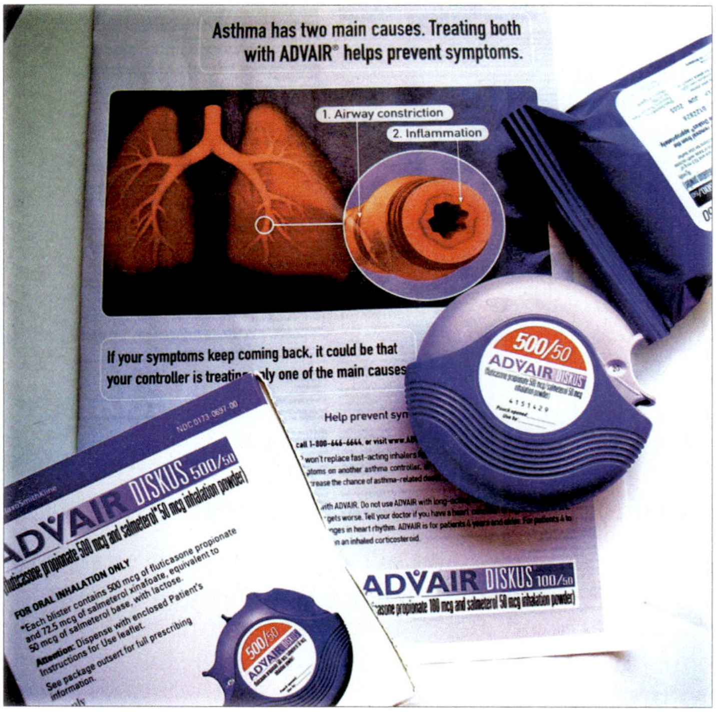

Source: GlaxoSmithKline. Used with permission.

Combinations of ICS and LABAs are used in the treatment of COPD (emphysema and chronic bronchitis); you will learn more about this in Chapter 13. Please see Table 7-9, which lists some combination drugs and their trade names and dosages.

TABLE 7-9 Commercially Available Combinations of ICS and LABA

Generic Names	Trade Name	Dosage
budesonide 160 mcg and formoterol 4.5 mcg	Symbicort®	Two inhalations twice daily
fluticasone 250 mcg and salmeterol 50 mcg	Advair®	One inhalation twice daily
fluticasone 100 mcg and vilanterol 25 mcg	Breo Elipta®	One inhalation once daily
mometasone 50 mcg and formoterol 5 mcg	Dulera®	Two inhalations twice daily

time for review

Do you start early or wait until later to administer corticosteroids? How do you decide what route to use? If using an inhaled bronchodilator in conjunction with an inhaled steroid, which do you give first and why?

7.2i Steroid Dependency

Clinical pearl

Additional uses of corticosteroids include stimulation of lung maturation in the fetus, relief from rheumatoid arthritis, and prevention of organ transplant rejection.

Steroid dependency can be classified into two forms. One is related to a psychological desire for the drug, and the other is related to physiologic steroid suppression of the normal functions of the HPA. Psychological dependence can occur because of the sense of well-being induced by these drugs as well as the effective symptom relief they provide.

Withdrawing patients from steroids quickly can lead to physiologic adrenal insufficiency symptoms from HPA suppression. Steroid withdrawal syndrome consists of anorexia, nausea, vomiting, lethargy, headache, and hypotension. Ways to avoid steroid dependence include alternate-day steroid administration and aerosol use.

7.3 ANTIASTHMATICS

7.3a Cromolyn and Nedocromil Sodium

Whereas corticosteroids are effective in treating an already established inflammatory process, mast cell membrane stabilizers can impair or prevent the inflammatory process from ever beginning by preventing rupture of mast cells. Cromolyn and nedocromil (Alocril®), a chemical derivative with similar pharmacology, are similar drugs whose main difference is potency. For this reason we will talk about the two drugs concurrently. They are used for allergic and nonallergic intermittent asthma and also for prevention of allergic rhinitis and exercise-induced bronchospasm (EIB).

Cromolyn is *not* a bronchodilator or inhibitor of action of the chemical mediators already released. The effect of cromolyn is prophylactic, and the drug must be used as a pretreatment. It is theorized that calcium influx into the mast cell is needed for microfilament contraction that then expels the contents of (*degranulates*) the mast cell. Cromolyn works to inhibit calcium influx into the mast cell, and this prevents release of inflammatory mediators. This is why the drug is called a mast cell stabilizer or mediator-release inhibitor (MRI). By inhibiting release of inflammatory mediators, it blunts early- and late-phase asthmatic reactions to antigens, and it inhibits mast cell degranulation produced by immunologic and nonimmunologic mechanisms.

These drugs inhibit immediate early asthmatic reaction (EAR) to allergic challenge and EIB. Even though the following effects have not been associated with mast cell mediator release, cromolyn has been shown to inhibit bronchoconstriction produced by inhalation of cold air and ultrasonically nebulized water. These drugs also inhibit late asthmatic reactions (LAR) and prevent subsequent bronchial hyperresponsiveness (BHR). Long-term treatment can prevent the rise in BHR that is associated in some patients with pollen seasons. Even though they have not been directly compared to inhaled corticosteroids in a clinical trial, it is widely believed that these drugs are less effective clinically.

Clinical Pearl

Cromolyn and nedocromil are not bronchodilators and must not be used for acute reversal of bronchospasm. They must be used regularly for maximum effectiveness, even during symptom-free periods.

7.3b Dosage Forms

Cromolyn and nedocromil are poorly absorbed from the gastrointestinal tract, so they only work when they are deposited directly into the airways by aerosol administration and are not effective in oral forms. Cromolyn is available as a solution for nebulization. Response and duration are both dose related. Cromolyn nebulized solution is compatible with β-agonist solutions, so they can be administered together. Nedocromil is available only as an MDI but is no longer available in the United States, and the prophylactic effect can take from 4 to 6 weeks to improve symptoms. The only way to know whether the drug will work is to try it for 4 to 6 weeks and check the response. A positive response is less frequency and/or severity of asthmatic episodes. Cromolyn may be an alternative for children who have side effects from theophylline.

7.3c Side Effects

Nedocromil and cromolyn are nontoxic drugs with no predilection for tolerance. Following inhalation, cough and wheeze have been reported as well as bad taste and headache. Significant adverse side effects occur in less than 1 in 10,000 patients.

7.4 PROSTAGLANDINS

7.4a Physiology

Prostaglandins are present in almost all tissues, including the lungs. Prostaglandins are yet another group of chemical mediators that modulate airway function and pulmonary hemodynamics. Anything that promotes release of prostaglandins in the lung can alter ventilation perfusion disturbances. Some examples of these factors are presented in Table 7-10.

Clinical pearl

Some drugs inhibit prostaglandin (PG) synthesis in the body. These are commonly known as nonsteroidal anti-inflammatory agents and include common medications such as ibuprofen, aspirin, and naproxen, which will be mentioned in the discussion of pain medications. Their inhibitory effect has been related to the induction of bronchospasm when used in some patients with asthma. It may be that aspirin-sensitive asthmatics differ from nonsensitive asthmatics by having a different reliance on the PG mechanism than the β-system to regulate airway tone.

TABLE 7-10 Factors That Affect Prostaglandin Release in the Lung

Pulmonary embolism
Lung edema
Hypoxia
Bradykinin
Histamine
Antigen–antibody reaction

Prostaglandins are classified on the basis of their chemical structure and are categorized alphabetically. They are synthesized upon stimuli and are released, not stored, once they are made. In addition they have very short half-lives (minutes). The type of prostaglandin that dominates depends on the tissue location. In the lung, $PGF_{2\alpha}$ is the most common prostaglandin, and when stimulated and produced, it causes bronchoconstriction and increased mucus production.

PGE_1 and PGE_2 are also considered important in airway muscle tone and can cause bronchodilation. Prostaglandins are mentioned here because they may have future applications for therapy. Table 7-11 lists pulmonary effects of prostaglandins $PGF_{2\alpha}$ PGE_1, and PGE_2 in the lung.

TABLE 7-11 Effects of Prostaglandins in the Lung

	Airway	Blood Vessels
$PGF_{2\alpha}$	Bronchoconstriction Increased mucus secretion	Contraction Increased vascular resistance
PGE_1	Bronchodilation	Relaxation/decreased resistance
PGE_2	Bronchodilation	Contraction/increased resistance

7.5 LEUKOTRIENE MODIFIERS

7.5a Physiology

Leukotriene modifiers are the most recent group of oral medications to be available for asthma treatment; they inhibit the leukotriene mediator cascade from arachidonic acid metabolism that leads to airway inflammation. Leukotrienes are potent mediators of inflammation involved in the pathogenesis of asthma. Leukotrienes are derived from arachidonic acid by the 5-lipoxygenase pathway. This pathway forms leukotrienes that cause contraction of airway smooth muscle, vasodilation, increased vascular permeability, increased mucus secretion, and decreased mucociliary clearance when they activate receptors. The three agents available are zafirlukast (Accolate®), montelukast (Singulair®), and zileuton (Zyflo®). Zileuton is rarely used because it may cause injury to the liver and must be monitored closely for this potentially serious adverse effect. Zafirlukast and montelukast are leukotriene antagonists. They both work by preventing harmful effects of leukotrienes.

At this time these drugs are considered alternatives to low-dose inhaled steroids, cromolyn, or nedocromil in patients with mild to persistent asthma; they are used for long-term control, not acute treatment. They are a logical drug choice on the basis of the role of leukotrienes in inflammation as discussed previously.

Zafirlukast is effective for allergen-induced asthma and early and late allergen responses. For best effects, the drug should be taken on an empty stomach. The only clinically important drug interaction is with warfarin. Zafirlukast may increase the effects of warfarin resulting in an increased prothrombin time. Side effects of zafirlukast include pharyngitis, headache, rhinitis, and gastritis. It may also decrease liver function.

Research results have shown that montelukast can decrease the number of puffs of β-agonists daily in children and increase the morning forced expiratory volume (FEV_1). It has also been shown to increase FEV_1 in adults. When it is used in combination with inhalational corticosteroids, montelukast decreases the dose of inhaled steroid needed. Side effects, however, include fatigue, fever, nasal congestion, cough, dizziness, and rash.

The clinical use of this drug class is primarily in patients with mild to moderate asthma. Some people with asthma respond better to leukotriene modifiers than others. This probably has to do with the relative importance of leukotriene production in a given patient with asthma. Therefore patients are generally given a 1-month trial with this class of drugs; if they experience no improvement of symptoms during that time, they should be classified as leukotriene nonresponders and switched to another controller medication.

7.6 TREATING UPPER-AIRWAY CONGESTION

Any process that causes upper-airway congestion will of course make it more difficult to breathe and therefore increase the work of breathing. In someone who does not have lung disease, the increased work of breathing may be barely noticeable and just an annoyance. However, in patients who have lung disease, it may be overwhelming and contribute to overall decreased alveolar ventilation. Therefore treatment of the common "head cold" in these patients is no trivial matter.

7.6a Allergic Rhinitis

Allergic rhinitis (runny nose) can be seasonal or perennial. It is characterized by an immunologic response that causes symptoms such as sneezing, rhinorrhea, nasal congestion, and pruritus. In addition to increasing the work of breathing, any upper-airway congestion will increase airway resistance and the likelihood of spreading infection (see Figure 7-6). Because allergic rhinitis involves the degranulation of mast cells in the nasal passageways, one logical treatment is to stabilize the mast cells.

Clinical pearl

Eye symptoms such as itching can also be a problem in allergic rhinitis. Ophthalmic corticosteroids or antihistamines are available for this indication.

FIGURE 7-6 Allergic Rhinitis

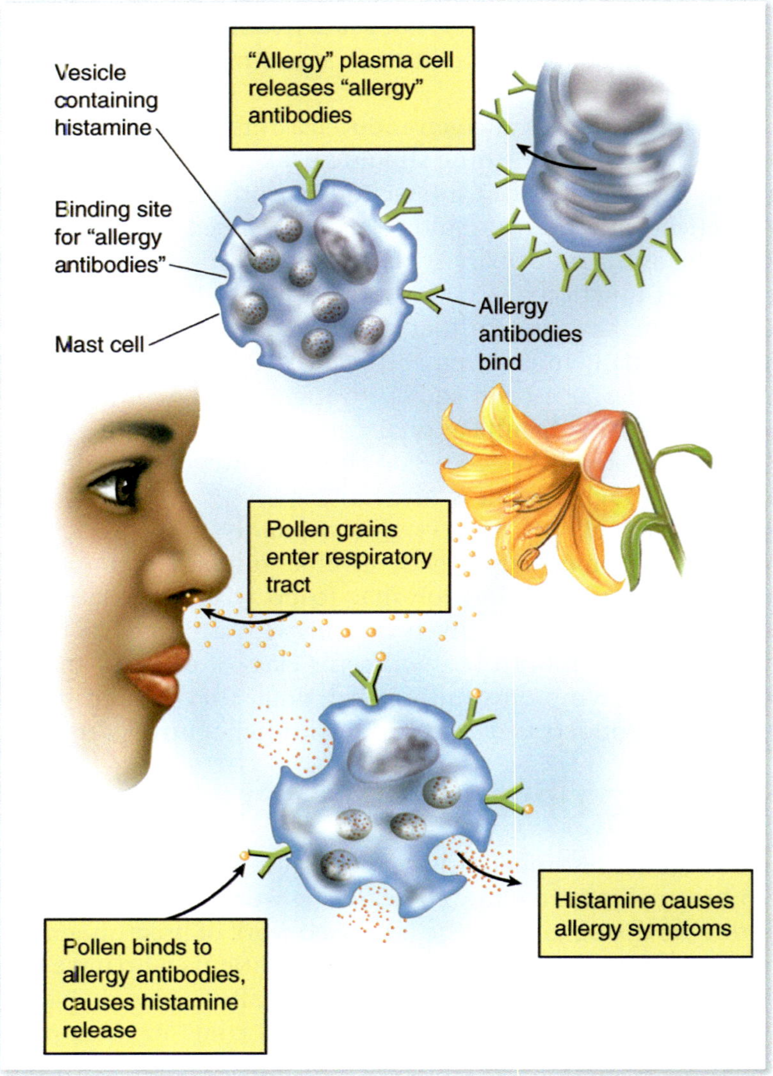

7.6b Intranasal Medications

Clinical pearl

Intranasal cromolyn may be beneficial when visiting a friend with a cat or on other occasions of one-time exposure to a known allergen if used 15 to 30 minutes before exposure.

Intranasal mast cell stabilizers are used for allergic rhinitis and are administered before the onset of pollen season. Cromolyn is available intranasally (Nasalcrom®) without a prescription and is effective for sneezing, rhinorrhea, and itching but not for preexisting nasal congestion. It must be given three to four times a day, and it takes 2 to 4 weeks to show full benefits. It is used most commonly in children with mild symptoms and whose parents wish to avoid intranasal corticosteroids.

Intranasal corticosteroids are also available. Intranasal corticosteroids inhibit cytokine release from nasal epithelial cells and inhibit leukotriene production. Intranasal corticosteroids also are beneficial in decreasing nasal congestion by decreasing function of mediators that affect vascular permeability. See Table 7-12 for common intranasal corticosteroids. This class of medications is the most effective treatment.

TABLE 7-12 Intranasal Corticosteroids

Generic Name	Brand Name
beclomethasone dipropionate	Beconase® AQ
budesonide	Rhinocort®
ciclesonide	Omnaris®
fluticasone propionate	Flonase®
triamcinolone	Nasacort®
mometasone furoate	Nasonex®

Intranasal corticosteroids can take 2 to 4 weeks to work, with 8 weeks being an adequate treatment trial for efficacy. Some of the newer products can work within 3 to 12 hours. Maximum effects can take up to 6 months. Products differ in their side effects (but not their efficacy), which include burning, stinging, irritation, and dry nose.

PATIENT & FAMILY EDUCATION

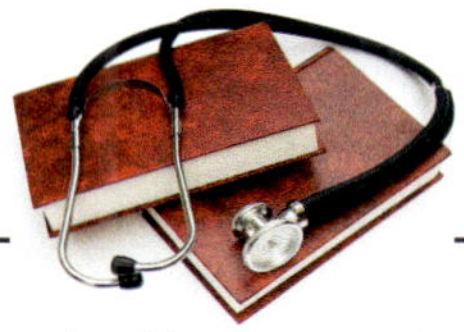

Therapy with intranasal medications should be started with the maximal dose for the patient's age. Once symptoms are controlled the dose should be reduced until the lowest effective dose is determined. If mucus crusting is present, it should be removed from the nose prior to use. Patients should position their head downward during administration to minimize drainage into the throat.

7.6c Antihistamines

Histamine is stored in tissue mast cells. In the lung, mast cells are located below the respiratory-tract mucosa in connective tissue. Scientific efforts have been made to identify factors that cause release of histamine from mast cell storage sites. These efforts have shown that the autonomic nervous system is involved through cholinergic and β- and α-receptor sites on mast cells. Histamine production is influenced by nonspecific stimuli to tissue such as chemical stimuli, physical injury, or allergy. Cigarette smoke and dust are examples of substances that can cause histamine release (see Table 7-13 for more examples).

BVT Lab

Improve your test scores. Practice quizzes are available at www.BVTLab.com.

TABLE 7-13 Factors That Influence Mediator Release from Mast Cells

Antigen–antibody IgE reactions
Mechanical tissue trauma
Tissue hypoxia
Drugs
Dust
Cigarette smoke

Histamine acts on two different receptors called histamine-1 and histamine-2. Histamine smooth muscle contraction is controlled by histamine-1 receptors. These receptors are activated by subepithelial irritant receptors, with a resultant increase in vagal activity. Drugs that antagonize histamine-1 receptors are called *antihistamines*.

Histamine release provokes airway obstruction. Airway obstruction can result from mucosal edema and inflammatory cell infiltration with eosinophils. This can be influenced by release of local mediators. See Table 7-14 for the pulmonary and systemic effects of histamine.

TABLE 7-14 Pulmonary and Systemic Effects of Histamine

Pulmonary Effect	Systemic Effect
Increased airway resistance	Vasodilation
Decreased maximum expiratory flow rate	Stimulation of adenyl cyclase in mast cells
Decreased diffusion capacity	Release of catecholamines from adrenal medulla
Increased total lung capacity	Increased vascular permeability
Increased mucus production	
Promotion of mucosal edema	

Clinical pearl

Even some drugs can cause histamine release. The itching that is frequently associated with use of opioids such as morphine is due to histamine release, although this does not necessarily imply that the patient is allergic to the drug. The effects on histamine release by neuromuscular-blocking drugs is one factor that influences the decision to use one drug instead of another.

The mechanisms involved in the release of histamine and other mediators during allergic response are complex and consist of many steps. The antigen–antibody interaction triggers many of the steps. Therapy for histamine release has been directed toward prevention or inhibition of mediator release from storage sites and antagonism of airway response to mediators.

Drugs used to prevent the release of histamine from mast cells include *β*-agonists, methylxanthines, and cholinergic blockers, as discussed in Chapter 5. In addition cromolyn and corticosteroids have a role in blocking histamine production, as discussed earlier in this chapter.

Antihistamines block the action of histamine at histamine-1 receptors. Here is the tricky part: They do this not by blocking the receptor but by inactivating the receptor. Sort of like when you "deactivate" by sitting down in front of the television after a long day of school or work. They do not prevent or block the release of histamine at histamine receptors in the GI system. They are not useful in acute asthma treatment, because so many other mediators are released in acute asthma episodes as well. Antihistamines are used basically for allergic rhinitis. Antihistamines prevent the onset of symptoms better than they reverse symptoms already present.

Clinical pearl

Histamine-2 receptors mediate actions of histamine on gastric secretion. Antagonists of this histamine are called H_2-blockers, not antihistamines, and drugs such as cimetidine (Tagamet®) are H_2-blockers, not antihistamines.

time for review

For predictable seasonal allergies, when would be the best time to start taking an antihistamine?

Side effects of antihistamines include dry mouth and throat, altered coordination, and sedation. One should not drive or operate dangerous machinery when under the influence of antihistamines (or anything else, for that matter). Some patients experience excitation rather than the expected sedation. Antihistamines can induce their own metabolism, which may present as what appears to be tolerance to the drug with chronic use.

Like cephalosporin antibiotics, there are first- and second-generation antihistamines. First-generation antihistamines are sedating, and second-generation are less so. Second-generation antihistamines have antiallergic and anti-inflammatory effects. Second-generation antihistamines are now the preferred agents, since the first-generation drugs impair CNS function and individuals consuming these OTC medications are considered to be under the influence of drugs. Improvement in symptoms with first-generation antihistamines occurs within 1 to 2 hours of the first dose, but maximum effects are not seen for weeks.

Clinical pearl

A histamine provocation test or challenge is based on airway hyperactivity. This test can provide not only information about an individual's response to therapeutic drugs but also diagnostic information.

Olopatadine and azelastine are antihistamine nasal sprays available by prescription. Azelastine can be administered as needed since it has a rapid onset (15 minutes) of action but can be sedating if swallowed. They may be useful in patients with mild or episodic symptoms (e.g., you are going to visit Uncle Charlie but are allergic to his dog).

Tolerance to the sedation effects may develop in 2 to 3 weeks; see Table 7-15 for common antihistamines.

Clinical pearl

First-generation antihistamines are very effective for symptom relief. However only about 30% of patients are satisfied with this treatment because of side effects, and they are considered second-line agents.

TABLE 7-15 Common Antihistamines

Generic Name	Brand Name
First Generation	
chlorpheniramine	Chlor-Trimeton®
diphenhydramine	Benadryl®
brompheniramine	J-Tan PD®
Second Generation	
loratidine	Claritin®
cetirizine	Zyrtec®
fexofenadine	Allegra®
desloratidine	Clarinex®
levocetirizine	Xyzal®

LIFE SPAN CONSIDERATIONS

First-generation antihistamines should be avoided in children and the elderly. Impairment of CNS function is well documented. In children, the first-generation antihistamines are associated with impaired school performance. Older adults are more susceptible to their anticholinergic effects such as blurred vision, confusion, and urinary hesitancy.

Clinical pearl

Regulations prevent some competitive athletes from taking oral stimulants such as decongestants. The over-the-counter decongestant phenylpropanolamine is no longer available because of its side effects.

7.6d Decongestants

Nasal decongestants are α-adrenergic drugs with corresponding vasoconstrictive properties. It is the vasoconstriction that reduces the blood flow and therefore the swelling of the nasal passages in the inflammatory process. Due to increasing pseudoephedrine (Sudafed®) abuse (used to produce methamphetamine and as an athletic "performance enhancer"), phenylephrine has been used as a replacement in most OTC combination antihistamine/decongestant preparations. It is less effective in reducing rhinitis symptoms and should be used cautiously in patients with diabetes, heart disease, hyperthyroidism, or glaucoma. Owing to its vasoconstrictive properties, blood pressure should also be monitored. Topical decongestants such as nasal sprays can be used, but not too frequently, or rebound nasal congestion occurs. Topical decongestants may be helpful for increasing absorption of intranasal corticosteroids by opening up the nasal passageways.

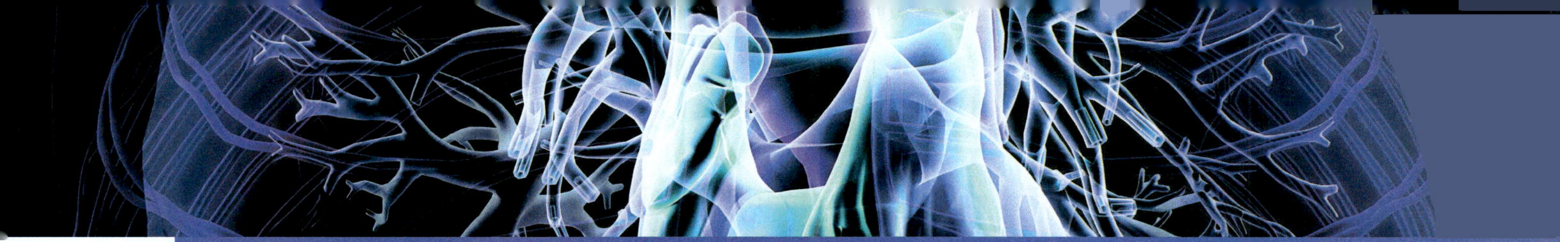

Summary

There are a variety of inflammatory pathways and mediators of inflammation. Anti-inflammatory drugs target these pathways to reduce the inflammatory response that leads to hyperactive airways, mucosal edema, and increased mucus production. Corticosteroids are among the mainstays of anti-inflammatory drugs. They vary in pharmacology and cardiorespiratory therapeutic applications. They have very important physiologic effects that must be balanced with their adverse effects. One method of achieving this balance is through careful attention to the route of administration and the dose and duration of use.

Antiasthmatic agents are used prophylactically to prevent the occurrence of the inflammatory response; their role is different than that of corticosteroids. Antiasthmatics include leukotriene modifiers and mast cell stabilizers.

Drugs that treat upper respiratory congestion are frequently used in combination with antiasthmatic and anti-inflammatory agents.

REVIEW QUESTIONS

1. The most common antibody involved in allergic asthma and rhinitis is
   (a) IgG
   (b) IgE
   (c) IgF
   (d) IgT
   (e) IgB
2. Corticosteroids can be classified as
   (a) mineralocorticoid
   (b) glucocorticoid
   (c) potassium sparing
   (d) glucose sparing
   (e) (a) and (b)
3. Routes used for corticosteroids include
   (a) inhalational
   (b) oral
   (c) intranasal
   (d) parenteral
   (e) all of the above

4. Check which indication would be appropriate for the following drugs.

prednisone	____ acute asthma treatment
	____ chronic asthma treatment
cromolyn	____ acute asthma treatment
	____ chronic asthma treatment
zileuton	____ acute asthma treatment
	____ chronic asthma treatment

5. Check which effect relates to each drug most closely.

β-agonists	____ block(s) histamine release
	____ block(s) histamine production
cromolyn	____ block(s) histamine release
	____ block(s) histamine production
corticosteroids	____ block(s) histamine release
	____ block(s) histamine production

6. Describe the early and late phases of inflammation and why they are important to pharmacotherapy.
7. Explain the role of the hypothalamic pituitary adrenal axis in terms the patient can understand.
8. List some factors that can influence mediator release from mast cells.
9. What are the important side effects of antihistamines?
10. A 57-year-old asthmatic presents with complaints of voice changes, hoarseness, white spots on his throat and tongue, and a "funny taste in his mouth." What type of medication and route do you suspect may be causing these complaints? What would the proposed treatment and follow-up education consist of?
11. A patient with a history of severe late-phase asthma response is prescribed an inhaled short-acting bronchodilator, corticosteroid, and mast cell stabilizer. Explain in lay terms when each of these drugs is indicated and highlight any special considerations concerning sequence, side effects, and what to expect as positive outcomes.

Case Study 1

A 24-year-old woman

A 24-year-old woman with persistent mild asthma has noticed that she is having more acute episodes, especially during the fall season. Her peak flows often drop to 50% of predicted during this period, and she has to use her quick-acting rescue bronchodilator frequently. This is the only respiratory medication she is taking. List other categories of respiratory medications that may help reduce the number and severity of her episodes. How and when would you suggest administering them?

Chapter 8

Antimicrobial Agents

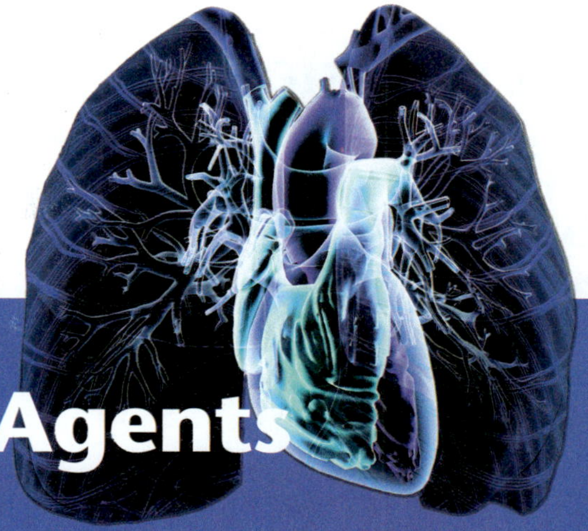

OBJECTIVES

Upon completion of this chapter you will be able to

- Understand the differentiation between gram-positive and gram-negative bacteria.
- Discuss implications of antimicrobial sensitivities and resistance patterns.
- Understand basic concepts of anti-infective therapy.
- Identify the basic classifications of antibiotic, antiviral, antitubercular, and antifungal drugs.
- Describe the role of aerosol anti-infective agents that may be administered directly into the lungs.

KEY TERMS

aerobic
anaerobic
antibiotic
bactericidal
bacteriostatic
broad-spectrum
chemotherapy
empiric
flora
Gram stain
narrow-spectrum
pathogen
resistance
susceptibility test

ABBREVIATIONS

AIDS	acquired immunodeficiency syndrome
ARDS	acute respiratory distress syndrome
CMV	cytomegalovirus
HIV	human immunodeficiency virus
MBC	minimum bactericidal concentration
MIC	minimum inhibitory concentration
MRSA	methicillin-resistant *Staphylococcus aureus*
NRTI	nucleoside reverse transcriptase inhibitor
NNRTI	non-nucleoside reverse transcriptase inhibitor
PBP	penicillin-binding protein
PJP	*Pneumocystis jiroveci* pneumonia (formerly called *Pneumocystis carinii pneumonia,* or PCP)
RSV	respiratory syncytial virus
SPAG	small-particle aerosol generator
TB	tuberculosis
TEM	transmission electron micrograph
VRE	vancomycin-resistant *Enterococcus*
WBC	white blood cell, or leukocyte

Clinical pearl

What's in a name? Antibiotics treat bacterial infections, so what about viral and fungal infections? A general and broader term for any agent used to treat infectious microorganisms is *anti-infective* or *antimicrobial,* and that comprises antibacterial, antiviral, and antifungal agents.

The antibiotic era began with the discovery of sulfanilamide in the early 1930s and, subsequently, penicillin in the 1940s. The availability and widespread use of antibiotics have been both a tremendous benefit and a burden to medical care. The beneficial effects are clear in the number of lives that have been spared from bacterial, viral, and fungal infections. The burden has presented itself with a vengeance in the last several decades with the evolution of pathogens that are able to resist the effects of many anti-infective agents.

This chapter provides a general overview of the principles of antibacterial, antiviral, and antifungal chemotherapy. Although this is a textbook on pharmacotherapy, it is still important to review basic microbiology principles and apply them to drug therapy, so they will be reviewed here. Although protozoa and algae are also microorganisms, the limited contact that most health professionals have with them will limit their discussion in this chapter. In Chapter 14 we will look at the "big picture" and discuss the applications of anti-infective agents for particular respiratory indications such as pneumonias, tuberculosis, cystic fibrosis, bronchitis, COPD, and human immunodeficiency virus (HIV).

8.1 GENERAL PRINCIPLES OF ANTI-INFECTIVE THERAPY

8.1a Terminology

Chemotherapy is the application of a chemical agent that has specific toxic effects on disease-producing organisms in a living animal. A chemotherapeutic substance derived from a living organism that kills microorganism growth is an **antibiotic.** *Antibiotic* is a general term derived from the Greek roots *anti-* (against) and *bios* (life). The term was originally used to distinguish chemical therapeutic agents from those that come from living organisms such as penicillin. Nowadays, drugs are made mainly in the lab, and we do not distinguish between chemical and naturally produced drugs. Traditionally, however, antibiotics are drugs used to treat bacterial infections.

8.1b The Infection Process

Before you make a decision about pharmacologic therapy for an infection, it is of course important to make sure an infection is present. Signs and symptoms of an infectious process in the respiratory system can include subjective complaints of dyspnea, malaise, weakness, pain, and fatigue. Objective findings of fever, hypoxemia, elevated white blood cell (WBC) count, changes on X-rays, and a dry or productive cough may also be present.

Once you have established the presence of an infectious process, you must determine where it is located. Is it a respiratory or urinary tract infection? Is it a localized or systemic infection? Infections can be localized to a certain area, such as the lungs, or may become systemic and spread via the bloodstream throughout the body. Systemic infections cause hemodynamic, hematologic, neurologic, cellular, and of course respiratory changes. For this discussion we are most interested in respiratory changes. These may include respiratory acidosis, tachypnea, hypoxemia, and even acute respiratory distress syndrome (ARDS). Systemic infections tend to require more aggressive treatment than local infections.

Clinical pearl

Fever alone is not diagnostic of a bacterial infection. Fever may be due to a virus or can even be caused by drugs or noninfectious processes such as inflammation. Elderly patients do not always exhibit a febrile response, or they may be on a drug that masks the fever. In older patients, one of the first clues to an infectious process may be a change in mental status.

8.1c Empiric Therapy

Pathogens are disease-causing microorganisms. What complicates the picture is that a microorganism may be present and not pathogenic in one individual but pathogenic in another. Likewise an organism in an individual may not normally be pathogenic, but changes in the person's immune system can make the same microorganism become a pathogen. Certain pathogens tend to be associated with certain sites of infection. See Table 8-1 for a list of pathogens that are common in respiratory infections. This knowledge can allow therapy to be **empiric**. "Empiric" implies that antibiotic therapy will be initiated on the basis of available data about the *most likely* cause of an infection in a given location (blood, skin, lungs, etc.).

Clinical pearl

Increased WBC count, or leukocytosis, can be a nonspecific sign of infection. Physicians frequently check to see if the patient has a "shift to the left." This refers to the presence of bands and immature neutrophils on the complete blood count (CBC) differential. This may suggest that the bone marrow is responding to an infection. It is important to remember that infection is not always associated with leukocytosis. Also the corticosteroid drugs frequently used in respiratory patients can mask infection.

TABLE 8-1 Suspected Respiratory Infection Pathogens

Infection	Suspected Pathogen
Pharyngitis	Group A *Streptococcus*
Bronchitis	Rhinovirus, influenza A and B
Acute sinusitis	*Streptococcus pneumoniae*
Chronic sinusitis	Anaerobes, *Staphylococcus aureus*
Pneumonia	
Community-acquired	*Streptococcus pneumoniae*
	Haemophilus influenzae
Health-care-associated	*Staphylococcus aureus*
	Gram-negative aerobic rods
Otitis media	*Streptococcus pneumoniae*
Epiglottitis	*Haemophilus influenzae*
Croup	Parainfluenza virus

The organism responsible for an infection may be a part of the patient's normal **flora**. Often these flora share a symbiotic relationship with the host. When something is altered that changes the symbiotic relationship, the organisms may flourish beyond the normal balance and become pathogenic. For example fungal overgrowth may result secondary to antimicrobial use (e.g., a vaginal yeast infection during or following a course of antimicrobial therapy for sinusitis), or secondary bacterial infection may result from a primary viral infection (e.g., *Streptococcus pneumoniae* pneumonia that develops following a primary infection with influenza). See Table 8-2 for a list of common flora found in a sputum sample.

TABLE 8-2 Common Normal Flora in Sputum Sample

Gram-Positive Cocci	Gram-Negative Bacilli	Gram-Negative Cocci
α-Hemolytic *Streptococci*	*Haemophilus influenzae*	*Moraxella catarrhalis*
Pneumococci		
Staphylococcus epidermidis		

time for review

What symptoms might lead you to suspect a pulmonary infection?

8.1d Classification of Bacteria

To understand bacterial pathogens, it is important to understand the classification of bacteria. One of the broadest classifications is based on need for oxygen. If a bacterium needs oxygen to survive, it is **aerobic**. If it does not, it is called **anaerobic**. Fewer antibiotic options are available to treat anaerobic infections, and those infections can be serious. Before you can determine which antibiotic should be used against a certain strain of bacteria, you must have a sample of the infected area tested in the laboratory, where it can be viewed under a microscope, allowing the bacteria to be further classified by its characteristic shape and staining properties. When you look under the microscope, bacteria can be round or rod-shaped and exhibit certain individual shapes that act like fingerprints to help you identify bacterial type. See Figure 8-1 for the various types of bacteria classified according to shape.

8.1e Identification of Pathogenic Organisms

In a clinical setting the physician may elect to collect samples of secretions or fluids from the suspected site of infection for microbiologic evaluation to identify the pathogen. Proper collection technique is important when collecting samples and can influence the validity of results. Even obtaining a sample (sputum, for example) from a patient can be harder than you might think. Starting an antibiotic before a proper sample is collected can hamper interpretation and identification of the pathogenic organism later on. Laboratory technicians can perform tests on these samples, such as the **Gram stain** and **susceptibility testing** (e.g., automated using machines such as the Vitek® 2), which can be used to guide treatment.

BVT Lab

Flashcards are available for this chapter at www.BVTLab.com.

FIGURE 8-1 Bacteria Morphology

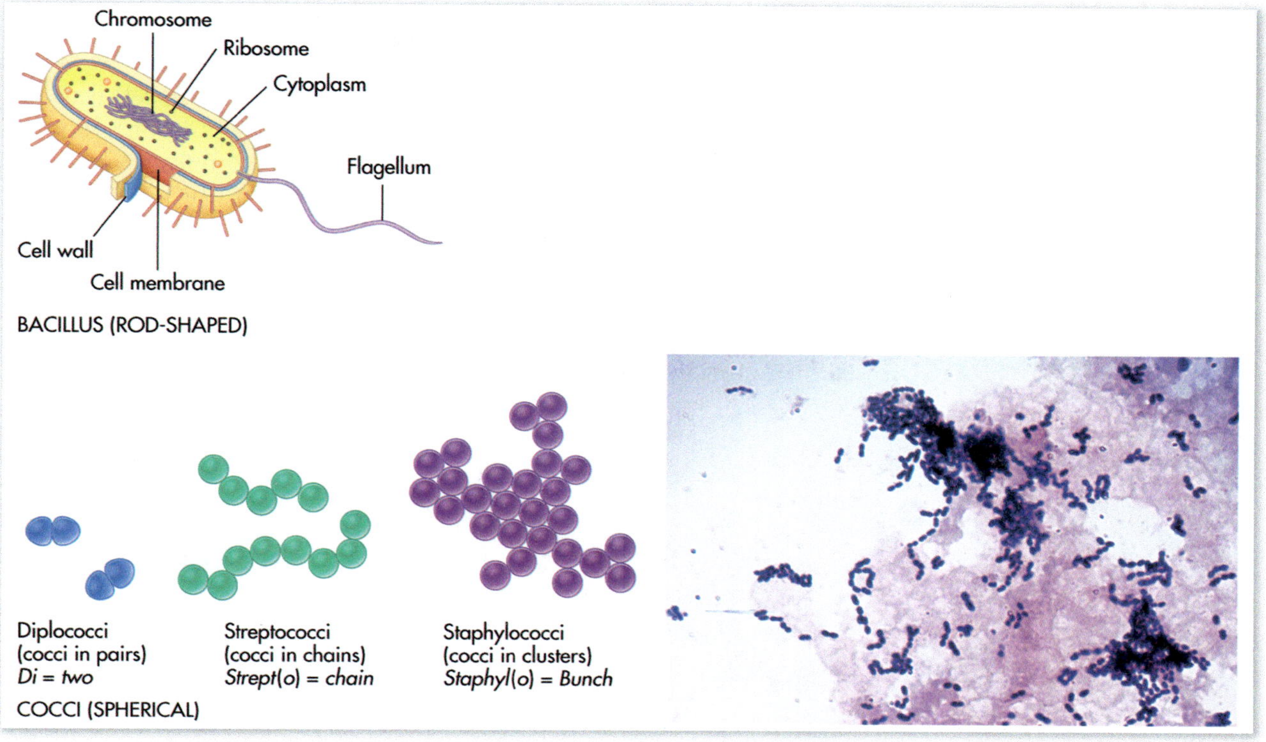

Gram Stain

The first test usually performed to classify bacteria is a Gram stain. Depending on their chemical makeup, microorganisms react differently when stained with colored dyes in a lab. Gram-positive bacteria stain purple, and gram-negative bacteria stain pink upon completion of the Gram stain procedure.

The Gram stain determines the basic characteristics of the pathogen (e.g., bacterial or not, shape, gram-positive or gram-negative). On the basis of this reaction, microorganisms are classified into broad categories as gram-positive [sometimes shown as Gram (+)] or gram-negative [Gram (–)]. See Table 8-3 for representative gram-positive and gram-negative bacteria.

TABLE 8-3 Representative Gram-Negative and Gram-Positive Bacteria

Gram-Negative Bacteria	Gram-Positive Bacteria
Pseudomonas	*Clostridia*
Bacteroides	*Listeria*
Campylobacter	*Streptococci*
Haemophilus	*Staphylococci*
Klebsiella	
Legionella	

The Gram stain allows differentiation between bacterial cell types on the basis of chemical differences in their cell walls. Gram-positive cell walls are composed of a uniform monolayer of peptidoglycans, while gram-negative cell walls are composed of multiple layers, including an outer lipopolysaccharide/lipoprotein membrane and an inner peptidoglycan layer. In all bacteria, the cell wall functions to maintain the integrity of the cell, allowing for growth in different environments. It also serves as the target and mechanism of action for several classes of antibacterial agents (e.g., β-lactams and glycopeptides). By knowing about the kind of cell wall, you are one step closer to customizing antibiotic treatment against the type of bacteria and the type of infection. See Figure 8-2 for the differences between gram-positive and gram-negative cell walls.

FIGURE 8-2 Bacterial Cell Walls

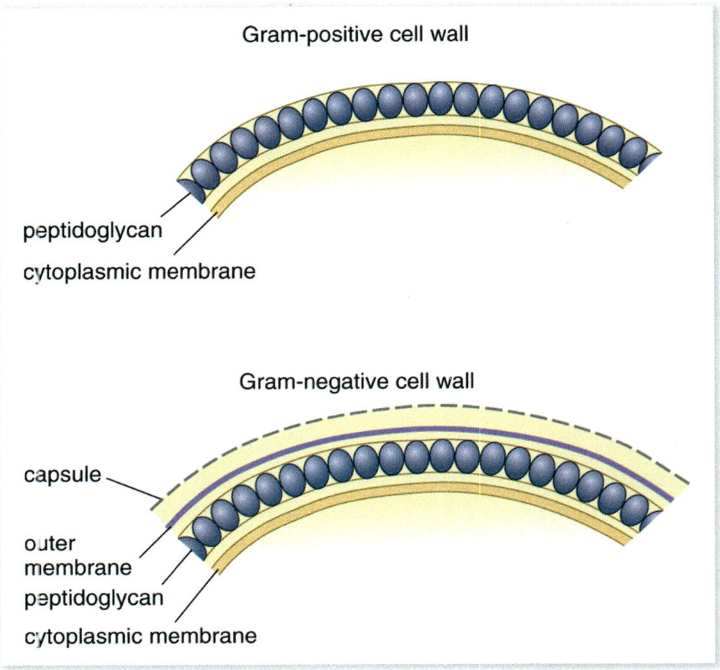

Clinical pearl

It is best to collect the sample of material from the infected area before an antibiotic is started; otherwise, you may not be able to grow and identify the pathogen. In patient care situations, antibiotics are often started before the results of laboratory tests are available. For serious infections it is important to start an antibiotic as soon as possible and to adjust the drug or dose once a more precise diagnosis is available.

Susceptibility Testing Methods

After an organism is identified, its susceptibility characteristics may be determined as a guide to antimicrobial therapy. If a microorganism is susceptible to an antibiotic, the antibiotic has a better chance of fighting the infection than if it is not susceptible. There are several methods by which microbial susceptibility may be determined. We will review disk diffusion and broth dilution methods.

Disk Diffusion This is a classic laboratory technique that provides qualitative information about susceptibility. The bacteria are cultured and grown on solid media (e.g., in a petri dish). Antibiotic-containing paper disks are then placed on the "lawn" of bacteria. After incubation, the areas without bacterial growth, known as the *zone of inhibition*, are measured and compared with established standards to determine whether it is sensitive (the antibiotic will work), intermediate (the antibiotic may or may not work), or resistant (the antibiotic will not work) (see Figure 8-3).

FIGURE 8-3 Disk Diffusion

Note: Notice the different sizes of the ring around each disc that was placed in the bacterial growth medium. The larger the ring of nongrowth, the more potent that drug is against that specific pathogen.

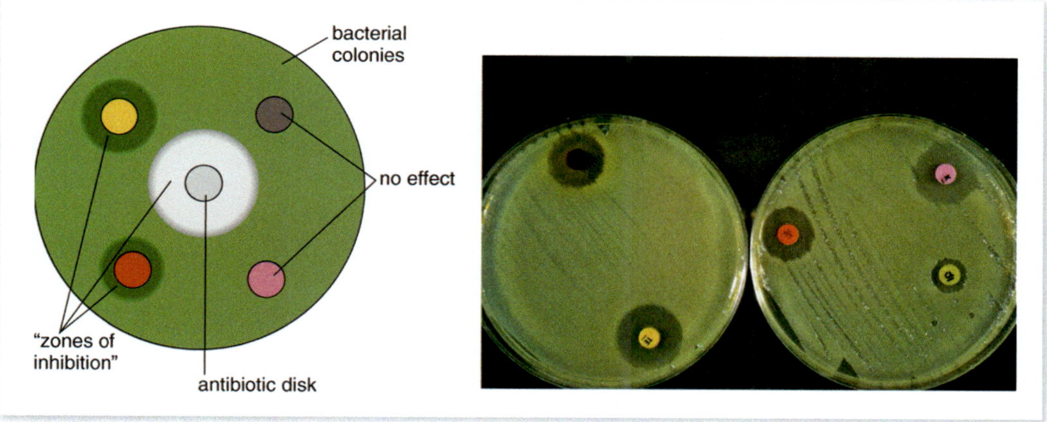

Broth Dilution There are two types of broth dilution broth macrodilution and broth microdilution. We will discuss the macro version first. Broth macrodilution is an uncommonly used clinical method for determining bacterial sensitivity to an antimicrobial agent. This type of testing is more quantitative than the disk diffusion method; that is, it can more accurately identify the concentration of a drug needed to inhibit organism growth. The organism is placed in various test tubes containing defined concentrations of an antimicrobial agent and a liquid growth medium (see Figure 8-4). The test tubes are incubated for a designated amount of time and inspected visually for organism growth. The test tube with the lowest concentration of antimicrobial agent that inhibits the growth of the organism is referred to as the *minimum inhibitory concentration* or MIC (test tube #4 in Figure 8-4). The MIC does not provide information about whether the organism is actually killed. The *minimum bactericidal concentration*, or MBC, determines this information. MBC determines the killing activity associated with an antimicrobial. The MBC is determined by taking a sample from each clear MIC tube and culturing it on agar plates. The concentration in which no significant bacterial growth is observed is the MBC. This method is labor intensive and prone to human error since the dilutions must be made manually.

The broth microdilution test uses commercially prepared panels or "wells" of different concentrations of antibiotics. The wells are inoculated with standard concentrations of bacteria and then incubated. Light diffusion through the broth may be inspected manually or by an automated photometer. The results are reported as an MIC. Since the wells are commercially available, this reduces the time involved and the potential for error.

FIGURE 8-4 Broth Dilution

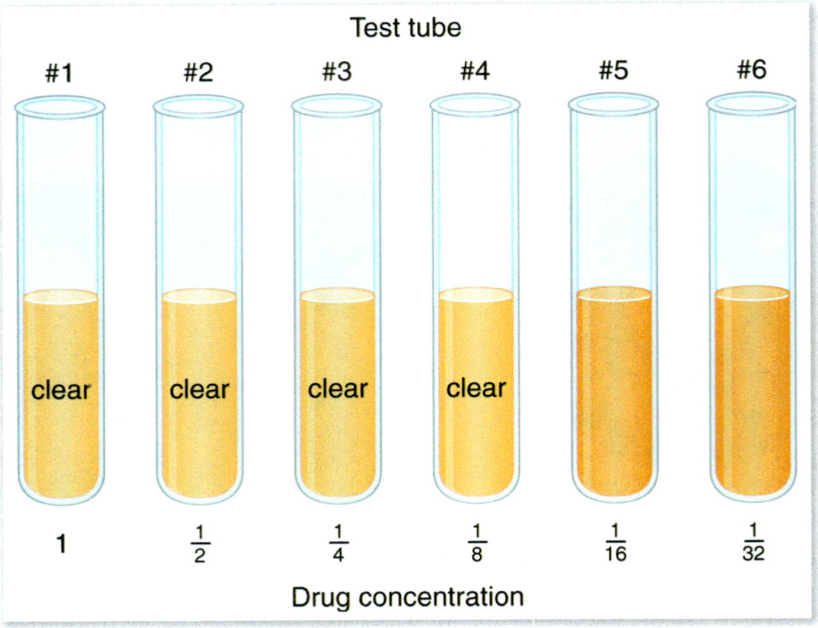

The concentrations of the antimicrobial agent used in these methods usually start several-fold higher than those concentrations that can safely be reached in the patient and are then serially diluted. If the MIC is identified at a concentration that cannot be achieved in the patient, then the organism is considered resistant. If the MIC is identified at a clinically achievable level, the organism is considered sensitive. If the MIC is identified at a level that may or may not be clinically achievable, the organism is considered intermediate.

Automated Instruments The FDA has approved four automated systems (e.g., Vitek® 2) that can provide susceptibility results faster than the preceding methods. The disadvantages of these systems include cost and the inability to detect certain types of bacterial resistance patterns.

8.1f Mechanisms of Resistance

The development of so-called *superbacteria* has been facilitated by the widespread misuse of antibacterial agents for infections of viral origin (e.g., common colds, influenza) and the continued use of **broad-spectrum** agents in the treatment of infections caused by single organisms, in which case a **narrow-spectrum** agent would do. Use of antibiotics that are effective against a wide range of microorganisms (broad-spectrum drugs) can result in overkill if a drug effective against fewer microorganisms (a narrow-spectrum drug) would be just as effective. Such use has resulted in selective evolution of bacteria that have adapted to become resistant to certain antibiotics, leaving physicians with limited options for the management of some infections. Viruses and fungi are also able to evolve into "superpathogens" when they are exposed to antivirals and antifungals, respectively.

Resistance to anti-infectives develops in many ways. For example the drug may actually be destroyed by bacterial enzymes. Bacteria that produce the enzyme β-lactamase can render cephalosporins and penicillins inactive. Another type of resistance occurs when some organisms develop alterations in the proteins that are binding sites for antibiotics. This prevents the attachment of the antibiotics to the bacteria.

Resistance also develops when patients take antibiotics when they are not clinically indicated. A rather common occurrence is for patients with acute bronchitis to be prescribed antibiotics even though the majority of cases are caused by viruses. Helping patients understand which infections require antibiotics (e.g., pneumonia, cellulitis) and which do not (e.g., acute bronchitis, colds) is an important role for every clinician.

Patient & Family Education

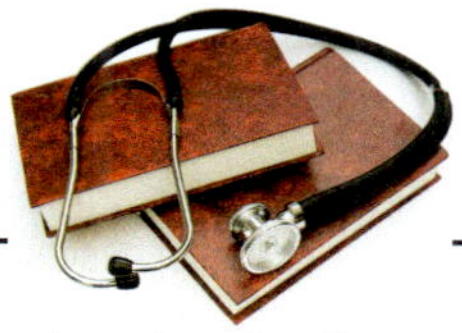

Every health-care professional should assist with educational efforts promoting the appropriate use of anti-infective drugs. Clinical development of this class of medications has slowed to a crawl. Companies are not willing to invest millions of dollars developing drugs that clinicians are told not to use until resistance becomes a problem.

time for review

What would you tell a patient who says she is disappointed with her physician who did not prescribe an antibiotic for her acute bronchitis?

8.1g Monitoring Anti-Infective Therapy

Anti-infective treatment can be monitored by clinical or microbiologic response. A clinical response means that the signs and symptoms of infection are gone, as evidenced by declining WBC count and fever elimination. A microbiologic response means the microorganism has been eliminated.

Following initiation of anti-infective therapy, it may be necessary to monitor drug levels for select agents. An example of an antibiotic class that is frequently monitored is the aminoglycosides. These agents have a narrow therapeutic index, meaning there is a fine line between therapeutic efficacy and toxicity.

time for review

What pulmonary signs and symptoms would you monitor to see whether an antibiotic therapy is being effective for a lung infection?

8.2 CLASSIFICATION OF ANTIBACTERIAL AGENTS

8.2a Bacteriostatic Versus Bactericidal

There are many ways to classify antibacterials. The first way relates back to the lab test discussion. Antibacterial drugs are classified as either bacteriostatic or bactericidal. **Bacteriostatic** agents inhibit the replication of microorganisms and prevent the growth of the organisms without destroying them. **Bactericidal** drugs actively kill bacteria. Most antibiotics are bacteriostatic at low concentrations, but at higher concentrations, bactericidal activity is more likely to be present. See Table 8-4 for some common bacteriostatic and bactericidal drugs.

TABLE 8-4 **Classes of Antibacterials**

Bactericidal	Bacteriostatic
penicillins	erythromycin
cephalosporins	tetracyclines
vancomycin	

8.2b Broad-Spectrum Versus Narrow-Spectrum

Antibacterials can also be classified according to whether they are broad- or narrow-spectrum. Broad-spectrum antibiotics are effective against a wider range of bacteria than are narrow-spectrum antibiotics. See Table 8-5 for examples of this classification system.

TABLE 8-5 **Antimicrobial Spectrum Classification**

Broad-Spectrum	Narrow-Spectrum
tetracyclines	penicillins
cefepime	erythromycin
meropenem	vancomycin

8.2c Based on Mechanism of Action

Just as there are many ways of classifying bacteria (aerobic/anaerobic, gram-positive or -negative), there are also multiple ways to classify antibacterial agents. One of the most commonly used antibacterial classifications is based on the mechanism of action of the anti-infective agent (see Table 8-6). Although this may seem most logical for pharmacology purposes, drugs are rarely selected clinically by their mechanism of action.

TABLE 8-6 Anti-Infective Classification Based on Mechanism of Action

Category	Mechanism of Action
I	Inhibit the synthesis of the bacterial cell wall or activate enzymes that disrupt the bacterial cell wall (penicillins, cephalosporins, vancomycin, antifungals)
II	Act directly on the cell membrane of the microorganism, causing leaking of the components of the cell (amphotericin B, nystatin)
III	Inhibit protein synthesis by disrupting functions of the bacterial ribosomes (macrolides, tetracyclines)
IV	Disrupt protein synthesis as well, but through a different process than category III (aminoglycosides)
V	Alter the synthesis and metabolism of nucleic acid (rifampin, metronidazole, quinolones)
VI	Inhibit metabolic processes fundamental to the microorganism (sulfonamides)
VII	Inhibit viral replication by binding to viral enzymes needed to make DNA (acyclovir)

8.2d Antibacterial Agents

Now we will give a brief description of each of the following antibacterial drug classifications: β-lactams, quinolones, aminoglycosides, glycopeptides, protein synthesis inhibitors, tetracyclines, folate inhibitors, oxazolidinones, quinupristin-dalfopristin, daptomycin, metronidazole, and antitubercular agents (see Table 8-7).

TABLE 8-7 Classes of Antibacterials

β-lactams	tetracyclines
aminoglycosides	glycopeptides
protein synthesis inhibitors	quinupristin-dalfopristin
folate inhibitors	metronidazole
quinolones	oxazolidinones
daptomycin	antitubercular agents

β-Lactams

β-Lactams include the following classes of drugs: penicillins, cephalosporins, monobactams (Azactam®), carbacephems, and carbapenems (imipenem, meropenem). All β-lactam antimicrobials act via inhibition of bacterial cell wall synthesis; to be effectively bactericidal, they require sensitive bacteria to be actively dividing. Their action is mediated through inhibition of enzymes that help build the bacteria's cell walls. These enzymes are generally referred to as penicillin-binding proteins (PBPs) and are located under the cell wall.

Bacteria have the ability to develop resistance to β-lactam antimicrobials via a number of mechanisms. One such mechanism of resistance is the production of β-lactamase (also known as penicillinase) enzymes, which destroy the β-lactam ring, rendering the drug inactive. This is because an intact chemical β-lactam ring is necessary for the antibiotics' bactericidal activity.

Clinical pearl

Penicillins are frequently used for prophylaxis to decrease the risk of infection in patients with conditions such as mechanical valves that may predispose them to infection. For example patients who have prosthetic heart valves should take amoxicillin 30 to 60 minutes before a dental procedure to prevent a cardiac infection. That infection could occur as a result of bacteria being spread through the blood from the mouth to a vulnerable site such as the heart with dental manipulation.

Penicillins The penicillins can be further subdivided into natural penicillins, penicillinase-resistant penicillins, aminopenicillins, extended-spectrum penicillins, and drugs combined with β-lactamase inhibitors. By changing the basic chemical structure, researchers have developed many penicillin derivatives. Combining a penicillin with a β-lactamase inhibitor prevents degradation of the penicillin by certain types of β-lactamases. Extended-spectrum penicillins are more resistant to inactivation by gram-negative bacteria. See Table 8-8 for commonly used penicillins.

Diarrhea is a main side effect of penicillins and most antibiotic classes. Otherwise penicillins have very little toxicity, although up to 10% of patients report an allergy to this drug class. In large studies, however, most people who report allergies to penicillins can still safely use them. The allergy can vary from an itchy, red, mild rash to wheezing and anaphylaxis.

Table 8-8 **Commonly Used Penicillins**

Type	Generic Name	Brand Name
natural penicillins	penicillin G	
	penicillin V	
aminopenicillins	ampicillin	
	amoxicillin	Moxatag®
penicillinase-resistant penicillins	dicloxacillin	
	nafcillin	Nallpen®
extended-spectrum penicillins	piperacillin	
drugs combined with β-lactamase inhibitors	amoxicillin-clavulanate	Augmentin®
	ampicillin-sulbactam	Unasyn®
	piperacillin-tazobactam	Zosyn®

Clinical pearl

A patient with a skin test–proven penicillin allergy has about a 2% possibility of also being allergic to a cephalosporin antibiotic.

Cephalosporins Cephalosporins basically have the same mechanism of action as penicillins. They differ from penicillins in their antibacterial spectrum, resistance to β-lactamase, and pharmacokinetics. One of the advantages of some cephalosporins over penicillins is that they have longer half-lives, which allows for infrequent outpatient parenteral dosing for chronic infections.

The cephalosporins are now divided into five generations. In general, as you move from one generation to the next, gram-negative activity increases while gram-positive activity declines. First-generation cephalosporins are used for community-acquired infections in ambulatory patients and mild to moderate infections in hospitalized patients. Second-generation cephalosporins are used for otitis media in pediatrics and for respiratory and urinary tract infections in hospitalized patients. Third-generation cephalosporins are used for serious community- and health care–associated infections. Because of their long half-lives, they are also used for ambulatory patients. Fourth- and fifth-generation cephalosporins are used for pneumonia, urinary tract infections, and skin infections that are acquired in health-care settings. Cephalosporins have the same side effects as penicillins and are less toxic than many antibiotics. See Table 8-9 for some commonly used cephalosporins.

Recently, the U.S. FDA approved two new cephalosporin-beta-lactamase inhibitor combinations to treat urinary tract and intra-abdominal infection. Ceftazidime-avibactam and ceftolozane-tazobactam have activity in the laboratory against aerobic gram-negative rods such as *Pseudomonas aeruginosa* as well as most extended-spectrum-beta-lactamase-producing gram-negative rods. Ceftazidime-avibactam also has activity against carbapenemase-producing gram-negative microbes. If these new combination cephalosporin drugs work well to combat infections against multidrug-resistant bacteria, they will be a welcome addition to our fight against multidrug-resistant organisms.

TABLE 8-9 Commonly Used Cephalosporins

Generation	Generic Name	Brand Name	Route of Administration
First	cephalexin	Keflex®	PO
	cefazolin	Ancef®	IM, IV
Second	cefaclor	Ceclor®	PO
	cefoxitin	Mefoxin®	IM, IV
	cefuroxime	Ceftin®, Zinacef®	PO, IM, IV
Third	ceftriaxone	Rocephin®	IM, IV
	ceftazidime	Fortaz®	IM, IV
	cefixime	Suprax®	PO
Fourth	cefepime	Maxipime®	IM, IV
Fifth	ceftaroline	Teflaro®	IV
Cephalosporin-beta-lactamase-inhibitors	ceftazidime-avibactam	Avycaz™	IV
	ceftolozane-tazobactam	Zerbaxa™	IV

Learning Hint

As indicated by the class name, monobactams have one (*mono*-) β-lactam ring.

Monobactams Aztreonam (Azactam®) is the only currently available antimicrobial in the new synthetic drug class called monobactams. Aztreonam is available parenterally and has a wide spectrum of activity against gram-negative organisms but little to none against gram-positive or anaerobic microorganisms. An advantage of this drug is its unlikely cross-allergenicity with other β-lactams. Side effects include swelling at the injection site, nausea, vomiting, and diarrhea.

Carbapenems Four carbapenems are currently available for use in the United States: imipenem (Primaxin®), meropenem (Merrem®), ertapenem (Invanz®), and doripenem (Doribax®). They are so similar in chemical class that they are frequently lumped together for discussion. They have the same pharmacologic activity as other β-lactam antibiotics and are broad-spectrum and active against many organisms that are resistant to penicillins, cephalosporins, and aminoglycosides. For this reason they are usually reserved for serious infections. Side effects include nausea, which may be related to the infusion rate, seizures, dizziness, and confusion.

Now that we have discussed the β-lactams in total, we can move on to another classification of antibacterials.

Quinolones

Quinolones are bactericidal. They block an enzyme responsible for DNA growth. Human cells do not have this enzyme, so the drug is specific for microorganisms. This drug class has been available for years as a quinolone called nalidixic acid (no longer available) that was used selectively for urinary tract infections caused by gram-negative pathogens.

There are many drug interactions with quinolones. These drugs should not be taken with antacids, because antacids may interfere with quinolone absorption. Quinolones may increase theophylline toxicity. Quinolones, like many antibiotics, are phototoxic, and patients should use sunscreen when taking them. Tendon rupture and tendonitis are reported uncommonly with the fluoroquinolones. The FDA recommends contacting a physician at the first sign of swelling, inflammation, or tendon pain. Other quinolone side effects include nausea, dizziness, and an unpleasant taste.

Common fluoroquinolones include

- ciprofloxacin (Cipro®)
- levofloxacin (Levaquin®)
- moxifloxacin (Avelox®)
- gemifloxacin (Factive®)

Clinical pearl

Newer quinolone agents have a fluorine group chemically attached and are called *fluoroquinolones*. The chemical change allows the antibiotic to penetrate bacteria better than plain quinolones can. Fluoroquinolones are used for lower respiratory tract infections.

Clinical pearl

Quinolones penetrate bone and are good for joint infections. They should not be used, or used only with caution, in children because they can inhibit cartilage formation.

Aminoglycosides

Aminoglycosides are used in many serious infections for gram-negative coverage. They are frequently used concurrently with another drug, such as ampicillin, to fight gram-positive organisms. They are bactericidal and dosed on the basis of weight, renal function, and serum blood levels. Because they are ototoxic and nephrotoxic, they are not used for infections that could be treated just as effectively with an alternative agent. Aerosolized tobramycin can improve lung function in cystic fibrosis patients who are chronically infected with *Pseudomonas aeruginosa*. Aminoglycosides may increase muscle weakness because of a potential blockage of signals at the neuromuscular junction. Examples of aminoglycosides include

- amikacin
- gentamicin (Garamycin®)
- tobramycin

Glycopeptides

Vancomycin (Vancocin®), dalbavancin (Dalvance®), oritavancin (Orbactiv®), and telavancin (Vibativ®) are bactericidal glycoprotein antibiotics. They bind to the cell walls of reproducing microorganisms and inhibit cell wall synthesis. The cell then becomes susceptible to lysis. This class of medications is indicated for infections caused by gram-positive cocci. They are frequently reserved for confirmed or suspected methicillin-resistant *Staphylococcus aureus* (MRSA) infections. Hospitals closely monitor their vancomycin sensitivity patterns, because there are few alternatives should resistance become prevalent. Vancomycin can cause side effects with intravenous administration such as hypotension, nephrotoxicity, and ototoxicity. Rapid infusion can cause a histamine release and flushed skin, or what is called "red man syndrome" (really!). Vancomycin is monitored by serum drug levels. The other drugs in this class have a similar side effect profile except they may cause an elevation in liver enzymes. It is worth mentioning that oritavancin has a very long half-life (245 hours) and is used as a single dose to treat skin infections.

Protein Synthesis Inhibitors

Protein synthesis inhibitors include macrolides and tetracyclines. Macrolides are commonly used to treat pulmonary infections. Erythromycin is in the macrolide class and may be bactericidal or bacteriostatic, depending on the organism's susceptibility and the drug concentration. Erythromycin may cause stomach distress and diarrhea, although the newer macrolide azithromycin causes less of this. Erythromycin interacts with theophylline to decrease theophylline metabolism; so doses of theophylline need to be adjusted when erythromycin is used concurrently. Because macrolides are commonly prescribed for respiratory infections, this interaction should be closely monitored. Common macrolides include

- erythromycin (E-mycin®)
- clarithromycin (Biaxin®)
- azithromycin (Zithromax®)
- telithromycin (Ketek®)

Tetracyclines

The tetracyclines have been available for approximately 50 years and have a relatively broad spectrum of activity, including against gram-positive and gram-negative aerobic and anaerobic bacteria as well as mycoplasmas, some mycobacteria, chlamydia, and spirochetes. They are produced by soil organisms and are bacteriostatic. Uses include treatment for acne, Rocky Mountain spotted fever, Lyme disease, and as part of a treatment regimen for peptic ulcer disease.

Tetracycline cannot be taken with antacids, iron, or dairy products, because they will bind with each other and not be absorbed. Pregnant women and children under the age of 9 years should not take tetracycline, because permanent tooth discoloration could result. Tigecycline (Tygacil®) is a new parenteral derivative of minocycline. Common tetracyclines include

- doxycycline (Vibramycin®)
- minocycline (Minocin®)
- tigecycline (Tygacil®)

Clinical pearl

Many people save antibiotics left over from a previous infection for another time. Most drugs simply lose effectiveness when they become out of date; tetracycline, however, can cause a serious renal problem if it is used after its expiration date.

Folate Inhibitors

Sulfonamides are classic examples of folate inhibitors and are considered bacteriostatic. They block a step in the synthesis of folic acid and destroy bacteria. The most common side effects are rash, drug fever, and blood complications. Their main use is in the treatment of uncomplicated urinary tract infections. Sulfonamides are frequently used in combination with trimethoprim for *Pneumocystis jiroveci*. This will be discussed more in Chapter 14. Common sulfonamides include

- sulfamethoxazole/trimethoprim (Bactrim®, Septra®)
- sulfadiazin

Clinical pearl

Patients taking sulfonamide antibiotics should drink six to eight glasses of water daily to prevent the drug from depositing as crystals in the urine or kidneys.

BVT Lab

Visit www.BVTLab.com to explore the student resources available for this chapter.

Oxazolidinones

Linezolid (Zyvox®) and tedizolid (Sivextro®) are the only oxazolidinones clinically available at present in the United States. The oxazolidinones are synthetic agents with a novel mechanism of action of inhibiting the bacterial translation (synthesis of essential proteins) process. This class is mainly bacteriostatic and active primarily against gram-positive agents. Linezolid is available orally and IV for treatment of vancomycin-resistant *Enterococcus faecium* infections, community-acquired pneumonia, nosocomial pneumonia (MRSA), and skin and soft tissue infections. Tedizolid currently only has skin and skin structure infections as FDA-approved indications. Complete blood counts should be monitored weekly in patients on either agent. Myelosuppression (anemia, leukopenia, pancytopenia, thrombocytopenia) has been reported especially in patients on prolonged therapy.

Quinupristin-Dalfopristin

Quinupristin-dalfopristin (Synercid®) is a parenteral product comprised of two drugs from the chemical class called streptogramins. Both are bacteriostatic against gram-positive bacteria. They can be bactericidal against *Staphylococci*, including the methicillin-resistant strains. They may have a role in infections associated with vancomycin-resistant *Enterococcus* (VRE).

Daptomycin

Daptomycin (Cubicin®) is a lipopetide bactericidal antibiotic that works by depolarizing the cell membrane. It is active against gram-positive organisms such as MRSA and VRE. It is useful to treat MRSA blood stream infections but cannot be used to treat pneumonias since its activity is inhibited by pulmonary surfactant. This drug may cause a peripheral neuropathy or myopathy, and close clinical monitoring for these conditions is warranted.

Metronidazole

Metronidazole (Flagyl®) is a synthetic drug with an anaerobic spectrum of activity (e.g., *Clostridium difficile*). It is part of one antibiotic treatment for peptic ulcer disease. Side effects include a metallic taste and intolerance to alcohol. Patients on metronidazole should not drink alcohol for up to 3 days after discontinuing the drug, to prevent adverse effects of nausea and flushing that may result from the combination. This is similar to the reaction alcoholics have if prescribed the alcohol-deterrent disulfiram (Antabuse®) as an aid to alcoholism recovery.

Clinical pearl

Rifampin, used to treat TB, can cause urine, feces, saliva or sputum, and tears to be colored red-orange. Patients should be warned to expect this and should be cautioned about staining soft contact lenses. Is it any wonder compliance may not be good with TB drugs, considering these side effects?

Antitubercular Agents

Tuberculosis (TB) is a disease that is usually confined to the lungs (see Figure 8-5 for an X-ray of a TB patient). For this reason it is an important part of this book and will be elaborated upon more in Chapter 14; we will merely introduce it here. TB can be symptomatic or asymptomatic, but it is a chronic disease requiring months of treatment with the appropriate anti-infective.

Drug-resistant TB can occur because of suboptimal treatment of tuberculosis. At diagnosis most TB is susceptible to the chosen drugs, but because of the long duration of treatment needed and resultant noncompliance with drugs, resistant TB often develops. This has the potential to become a public health emergency, especially because there are currently no new drugs for TB in clinical research trials.

FIGURE 8-5 **Chest X-ray Showing Tuberculosis**

Tubercular nodular lesions can be seen in the right upper lobe.

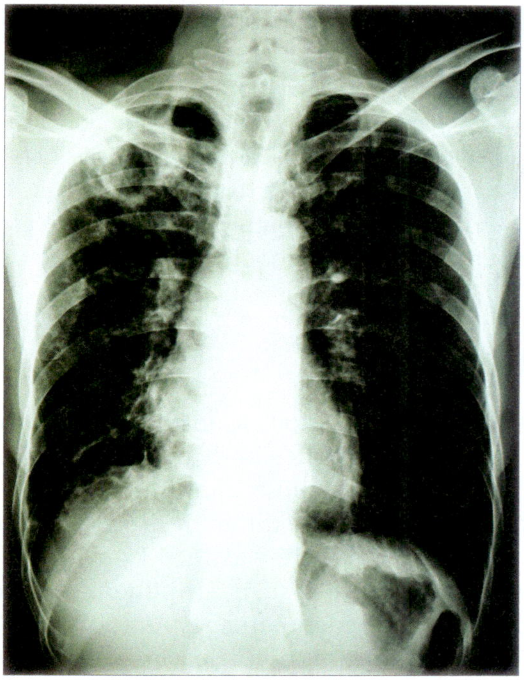

Source: Thinkstock

TB treatment consists of a combination of drugs categorized as first-line drugs. Second-line drugs are reserved for treatment-resistant TB or drug intolerance. Second-line drugs are secondary because they are either more toxic or have limited clinical experience in TB treatment. See Table 8-10 for a list of drugs used to treat TB.

TABLE 8-10 **Drugs Used to Treat Tuberculosis**

	Generic Name	Brand Name
Primary	isoniazid	
	rifampin	Rimactane®
	pyrazinamide	Tebrazid®
	ethambutol	Myambutol®
	rifabutin	Mycobutin®
	bedaquiline	Sirturo®
Secondary	streptomycin	
	cycloserine	Seromycin®
	ethionamide	Trecator®

Isoniazid can cause liver toxicity, which is enhanced when alcohol is used concurrently. Patients frequently complain of a peripheral neuropathy with isoniazid or ethionamide. Ethambutol may cause optic changes. Bedaquiline is a recently approved addition to our anti-TB armamentarium. It has unique activity to help combat pulmonary multidrug-resistant TB as part of combination therapy.

Life Span Considerations

Young and old patients alike should keep up-to-date lists of true medication allergies. If a patient states that he or she is allergic to a particular antibiotic, for example, asking a few additional questions may help clarify the reaction as an adverse effect or intolerability rather than a true allergy. Hives, hypotension, and difficulty breathing should be taken seriously. Patient reports of nausea, vomiting, and diarrhea are adverse reactions and not true allergies.

8.3 ANTIVIRALS

Clinical pearl

Herpes and HIV can be in the cell, latent and undetectable, and surface long after the initial transmission. The role of antivirals is to search for and destroy the virus in its host cell while not interfering with the normal function of that host cell.

Viruses are the most common infectious agents in humans. A virus is an *obligate* parasite, which means it can only live and replicate in a living host cell. This makes it difficult to kill the virus without harming the host cell. Because this is a different situation than with bacteria, different drugs are needed to treat viruses than are used for bacteria. Viruses are classified by whether they contain RNA or DNA. RNA viruses cause diseases such as influenza, polio, HIV, rabies, and encephalitis. DNA viruses cause adenovirus respiratory disease, papilloma warts, herpes simplex, and Epstein–Barr mononucleosis (see Figure 8-6).

Immunization has been the mainstay treatment of many of the viral infections such as influenza, measles, mumps, polio, and rubella. Only recently have more antiviral drugs become available for diseases such as influenza. Viral infections are classified by their severity, length of time present, and body parts affected. Infections such as the common cold and influenza can be acute and resolve quickly; other infections can be slow and have a progressive course, as with HIV. Viral infections can be local and affect just the respiratory tract, for example, or generalized and spread throughout the bloodstream. Some viruses can be dormant and then under certain conditions reproduce again. This is called *latency* and implies that a disease may surface years after transmission or after the initial breakout.

FIGURE 8-6 A Virus

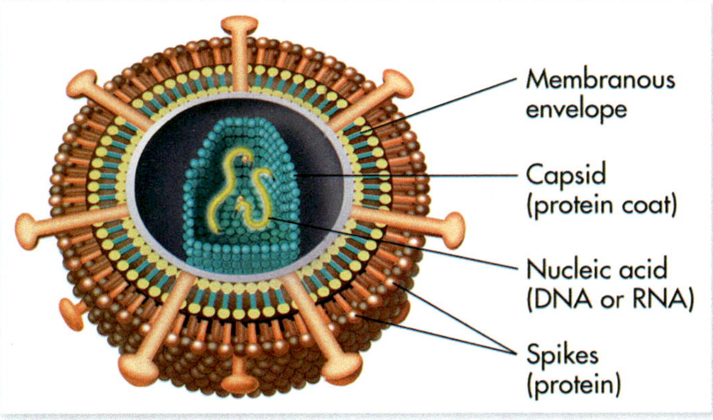

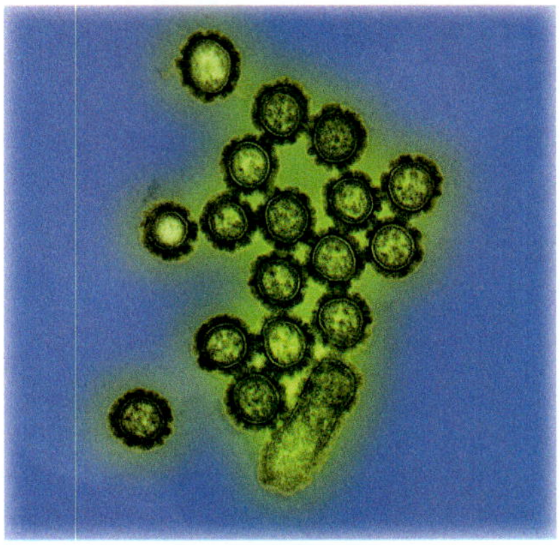

H1N1 Virus
Source: National Institute of Allergy and Infectious Diseases

8.3a Antivirals to Treat Herpes

Herpes is a DNA virus that can cause the vesicular skin eruptions most people know as fever blisters or cold sores. It can also cause genital herpes, which can be spread by sexual contact with an infected person. The main drugs to treat herpes are acyclovir (Zovirax®), famciclovir (Famvir®), and valcyclovir (Valtrex®). These drugs interfere with viral DNA and inhibit viral replication. They are also used to treat post-herpetic neuralgia, or shingles.

Zanamivir and oseltamivir have been marketed as drugs to cut the duration of the flu by at least 1 day and maybe 3. These two drugs are called neuraminidase inhibitors. They are indicated for treatment of both influenza A and influenza B. Zanamivir is available as an inhaled medication delivered by a breath-activated "diskhaler." It has been associated with adverse respiratory effects in patients with airway disease. These agents are most effective in preventing influenza if started within 30 hours of symptoms or exposure.

Clinical Pearl

Oral or inhaled medications to treat flu do not replace vaccination. In cases when the flu isolates are the same ones covered by the vaccine, flu treatment with these antivirals may be less significant.

8.3b Antivirals to Treat Respiratory Syncytial Virus

Respiratory syncytial virus (RSV) is a pathogen that causes bronchiolitis and pneumonia and is a major cause of acute respiratory disease in children (see Figure 8-7). Ribavirin is an antiviral with inhibitory activity against RSV, influenzas A and B, and herpes simplex. Although its mechanism is not known for sure, it inhibits essential nucleic acid formation in viral particles. Severe cases of RSV are treated with aerosolized ribavarin (Virazole®). Ribavirin is administered through a small-particle aerosol generator (SPAG-2). It can be given as a continuous aerosolization by mixing 6 g of ribavirin with 300 ml of preservative-free sterile water or normal saline and nebulized for 12 to 18 hours daily for 3 to 7 days. Because aerosolized ribavirin can escape into the air around the patient, visitors and staff may be exposed to the drug, and because of its teratogenicity, this is a concern. The American Academy of Pediatrics only recommends ribavirin for immunosuppressed patients with severe RSV disease. It should not be mixed with any other aerosol medications. See Table 8-11 for common antivirals used to treat herpes, influenza, and RSV.

Clinical Pearl

Sometimes worsening of respiratory status occurs with ribavirin. For patients who require assisted ventilation, drug deposition in the ventilator circuit and valves may interfere with ventilation.

FIGURE 8-7 Respiratory Syncytial Virus

Colorized transmission electron micrograph (TEM) of the respiratory syncytial virus (RSV).

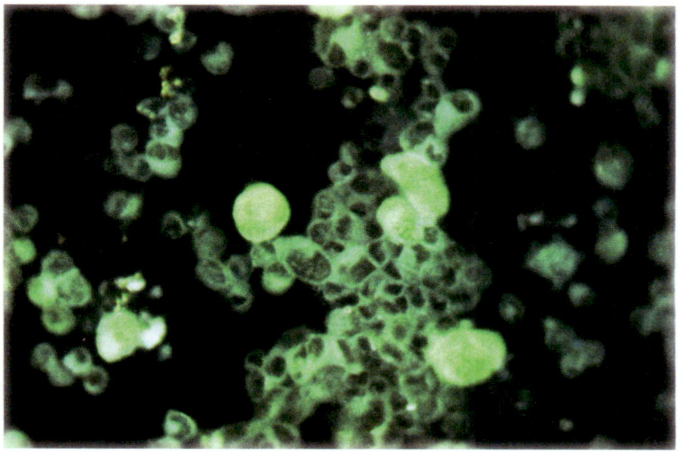

Source: CDC/ Dr. Craig Lyerla

TABLE 8-11 Common Antivirals

Disease	Generic Name	Brand Name
Herpes	acyclovir	Zovirax®
	famciclovir	Famvir®
	valcyclovir	Valtrex®
Influenza	zanamivir (inhaled)	Relenza®
	oseltamivir	Tamiflu®
	amantadine	Symmetrel®
	rimantidine	Flumadine®
RSV	ribavirin	Virazole®

8.3c Antivirals to Treat Acquired Immunodeficiency Syndrome (AIDS)

Learning Hint

Even though PJP is discussed with AIDS in this book, always remember that PJP can occur in non-AIDS patients as well.

Untreated, AIDS is a progressively fatal disease caused by the retrovirus, human immunodeficiency virus (HIV). Treatment of HIV comprises several different drugs to suppress the virus. These drugs are termed *antiretrovirals*. Pharmacologic classes include nucleoside reverse transcriptase inhibitors, non-nucleoside reverse transcriptase inhibitors, protease inhibitors, integrase strand transfer inhibitor, fusion inhibitor, and CCR5 antagonists (see Table 8-12). In addition several HIV vaccines are undergoing clinical testing. AIDS depresses the immune system and allows infections to develop. These can include herpes simplex virus, cytomegalovirus (CMV), malignant Kaposi sarcoma, and commonly *Pneumocystis jiroveci*, which can lead to severe pneumonia in AIDS patients. Because of their relationship to the respiratory system, AIDS and *Pneumocystis jiroveci* pneumonia (PJP) are discussed in Chapter 14.

TABLE 8-12 Common Antiretrovirals (for a more complete listing visit www.aidsinfo.gov)

Antiretroviral	Generic Name	Brand Name
Nucleoside reverse transcriptase inhibitors (NRTIs)	abacavir	Ziagen®
	didanosine (ddI)	Videx®
	lamivudine (3TC)	Epivir®
	zidovudine (AZT)	Retrovir®
Non-nucleoside reverse transcriptase inhibitors (NNRTIs)	efavirenz	Sustiva®
	nevirapine	Viramune®
Protease inhibitors	indinavir	Crixivan®
	ritonavir	Norvir®
	atazanavir	Reyataz®

8.4 ANTIFUNGALS

A fungus is reproduced by spores, has a rigid cell wall, and has no chlorophyll. Fungi include mushrooms, yeasts, and molds. Fungi have ergosterol instead of the cholesterol found in human cells. Antifungals work by preventing the making of ergosterol, which is a building block for the cell membranes. Fungal infections are most likely to develop in patients with impaired immune systems. In addition antibiotics can destroy the body's natural flora, which can result in an opportunistic fungal infection.

Some examples of fungal infections include ringworm, athlete's foot, and "jock itch," all of which can be treated with topical antifungal creams. More serious fungal infections include histoplasmosis within the lung and *Candida albicans* (thrush) in the oral cavity. These can progress to systemic infections (see Figure 8-8).

Clinical pearl

There's a fungus among us. Fungal infections are frequently asymptomatic and may be more of a cosmetic issue than a health-care issue, as in the case of nail infections.

FIGURE 8-8 Types of Fungi and a Newborn with Oral Thrush

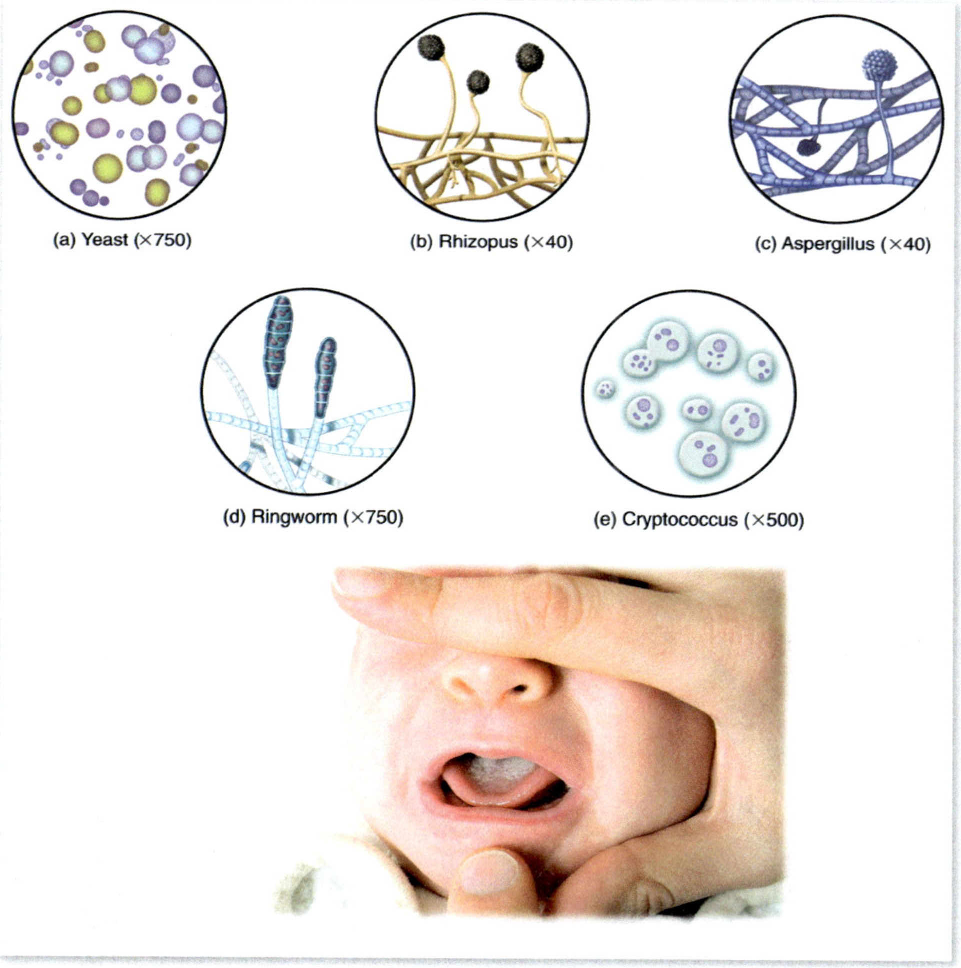

Nystatin is an antifungal agent available as an oral suspension and as a topical cream; it is used to treat *Candida albicans* and skin fungal infections. Azole antifungal agents include miconazole (Monistat®), which is used as a topical treatment for superficial or vaginal yeast infections, and fluconazole (Diflucan®) or voriconazole (Vfend®), which can be administered IV or orally for systemic fungal infections. Other systemic antifungal agents include the echinocandins caspofungin (Cancidas®), anidulafungin (Eraxis®), and micafungin (Mycamine®).

The echinocandins are generally reserved for *Candida* species that are resistant to fluconazole.

Amphotericin B deoxycholate was used for decades as the standard drug treatment for serious *Candida* infections. When amphotericin B is given intravenously, it requires close clinical monitoring. Toxicity can include electrolyte abnormalities and renal damage. Due to this toxicity several lipid-based products were developed that have much less toxicity but are significantly more expensive. See Table 8-13 for some common antifungal agents.

Clinical pearl

It's easy to remember the class of antifungals by just looking at the generic name. Note that the azoles end in *-azole* and the echinocandins end in *-fungin*.

TABLE 8-13 Common Antifungals

Generic Name	Brand Name	Indication/Route
nystatin		Topical for skin candidiasis or oral thrush
miconazole	Monistat®	Topical preparations for cutaneous yeast or vaginitis infections
amphotericin B		IV
liposomal amphotericin B	AmBisome®	IV
fluconazole	Diflucan®	PO and IV
voriconazole	Vfend®	PO and IV
ketoconazole	Nizoral®	Local scalp shampoo or PO
caspofungin	Cancidas®	IV
anidulafungin	Eraxis®	IV
micafungin	Mycamine®	IV

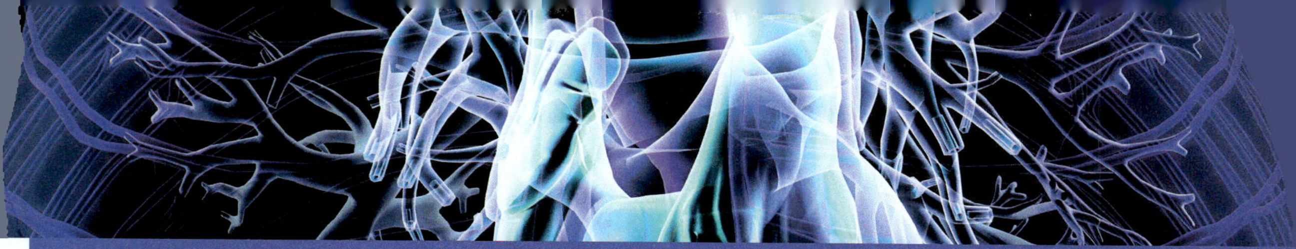

Summary

Health-care practitioners must be able to identify signs and symptoms of infection and be familiar with medical indications for antibiotics. Just as important, if not more important, is knowledge of indications *not* to use antibiotics. Currently available drugs to prevent or treat infection fall into several different classifications and vary in their degree of effectiveness against different microorganisms. Several factors are involved in appropriate antibiotic drug selection, some of which require incorporation of microbiologic principles and effective patient monitoring of signs and symptoms. This chapter provides a foundation for applying these drugs to clinical practice in the treatment of respiratory infectious diseases, which will be presented in more detail in Chapter 14.

REVIEW QUESTIONS

1. Bacteria are classified on the basis of
   (a) dilution of serum
   (b) staining properties
   (c) need for water to survive
   (d) location in the body
   (e) resistance patterns
2. β-Lactam antibiotics include
   (a) penicillins
   (b) cephalosporins
   (c) monobactams
   (d) carbapenems
   (e) all of the above
3. Antivirals for flu treatment
   (a) replace vaccination
   (b) are only administered IV
   (c) are most effective 3 days after flu presentation
   (d) may decrease the duration of the flu
   (e) also treat RSV
4. Viruses
   (a) are the least common infectious agents in humans
   (b) are classified by cell wall type and shape
   (c) are responsible for symptomatic TB
   (d) can be dormant or latent
   (e) inhibit further viral replication

5. White blood cell (WBC) count elevation
   (a) is always associated with an infection
   (b) equals normal flora in sputum
   (c) can be present without an infectious process
   (d) determines the need for bactericidal or bacteriostatic therapy
   (e) is always associated with TB
6. How do a bactericidal and a bacteriostatic antibiotics differ?
7. Why is resistance a problem with antibiotics?
8. Describe the role of empiric antimicrobial therapy.
9. How would you explain the difference between a broad-spectrum and a narrow-spectrum antibiotic?

Case Study 1

A 68-year-old man

A 68-year-old man is hospitalized for possible pneumonia. His past medical history is significant for three outpatient courses of antibiotics over the last 2 months with tetracycline, erythromycin, and levofloxacin. However he has stated that on some occasions he stopped taking the antibiotic prematurely because he felt better, and on other occasions he discontinued antibiotic use owing to an upset stomach. What type of education would you give this patient? What signs and symptoms would you expect with his pneumonia? What lab and diagnostic tests would confirm the pneumonia? Finally why may this patient be more difficult to treat with anti-infective agents?

Chapter 9

Cardiac Agents

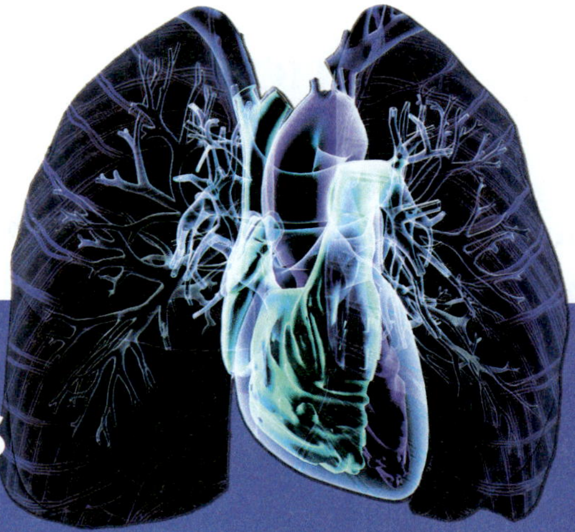

OBJECTIVES

Upon completion of this chapter you will be able to

- Define key terms related to cardiac agents.
- Relate cardiovascular physiology to pharmacologic treatments.
- Describe indications and pharmacologic effects of antiarrhythmics, ACE inhibitors, angiotensin-receptor blockers, inotropic agents, antidiabetic agents, antilipidemics, and vasodilators.
- Understand the role of pharmacologic therapy in arrhythmias, heart failure, acute coronary syndrome, myocardial infarction, hyperlipidemia, diabetes, and angina.
- Discuss the relationship between diabetes and cardiovascular disease.
- Describe the pharmacologic treatment for diabetes.

KEY TERMS

action potential
afterload
angina
arrhythmia
automaticity
chronotropic
conduction
dromotropic
inotropic
preload
proarrhythmia
refractory period
vasodilator

ABBREVIATIONS

ACC American College of Cardiology
ACE angiotensin-converting enzyme
ACLS Advanced Cardiac Life Support
ACS acute coronary syndrome
AHA American Heart Association
ARB angiotensin-receptor blocker
AV atrioventricular
BAR bile acid resin
BNP β-natriuretic peptide
Ca calcium
CHD cardiovascular heart disease
DPP dipeptidyl peptidase
EDRF endothelium-derived relaxing factor
ECG/EKG electrocardiogram
GLP glucagon-like peptide
HDL high-density lipoprotein
HF heart failure
HR heart rate
ICD implantable cardioverter-defibrillator
ISDN isosorbide dinitrate
ISMN isosorbide mononitrate
K potassium
LDL low-density lipoprotein
MI myocardial infarction
Na sodium
NCEP National Cholesterol Education Program
NPH neutral protamine of Hagedorn
PCI percutaneous coronary intervention
PVC premature ventricular contraction
SA sinoatrial
TLC therapeutic lifestyle change (also means "tender loving care"—which is what you should provide for your heart)

The heart, lungs, and kidneys are intricately related, which explains the need for and cohesiveness of a textbook on cardiopulmonary pharmacology. For example patients with chronic lung disease often have chronic hypoxemia. The heart must compensate for the low levels of oxygen by several mechanisms that all increase the cardiac workload. Over time this can lead to heart disease secondary to the underlying lung disease.

The renal system is intricately related to the heart and lungs. The kidneys' regulation of fluid balance can affect the fluid volume and thus the pressures within the cardiovascular system. Too much fluid retention can build up and eventually back up into the lungs and severely impair vital diffusion of oxygen. If the kidneys do not maintain proper acid–base or electrolyte balance, serious cardiac arrhythmias may develop.

If the lungs do not maintain adequate oxygen levels, the heart may not function properly and cardiac output may decrease. Because the kidneys require adequate blood supply (perfusion) to function properly, they may be severely affected. As you can see any dysfunction in the heart, lungs, or kidneys may have major implications for other systems.

The cardiovascular system's primary role is to ensure the vital circulation of blood throughout the body. To accomplish this, three basic components are required. First a strong, functioning pump (the heart) must generate the pressure needed to push the blood through the system. Second a piping system (the vessels) must be able to transport the blood and appropriately handle and react to changes of pressures within the system. Finally the blood itself must flow freely through blood vessels and clot when the need occurs. This chapter focuses on pharmacologic agents that can ensure proper functioning of the heart and related systems. Chapter 10 focuses on drugs that affect the blood vessels and blood itself.

This chapter discusses the most common cardiopulmonary pharmacotherapies. The emphasis is on the treatment of the most common cardiac conditions: heart failure (HF), cardiac arrhythmias, myocardial infarction (MI), and angina. Pharmacologic classes discussed include antiarrhythmics, angiotensin-converting enzyme inhibitors, angiotensin-receptor blockers, inotropes, vasodilators, antidiabetic agents, and antilipidemics. The use of diuretics with heart failure is discussed in this chapter, with more information on the use of diuretics with hypertension provided in Chapter 10. Information on diabetes and its impact on the cardiovascular system is also presented.

9.1 CARDIOVASCULAR OVERVIEW

9.1a Basic Terminology

For the heart to function optimally, it must maintain an appropriate rate, rhythm, and force of contraction. Pharmacologic agents for the heart can affect these three variables either positively or negatively. **Chronotropic** drugs affect the rate of the heart and can either increase its rate (positive chronotropic effect) or decrease its rate (negative chronotropic effect). **Inotropic** drugs affect the force of contraction and again can be either positive or negative. **Dromotropic** drugs alter the rhythm or electrical conduction through the heart muscle. Positive dromotropic drugs enhance the electrical conduction of signals in certain parts of the heart, whereas negative dromotropic drugs slow conduction.

9.1b Cardiac Circulation

The heart is divided into four chambers (two ventricles and two atria). The atria sit above the ventricles and are reservoirs that allow blood to flow into the ventricles when the valves between them open. The tricuspid valve separates the right atrium and right ventricle. The mitral valve separates the left atrium and left ventricle. The heart can be considered as two separate pumps. The right side of the heart receives deoxygenated blood from all parts of the body and pumps this blood through the pulmonary system to become oxygenated. The left side of the heart receives the oxygenated blood and pumps it throughout the body (see Figure 9-1, which shows the cardiac circulation).

The heart's contractility is what supplies the pressure to force blood through the various vessels and supply perfusion throughout the body. The heart is functionally comprised of cardiac muscle. The heart, like any muscle, needs to be supplied with oxygen and vital nutrients to function properly. The coronary arteries supply blood to the heart, and coronary veins carry away the metabolic waste products.

Learning Hint

To remember the difference between the right and left heart, try to associate the letter "R" in "right" with the following: The right heart has the tricuspid valve and receives deoxygenated blood from the veins. Also, the right heart pumps into the respiratory system. Therefore the left heart must have the mitral valve and pumps oxygenated blood throughout the body.

time for review

How do you think blockage of coronary arteries will affect the heart's contractility?

FIGURE 9-1 Cardiac Circulation

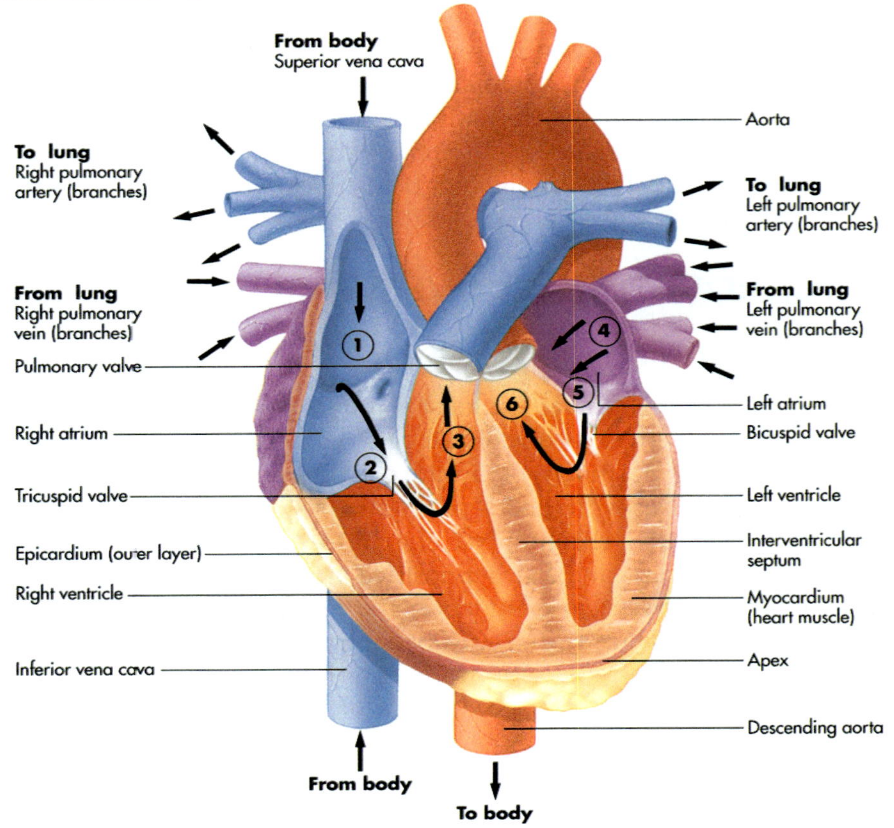

RIGHT HEART PUMP

1. Deoxygenated blood returns from the upper and lower body to fill the right atrium of the heart creating a pressure against the atrioventricular (AV) or tricuspid valve.
2. This pressure of the returning blood forces the AV valve open and begins filling the ventricle. The final filling of the ventricle is achieved by the contracting of the right atrium.
3. The right ventricle contracts increasing the internal pressure. This pressure closes the tricuspid valve and forces open the pulmonary valve thus sending blood toward the lung via the pulmonary artery. This blood will become oxygenated as it travels through the capillary beds of the lung and then returns to the left side of the heart.

LEFT HEART PUMP

4. Oxygenated blood returns from the lung via the pulmonary vein and fills the left atrium creating a pressure against the bicuspid valve.
5. This pressure of returning blood forces the bicuspid valve open and begins filling the left ventricle. The final filling of the left ventricle is achieved by the contracting of the left atrium.
6. The left ventricle contracts increasing internal pressure. This pressure closes the bicuspid valve and forces open the aortic valve causing oxygenated blood to flow through the aorta to deliver oxygen throughout the body.

9.1c Cardiac Conduction

For the heart to pump blood effectively, it must contract in a highly integrated and coordinated fashion. The right and left atria must contract at the same time, sending blood into the right and left ventricle, respectively. There must next be a slight contractile pause to allow the ventricles adequate filling time. Then the ventricles must contract simultaneously, the right sending its deoxygenated blood into the pulmonary system and the left sending its oxygenated blood through the aorta and out to the entire body.

Both electrical and mechanical properties of the heart are relevant to cardiovascular pharmacology. The heart muscle contraction and subsequent pumping represent a mechanical action. However, this mechanical action must be initiated by an electrical response. Muscle contraction is characterized electrically by a change in action potential, which is the basis for electrocardiogram (ECG) monitoring. In the heart, an intricate electric **conduction** system maintains regular rate and rhythm.

Cardiac activity depends on generation of an electrical impulse in the sinoatrial (SA) node, which is considered the normal pacemaker for the heart. The SA node is innervated by both parasympathetic and sympathetic nerves, which set the heart rate. In review, the sympathetic nerves release norepinephrine (NE) and cause adrenergic responses, and the parasympathetic nerves release acetylcholine (ACh) and cause cholinergic responses. NE increases heart rate and force of contraction, and ACh causes the opposite, so a balance is maintained. See Table 9-1 for the adrenergic and cholinergic effects on the heart.

Table 9-1 **Adrenergic and Cholinergic Effects on the Heart**

Sympathetic–Adrenergic	Parasympathetic–Cholinergic
↑ HR	Cardiac slowing
↑ force of contraction	↓ force of contraction
↑ automaticity	↓ automaticity
↑ AV conduction	Inhibition of AV conduction

The SA node paces the heart by depolarizing and stimulating the conducting tissues of the heart. The impulse then spreads through the atria. After the atria contract, the electrical impulse travels to the node between the atria and the ventricles, called the atrioventricular or AV node. There is a slight delay (approximately 0.20 second) to allow the ventricles to fill with blood. The impulse then travels through the *bundle of His*, located in the septal wall between the ventricles, and branches into the right bundle branch, going to the right ventricle, and the left bundle branch, going to the left ventricle. The bundle of His consists of a thick bunch of conducting fibers that carry current to the end of the conduction system, or the *Purkinje fibers*. From there, conduction proceeds through the Purkinje conduction system located throughout the ventricular muscle, depolarizing the ventricles, thus causing contraction. See Figure 9-2, which shows the electrical pathway of conduction through the heart.

9.1d Ion Influence

Now that we have discussed the mechanics of myocardial contraction, we can look at the physiologic processes that start it. The cardiac **action potential** is related to contraction and relaxation of the heart. This action potential is controlled at the cellular level by ions transporting in and out of cells. Different ionic currents generate different phases of the action potential. In each of the phases, an electrical gradient occurs between the inside and the outside of the cell membrane. Cells cycle among resting, activation, and inactivation states.

Specifically the pacemaking and conduction throughout the heart are driven by action potentials that are dependent on sodium (Na), calcium (Ca), and potassium (K) activity, and their passages through certain ionic channels within the membranes of the myocardial cells. Potassium moves out of the cell while sodium moves in for a process called depolarization, which precedes the mechanical contraction. The muscle must now return to its resting potential or repolarize, with potassium moving back into the cell and sodium back out.

FIGURE 9-2 Electrical Conduction Through the Heart

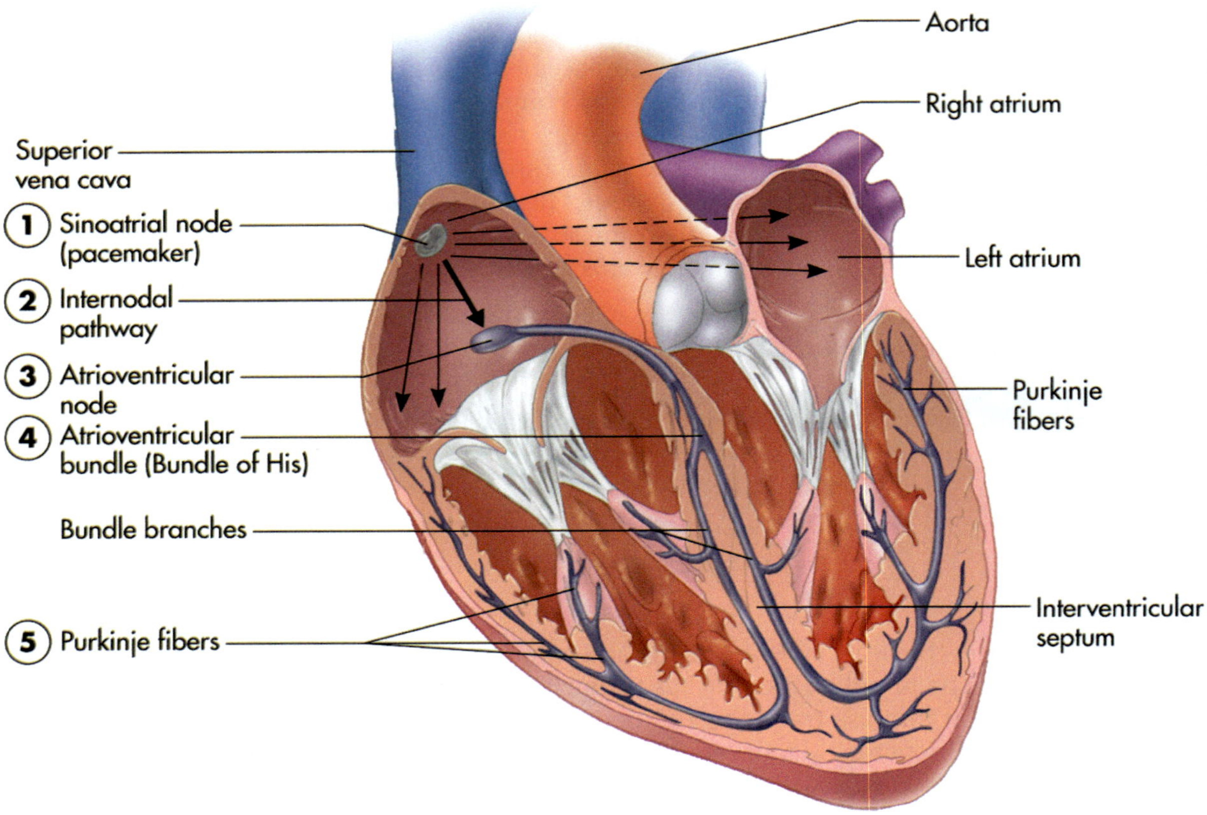

1. The sinoatrial (SA) node fires a stimulus across the walls of both left and right atria causing them to contract.
2. The stimulus arrives at the atrioventricular (AV) node.
3. The stimulus is directed to follow the AV bundle (Bundle of His).
4. The stimulus now travels through the apex of the heart through the bundle branches.
5. The Purkinje fibers distribute the stimulus across both ventricles causing ventricular contraction.

In addition calcium is needed for the actual muscle contraction to occur. Calcium influences actin and myosin, which control cardiac cell length and muscle contraction.

Some ionic channels cannot be reactivated or opened until a certain phase of the action potential occurs. The time when cells cannot be excited after electrical stimulation is called the **refractory period.** Some cardiac cells must wait for a stimulus, whereas others have spontaneous self-excitability capabilities. During some phases, different levels of refractoriness are present, which means that electrical stimulation cannot occur or can occur only with a very strong stimulus. Different tissues depend on different ions, have differences in recovery of tissue excitability, and are affected differently by drugs that influence their conduction properties.

time for review

Can you explain why it is important to monitor levels of the ions (electrolytes) sodium, potassium, and calcium through lab tests?

9.1e The ECG Tracing

Electrocardiograms record the electrical activity of the heart as deflection points represented by the letters P, Q, R, S, and T. Each of these letters represents either the depolarization or the repolarization process that occurs within various parts of the heart (see Figure 9-3, which shows a normal ECG tracing).

FIGURE 9-3 Normal ECG Tracing

Note: Atria repolarization normally occurs during QRS.

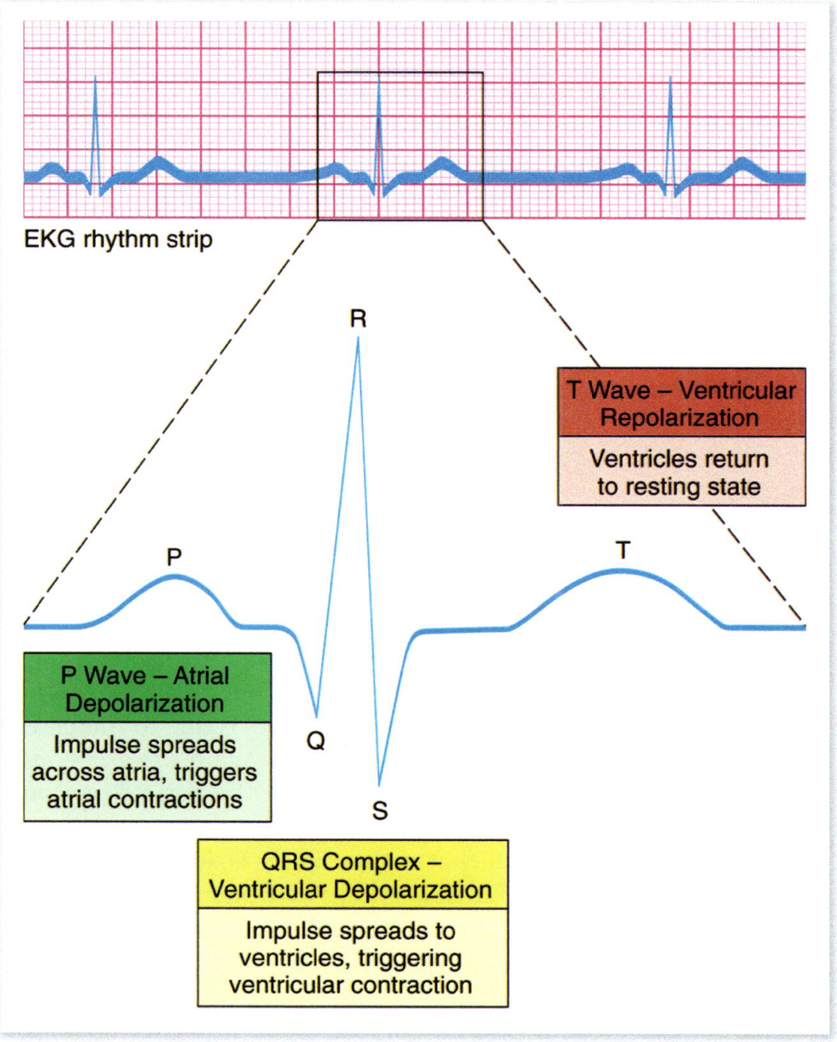

Learning Hint

The interval from the beginning of the P wave to the beginning of the QRS shows how long the impulse takes to travel from the atria to the ventricle. If that interval is too long, an atrioventricular conduction problem exists.

The P wave represents the atrial depolarization, which is normally followed by the mechanical contraction of the right and left atria. The QRS complex shows ventricular depolarization, which is followed by the mechanical contraction of the right and left ventricles. The T wave shows the repolarization (back to resting potential) of the ventricles so that they are ready for another stimulus. The atria must also return to resting or repolarize, and this normally occurs at the same time as the ventricles are depolarizing. Because the ventricles are much larger and generate a greater electrical deflection (QRS), you normally do not see the small deflection of atrial repolarization hidden in the QRS complex.

9.1f Arrhythmias

Any deviation from the normal ECG tracing is termed an **arrhythmia.** The mechanisms of cardiac arrhythmias include disorders of automaticity and/or conduction. **Automaticity** is the ability to generate pacemaking activity and is normal when pacemaker activity originates in the SA node. If the SA node fails, one of the other potential pacemakers may assume pacemaking activity. These other potential pacemakers are located in the atria, AV junction, and the ventricles. Arrhythmias occur mainly because the pacemaker originates somewhere other than the SA node (abnormal automaticity), or the impulse does not follow normal conduction pathway and so abnormal conduction occurs. When the SA node is altered and conduction is interrupted, other areas of the heart may assume the pacing function. These potential pacemaker cells can now become automatic and fire, thus causing a contraction to occur out of sequence, adversely affecting cardiac output.

Cells can become excited if there is an oxygen deficit, as in ischemia or infarction, or if an electrolyte imbalance occurs. Because these conditions can be transient and unpredictable, arrhythmia occurrence can be variable. Arrhythmias can occur in hearts with abnormal function or even in a normally functioning heart if it is influenced adversely by exercise, diet, or electrolyte changes.

Arrhythmias are diagnosed and treatment decisions are made on the basis of objective ECG data and subjective patient clinical signs and symptoms. By affecting cardiac conduction and the autonomic nervous system pharmacologically, drugs can assist in managing arrhythmias. Arrhythmias, regardless of where they originate, may cause no symptoms or may be life-threatening. Sometimes arrhythmias are rated according to their outcome potential as benign, potentially malignant, or malignant. This rating helps in making individualized decisions about whom to treat and with what drug to treat them, as well as what the benefit versus the risk is. Because underlying arrhythmias are variable by nature, **proarrhythmias**, or arrhythmias induced by the drugs themselves, can be difficult to diagnose, so awareness among health-care professionals is important. Decreased use of antiarrhythmics in the last few years is due to increased awareness of the proarrhythmic activity of these drugs. Again *proarrhythmic* means that the drugs may cause arrhythmias, which is not the desired outcome when you are giving them to decrease arrhythmias. Arrhythmias can even be a sign of antiarrhythmic drug toxicity. If that is the case, it is an indication to change the drug dosage rather than add a new antiarrhythmic to treat a symptom of antiarrhythmic toxicity. The antiarrhythmic digoxin is an example of a drug that can cause arrhythmias when it is given in toxic doses. Antiarrhythmic treatment is warranted when hemodynamic compromise occurs, when an increase in myocardial oxygen demand occurs, or when the arrhythmias may lead to malignant ventricular arrhythmias.

During the last several decades, the use of devices, surgery, and specialized heart catheterization procedures has assumed a more important role in the management of arrhythmias. Implantable cardioverter-defibrillators (ICDs) are now widely used in survivors of a cardiac arrest and in patients with heart failure who meet certain criteria to prevent death and hospitalizations.

9.1g Sites of Arrhythmias

Arrhythmias can develop in the atria or ventricles. They can happen in the critical care unit or while sitting at home in a recliner. Arrhythmias requiring drug treatment can be divided into supraventricular (above the ventricles) and ventricular on the basis of where in the heart the arrhythmias originate. The common supraventricular arrhythmias are atrial fibrillation or flutter, paroxysmal supraventricular tachycardia, and autonomic atrial tachycardias. The ventricular arrhythmias include premature ventricular contractions (PVCs), ventricular tachycardia, torsades de pointes, and ventricular fibrillation.

Potential arrhythmia outcomes can range from mild discomfort to sudden death. Recurrence of the arrhythmia is best documented by ECG or Holter test cardiac monitoring and should include not only time but also frequency of recurrence and any related activity. Symptoms tolerance, blood pressure, heart rate, side effects, quality of life, and economics are all considered in the benefit–risk decision to use an antiarrhythmic drug.

Learning Hint

Ventricular arrhythmias are typically more life-threatening than atrial arrhythmias. The ventricles are required to pump much longer distances than the atria, so conduction problems in the ventricles can lead to a more serious drop in cardiac output (left ventricle) or pulmonary perfusion (right ventricle).

9.2 ANTIARRHYTHMIC AGENTS

9.2a Therapeutic Goals

Goals for drugs used for cardiac arrhythmias include restoring and maintaining normal sinus rhythm in which the electrical impulse that begins cardiac conduction should occur at the SA node. In addition antiarrhythmic treatment attempts to suppress those excitable areas of the heart that fire outside of the normal conduction pathway and impair cardiac output. These areas are referred to as *ectopic* foci. Finally antiarrhythmic agents attempt to control ventricular rate and optimize cardiac output.

Learning Hint

Ectopic means "in an abnormal position." An ectopic pregnancy, for example, occurs when the fertilized egg implants outside the uterine cavity. An ectopic beat is the electrical stimulation of cardiac contraction beginning at another point or outside the normal conduction pathway.

9.2b Mechanism of Action

Antiarrhythmics' mechanism of action is both pharmacologic and electrophysiologic. They basically work to alter conduction through the atria or ventricles. They may do so in several ways. One way is to depress automatic properties of abnormal pacemaker cells. The drugs can accomplish this electrophysiologically by affecting depolarization and the threshold level of these excitable cells. Another way is to alter conduction characteristics within the heart by either facilitating or depressing conduction.

9.2c Classification of Antiarrhythmic Drugs

Antiarrhythmic drugs are described by four classes, with subclasses for Class I (see Table 9-2). This classification is based on electrophysiologic actions in vitro (in the lab), where the different drug classes affect different phases of the action potential or ionic channels. These drugs affect calcium, potassium, and sodium

Clinical pearl

Side effects of quinidine are related mainly to the drug's source of origin, which is tree bark. Quinidine is an example of a serendipitous drug. Its antiarrhythmic use was discovered when patients taking quinine for malaria found their atrial arrhythmias converted to normal cardiac rhythm.

TABLE 9-2 Antiarrhythmic Drug Classes with Representative Drugs*

Class	Function	Generic Name	Brand Name
IA	Na-channel blockers (moderate)	quinidine	Quinaglute®
		procainamide	Pronestyl®
		disopyramide	Norpace®
IB	Na-channel blockers (weak)	lidocaine	Xylocaine®
		mexiletine	Mexitil®
IC	Na-channel blockers (strong)	flecainide	Tambocor®
		propafenone	Rythmol®
II	*β*-adrenergic blockers*	propranolol	Inderal®
		esmolol	Brevibloc®
III	Drugs to prolong repolarization	amiodarone	Cordarone®
	K-channel blockers	sotalol	Betapace®
		dofetilide	Tikosyn®
		ibutilidez	Corvert®
		dronedarone	Multaq®
IV	Ca-channel blockers	verapamil	Isoptin®
		diltiazem	Cardizem®

** This is a representative sample, not a complete list.*

channels, prolong the repolarization phase, or block β-adrenergic activity, and they are classified accordingly.

It is important to notice that some of the most useful drugs for treating arrhythmias are not included in this classification system (e.g., atropine for bradycardia, epinephrine for asystole); these will be discussed in detail in Chapter 15 as part of the discussion of Advanced Cardiac Life Support (ACLS).

In addition this classification doesn't have a place for all drugs (such as digoxin). Adding to the confusion, drugs in the same class don't necessarily have the same medical indications or treat the same arrhythmias, and therefore drugs within each class cannot necessarily be substituted for each other. For example the antiarrhythmic ibutilide (Class III) may be effective to convert atrial fibrillation or flutter to sinus rhythm but would not be recommended to treat ventricular tachycardia. Many drugs also have properties of more than one antiarrhythmic class. This validates that what happens in the lab (in vitro) does not always translate directly to what happens in the human body (in vivo). Because the use of antiarrhythmic drugs is declining, the only antiarrhythmic drugs that are discussed in this section are the two unclassified agents digoxin (Lanoxin®) and adenosine (Adenocard®). These two antiarrhythmics and others will also be discussed in Chapter 15.

Although it would be nice to have a cookbook approach to arrhythmias, from the information presented so far, you can see why this is not possible. Likewise it is not possible to provide a simple table that matches type of arrhythmia with drug or antiarrhythmic drug class. The most specific antiarrhythmic drug use information that matches arrhythmia with drugs is found in the ACLS guidelines and will be covered in Chapter 15.

Digoxin

Digoxin (Lanoxin®) is an unclassified antiarrhythmic that inhibits the sodium/potassium exchange pump in the heart, which then leads to increased intracellular sodium and calcium. The increased total calcium available for release by the action potential causes an increase in the contractility of the heart. It also augments parasympathetic tone by inhibiting sympathetic outflow. This is how digoxin is capable of slowing the ventricular response in patients with atrial fibrillation or flutter. Digoxin has a half-life of 36 hours or longer, so frequently a loading dose is used.

Digoxin does not convert atrial fibrillation to normal sinus rhythm, but it does slow the ventricular rate. Atrial fibrillation is probably one of the more common types of dysrhythmias, which is why digoxin merits attention. Some side effects of digoxin include anorexia, visual disturbances, fatigue, and life-threatening arrhythmias. Serum levels of digoxin can guide dose adjustments. Drug interactions occur with drugs that affect serum electrolytes, and changes in renal function can affect digoxin excretion.

Clinical pearl

Digoxin is discussed further in relation to the treatment of heart failure, in which the prolongation of the PR interval (more filling time) coupled with increased myocardial contraction both help treat the disease.

Clinical pearl

Conversion of atrial fibrillation is considered only when it is documented that the arrhythmia has been present for less than 48 hours or if the patient is unstable. If it has been present for longer, hemodynamically stable patients must be anticoagulated before conversion is attempted.

LIFE SPAN CONSIDERATIONS

An irregular heart rate is not an uncommon problem in children. A thorough evaluation is important since these irregular heart rates can range from benign to potentially deadly.

The most common dysrhythmia in older adults is atrial fibrillation. This is an important problem in the elderly since it contributes to progressive left-sided heart failure and stroke.

Adenosine

Adenosine (Adenocard®) is an unclassified antiarrhythmic used to convert supraventricular tachycardia to a sinus rhythm, and at times it aids in the diagnosis of the rhythm disorders. It slows conduction through the AV and SA nodes and commonly causes a brief cardiac standstill that generally scares everyone involved in its administration (except for people like you who read this book and know what might be coming). The drug is used intravenously and has a very short half-life. Side effects include transient facial flushing and dyspnea. It should be used cautiously in asthmatics; theophylline blocks the electrophysiologic effects of adenosine.

9.3 HEART FAILURE

9.3a Pathophysiology

Heart failure used to be referred to as congestive heart failure (CHF). The name was changed because a patient can have heart failure without symptoms of congestion. Heart failure (HF) is one of the more common hospital discharge diagnoses in patients over age 65. Heart failure occurs when ventricles are not able to pump enough blood to supply the body. The loss of contractility or pump efficiency makes the blood volume increase within the heart, and the heart

BVT Lab

Visit www.BVTLab.com to explore the student resources available for this chapter.

eventually enlarges. This means that less blood gets to other parts of the body where it is needed and also causes the kidney to change fluid regulation. The kidneys, sensing a lack of perfusion, retain fluid to increase vascular volume to attempt to increase perfusion. This puts more stress on the heart and exacerbates the HF and edema. As a result edema occurs in the gravity-dependent extremities such as the ankles, and if HF is left untreated, fluid builds up in the lungs and can result in pulmonary edema.

HF can be right- or left-sided heart failure, and symptoms may vary for each. Because drugs can cause HF by inhibiting myocardial contractility or expanding plasma volume, drug-induced HF must be ruled out before treatment is started.

HF may be caused by an abnormality in systolic or diastolic function or both. Most of the drugs used to treat systolic HF are the same as for diastolic HF, but doses may be different. Systolic dysfunction is primarily decreased contractility. Diastolic dysfunction is primarily a restriction in ventricular filling.

9.3b Drugs to Treat Heart Failure

Pharmacologic treatment for HF consists of removing sodium and water with diuretics, increasing contraction of the heart with positive inotropic activity, and decreasing vascular resistance with vasodilators. **Afterload** is the force against which the heart must pump, and **preload** is the amount of blood in the ventricles before contraction. When volume increases secondary to sodium and water retention, the preload increases. Afterload increases can be caused by peripheral vasoconstriction. By decreasing preload and afterload, vasodilators can be effective treatment for HF. In essence they open up the pipes (vessels), thus decreasing the resistance to blood flow. Basically, drugs for HF improve heart contractility and decrease the heart's work (see Figure 9-4).

9.3c Digoxin for Heart Failure

Digoxin is one of the oldest inotropic drugs known. This is the same drug previously described as an unclassified antiarrhythmic. Inotropes increase the peak tension produced by the heart during systolic contraction. This allows the heart to pump blood more effectively. As mentioned previously in this chapter, digoxin increases calcium availability for contracting, which leads to enhanced force of contraction.

Digoxin has both mechanical and electrical effects in the heart. Digoxin's electrical effects occur because an increase in parasympathetic stimulation in the heart decreases firing in the AV node (negative dromotropic effect). This is beneficial because it allows for more effective ventricular filling time. Concurrently the mechanical action of digoxin increases cardiac contractility, so the heart pumps more strongly. This increased cardiac contractility coupled with better filling volume results in increased ventricular ejection, increased cardiac output, and increased renal blood flow. This also results in decreased compensatory sympathetic (reductions in plasma norepinephrine levels) and renal response, because the kidneys now are better perfused.

FIGURE 9-4 Sites of Action of Drugs to Treat HF

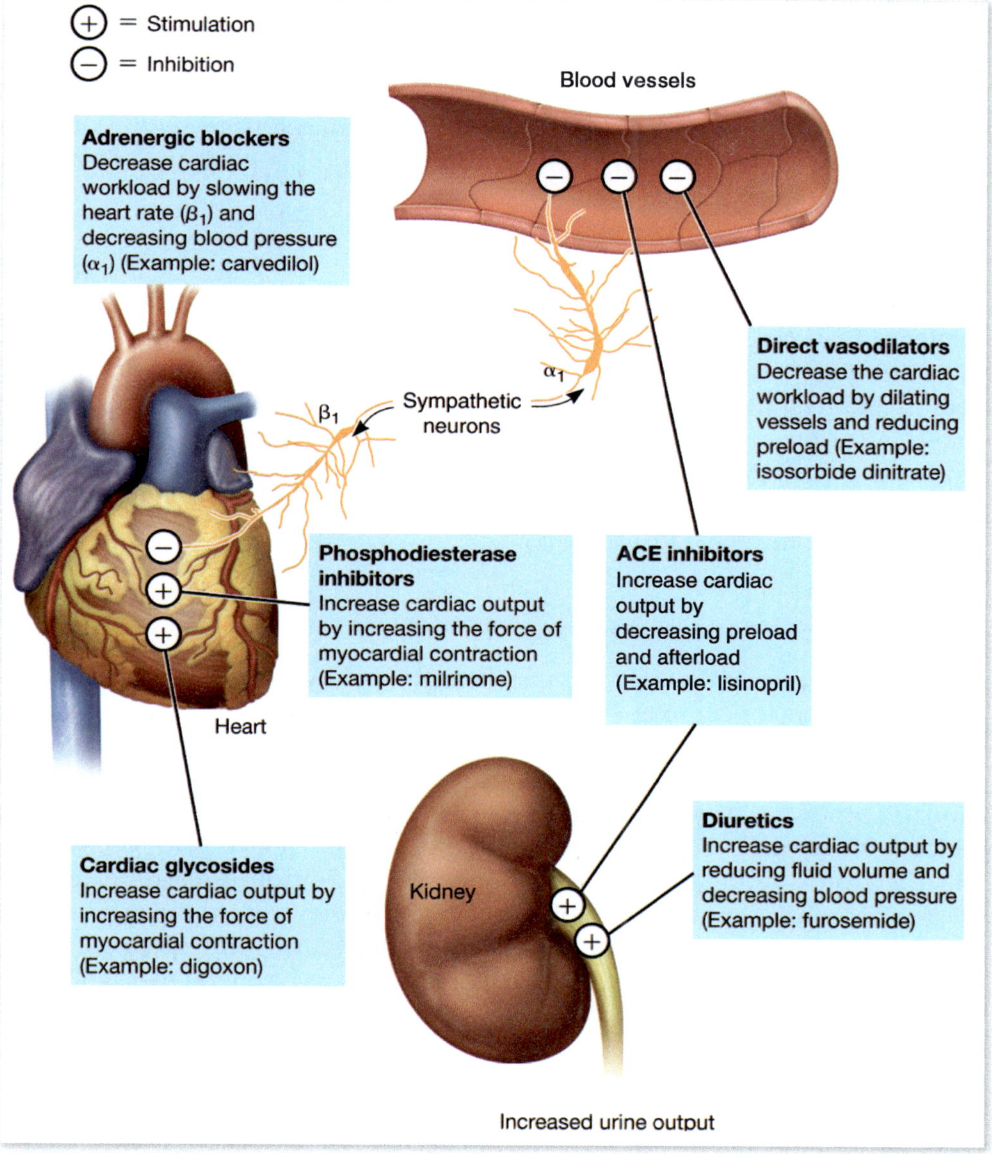

9.3d ACE Inhibitors for Heart Failure

Angiotensin-converting enzyme (ACE) inhibitors decrease blood levels of angiotensin II. Angiotensin II is a vasoconstrictor, and therefore blocking its production induces vasodilation. Angiotensin II also promotes sodium retention and increases norepinephrine release. Because vasoconstriction increases systemic vascular resistance in heart failure and causes an increased workload, promoting vasodilation by inhibiting angiotensin II is beneficial.

ACE inhibitors have no direct positive inotropic effects, but they decrease aldosterone secretion, salt and water retention, and vascular resistance. ACE inhibitors are beneficial to patients with systolic heart failure because they decrease afterload and attenuate the remodeling or structural changes that can occur in the congested heart due to heart failure. In addition they decrease symptoms and are shown to prolong life in patients with HF. Side effects of

ACE inhibitors include dry, nonproductive cough, worsening of renal function, proteinuria, and hyperkalemia. The increased potassium can be beneficial when ACE inhibitors are used concurrently with a diuretic for HF, which may lower serum potassium levels. ACE inhibitors have favorable effects on hemodynamics, clinical status, and symptoms in patients with heart failure. These effects are beneficial in patients with established HF as well as for prevention of heart failure. Examples of ACE inhibitors include captopril, benazepril (Lotensin®), and enalapril (Vasotec®).

Clinical pearl

The most recent treatment guidelines (ACC/AHA) for chronic heart failure include a new staging system that emphasizes risk-factor modification and preventive treatment strategies.

9.3e ARBs for Heart Failure

Angiotensin II–receptor blockers (ARBs) are used for hypertension and for HF. ARBs can block angiotensin II regardless of its origin and not affect bradykinin. Because bradykinin may be the cause of adverse effects such as angioedema and cough, ARBs may have a role in patients who are intolerant of ACE inhibitors. Blockade by ACE inhibitors can be incomplete, so ARBs and ACE inhibitors may be used together. ARBs cause side effects similar to ACE inhibitors: hypotension, hyperkalemia, and renal insufficiency.

9.3f β-Antagonists for Heart Failure

Learning Hint

Remember a previous learning hint that you have one heart (β_1) and two lungs (β_2)? Therefore, if the β-blocker for the heart condition also binds with and blocks the β_2-receptors in the lungs, bronchoconstriction may occur.

β-Blockers are also used for HF and may be beneficial by slowing the heart rate to allow more time for complete ventricular filling, blocking the deleterious effects of norepinephrine on the failing heart, reducing myocardial oxygen demand, and controlling blood pressure. The body's normal physiologic response to decreased cardiac output is activation of the sympathetic nervous system, so the use of β-blockers may make sense. Carvedilol (Coreg®) is a β-blocker with α-blocking, and therefore vasodilator, properties. Metoprolol controlled-release/extended-release (Toprol-XL®) and bisoprolol (Zebeta®) have been studied the most for HF. Symptom worsening due to the negative inotropic effects of β-blockers occurs unless doses are titrated slowly. ACC/AHA guidelines recommend that β-blockers be prescribed for all patients with stable systolic heart failure.

9.3g Vasodilators for Heart Failure

Vasodilators can greatly reduce the afterload forces on the heart. Three classes of vasodilators are used. Vasodilators decrease afterload by:

- Dilating arterial vessels (hydralazine)
- Dilating venous vessels and decreasing preload (isosorbide dinitrate, nitrates)
- Affecting both arterial and venous vessels (ACE inhibitors)

Clinical pearl

African Americans respond better to hydralazine and isosorbide for HF management. These two drugs are the first drugs approved by the FDA for a specific race of patients, and they are available commercially as a single-pill drug combination.

Hydralazine, the prototype arteriole dilator, is especially beneficial in reducing pulmonary vascular resistance in patients with severe pulmonary hypertension. Hydralazine can cause some fluid retention, which may result in the need for increased diuretic doses. It can also cause a reflex tachycardia, which may benefit from concurrent use of a β-blocker.

Nitrates complement hydralazine and are used topically or orally. The vasodilator nitroglycerin dilates arterioles (reducing afterload) and increases efficiency by affecting venous return (reducing preload returning to heart). By decreasing afterload and preload simultaneously, it increases cardiac output by decreasing systemic vascular resistance, and it relieves ventricular congestion through decreased venous return. Combination use of hydralazine–isosorbide dinitrate is a therapeutic option in patients who are not able to tolerate an ACE inhibitor or ARB or who remain symptomatic despite optimal treatment with ACE inhibitor/ARB, β-blocker, and diuretic.

As already described, ACE inhibitors inhibit angiotensin-converting enzyme. That enzyme is responsible for degradation of bradykinin and other vasodilators. Beneficial effects of lower pulmonary capillary wedge pressure and systemic vascular resistance result, as well as an increased cardiac index. Although hemodynamic tolerance occurs with other vasodilators, ACE inhibitors usually produce a greater response with time.

Calcium-channel blockers, in general, are not recommended for use in patients with HF. However amlodipine and felodipine are safe and well tolerated and can be used as add-on therapy to treat angina or hypertension in patients who require them in addition to preferred medications for HF.

Learning Hint

Because venous blood returns to fill the heart, it contributes to preload.

9.3h Diuretics for Heart Failure

Diuretic therapy is recommended for all patients with fluid retention and HF to get rid of excess volume that increases the workload of the heart. Loop diuretics (e.g., furosemide, bumetanide, torsemide) are the class of diuretics most frequently used to remove salt and water because they are the most potent. The risk of diuresis in HF is volume depletion and decreased cardiac output. Side effects of diuretics can include azotemia, dehydration, hypokalemia, hyponatremia, hypochloremic alkalosis, hypomagnesemia, hyperglycemia, and hyperuricemia. Despite the risk of hypokalemia, not all patients require potassium supplements. Automatically initiating potassium concurrently with a diuretic is therefore not recommended. Hyperkalemia can be just as dangerous as hypokalemia.

IV diuretics are frequently used for severe or unstable disease while oral dosage forms are used for chronic management. Diuretic doses are usually given early in the day to prevent nocturnal diuresis. Objective monitoring of diuretics in HF includes weight loss as well as decrease in edema and breath sounds associated with pulmonary edema. Because different diuretics may have different mechanisms of action, as discussed later in Chapter 10, combination use of two diuretics concurrently may be rational. See Figure 9-5 for a breakdown of the drugs used to treat HF.

Clinical pearl

Signs and symptoms that fluid is accumulating in the lungs include crackles on auscultation, low arterial oxygen levels due to diffusion impairment, changes on X-rays, and dyspnea.

FIGURE 9-5 Subgroups of Drugs for HF

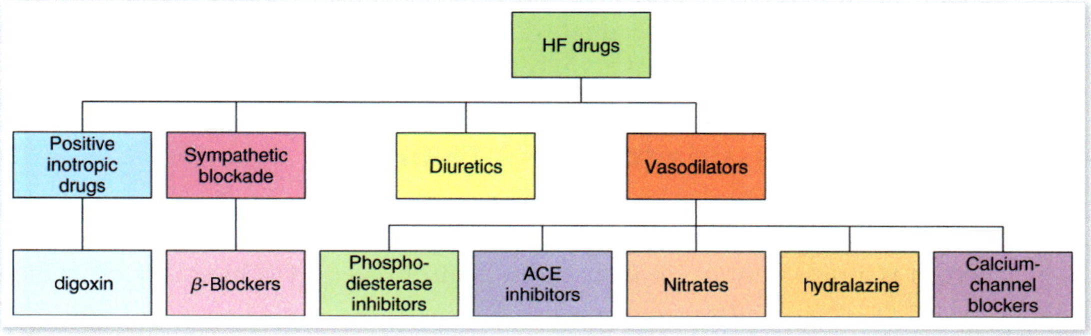

Patient & Family Education

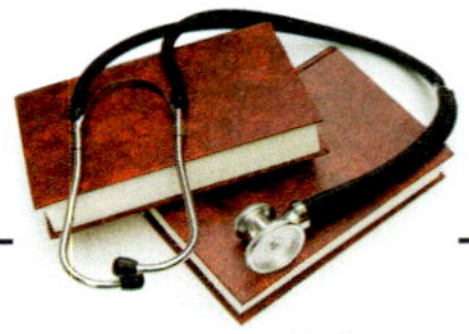

Patients with heart failure should be taught to weigh themselves daily. Diuretic doses can then be adjusted by the patient based upon specific weight increases or decreases. This is similar to how a patient with diabetes would adjust his or her insulin regimen to treat fluctuating glucose levels. Restricting sodium in the diet to 2–3 g or less will also help prevent the accumulation of fluid in the lungs and lower extremities.

9.3i Aldosterone Antagonists for Heart Failure

Aldosterone antagonists are beneficial in HF because of their inhibition of neurohormones that may contribute to adverse cardiac enlargement and fibrosis and their inhibition of potassium loss that may contribute to arrhythmias. Examples are spironolactone (Aldactone®) and eplerenone (Inspra®). These drugs have minimal diuretic effect even though they are classed as diuretics. Because these drugs are potassium-sparing, they may be advantageous for patients who require potassium supplementation.

9.3j Intravenous Inotropes for Heart Failure

β_1-Agonists, such as dobutamine, and phosphodiesterase inhibitors, such as milrinone, are often prescribed for patients with acute heart failure. Dobutamine is a β_1-agonist with some β_2-adrenergic activity that was developed because the β_1-agonist isoproterenol caused too many arrhythmias. Milrinone prevents the degradation of cyclic AMP by inhibiting phosphodiesterase, resulting in a reduction in vascular resistance and an increase in cardiac inotropy. Both drugs increase cardiac output and decrease left ventricular filling pressure. Both medications are available only for intravenous administration. The dosage of milrinone must be adjusted in patients with reduced renal function. A decrease in dobutamine's hemodynamic effects after 72 hours of continuous infusion may be due to downregulation of β_1-receptors.

9.3k Dopamine for Heart Failure

Dopamine is a precursor of norepinephrine and releases endogenous norepinephrine. Depending on the dose, dopamine stimulates dopaminergic and β_1- and α-adrenergic receptors. Dopamine affects dopamine receptors at low doses to improve renal blood flow. At high doses, it acts as an inotrope by stimulating β_1-receptors. Dopamine infusions may need to be tapered prior to discontinuation.

9.3l Nitroprusside for Heart Failure

Intravenous nitroprusside dilates both arterial and venous vessels, so it decreases afterload and preload. The drug is not stable in the presence of heat or light, which is a disadvantage in its use. The main side effect is hypotension, which decreases cardiac output.

9.3m Nitroglycerin for Heart Failure

For severe heart failure, intravenous nitroglycerin is used for preload reduction. With higher doses, nitroglycerin has beneficial coronary vasodilating properties that help with myocardial oxygen supply and demand. Hypotension can be rate-limiting, and tolerance may develop to the hemodynamic effects. Nitroglycerin may worsen cerebral edema if elevated cranial pressure is present.

9.3n Nesiritide for Heart Failure

Nesiritide (Natrecor®) is a recombinant manufactured drug identical to endogenous human β-natriuretic peptide (BNP). It acts like endogenous human BNP secreted by the ventricular myocardium, resulting in vasodilation and natriuretic effects. Nesiritide has been shown to improve hemodynamics and symptoms, but its use is infrequent due to evidence that it causes more deaths and deterioration in renal function when compared to intravenous nitroglycerin.

9.4 MANAGEMENT OF SHOCK

Shock is a potentially fatal condition in which tissues are poorly perfused. Treatment consists of oxygenation, blood pressure support, and maintaining acid–base balance. Different kinds of shock, such as cardiogenic or hypovolemic, may be treated differently. Some of the same drugs discussed for HF are used to treat shock. Vasopressors (agents that vasoconstrict) improve cardiac function by stimulating adrenergic receptors. When peripheral vasoconstriction occurs, blood is shunted to the heart and lungs. You will find more on the treatment of shock in Chapter 15, as part of the discussion of Advanced Cardiac Life Support.

time for review

Does it seem odd that a vasoconstrictor can be used to treat a condition characterized by poor tissue perfusion? The price paid for this may be ischemic damage peripherally. Can you explain why?

9.5 ANGINA

9.5a Pathophysiology of Angina

Angina or chest pain is a symptom of myocardial ischemia, or lack of oxygen, which occurs when oxygen supply and demand in the heart are unbalanced. The heart, like any muscle, needs oxygen and vital nutrients to function; these are supplied by the coronary arteries. Coronary blood flow is closely related to myocardial oxygen consumption. It is regulated physiologically by physical factors and vascular, neural, and humoral control. If the heart cannot respond to changes in demand or supply through increased blood flow because of occlusion of a coronary artery, a heart attack occurs. Drug therapy of angina is aimed at decreasing consumption of oxygen by the heart or increasing the delivery of oxygen to the heart. How much oxygen the heart needs is determined by contractility, rate of contraction, and the heart wall tension.

Clinical pearl

Not all chest pain is a heart attack. Patients with lung conditions such as pleurisy or trauma to the thorax may present with chest pain. Pleuritic chest pain (i.e., associated with the lungs) is usually sharp and stabbing in nature and located laterally or posteriorly. Nonpleuritic chest pain (not associated with the lungs) is usually centrally located and dull. This type of pain can also be from indigestion and is why some people deny heart attacks and claim indigestion. One of the main differentiating factors is that pleuritic chest pain will naturally get worse with deep breathing and cough, whereas nonpleuritic pain will be relatively unaffected.

9.5b Pharmacologic Treatment of Angina

Pharmacologic treatment of angina is aimed at pain relief and prevention of recurrent pain. Nitroglycerin administered sublingually is used for fast relief, because drug absorption is rapid by this route. Nitrates such as nitroglycerin reduce preload and afterload by dilating both veins and arteries, thus decreasing cardiac workload. Prophylactic treatment of chronic, stable angina is given by calcium entry blockers, β-blockers, nitrates, and/or ranolazine (Ranexa®). Myocardial ischemia can result from different mechanisms, so it makes sense to use antianginals that work by different mechanisms, and these drugs are often used together to achieve adequate relief. See Figure 9-6 for a breakdown of the drug groups used to treat angina.

FIGURE 9-6 Subgroups of Drugs for Angina

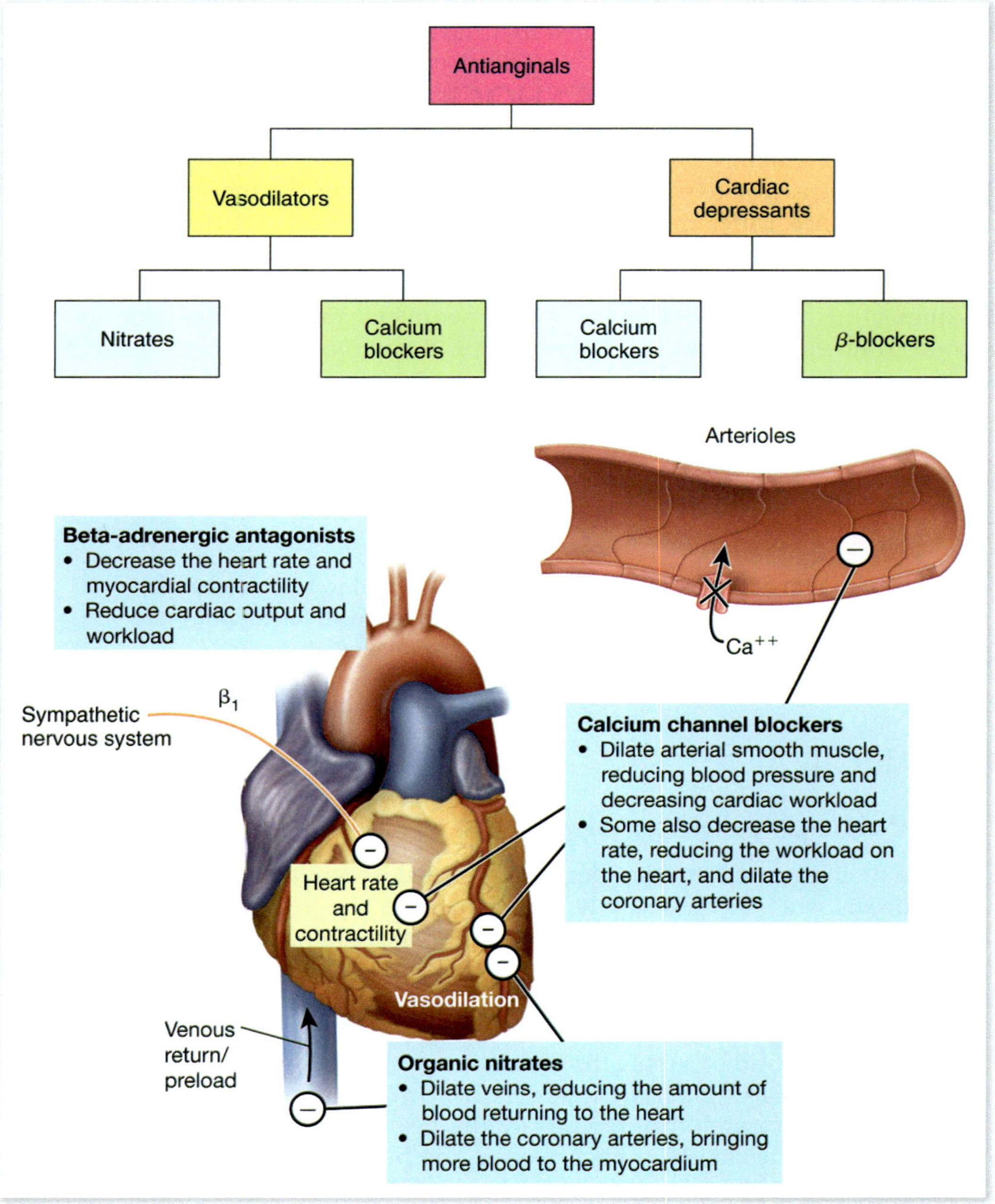

9.5c β-Blockers as Antianginals

β-Receptors are connected to adenyl cyclase by a G protein. When a β-agonist binds with the receptor, the G protein tells adenyl cyclase to make cyclic adenosine monophosphate (cAMP). The new molecule then acts like a messenger in the cell and can cause hyperpolarization of some parts of the heart. This can be a problem if the heart is damaged or hypoxic. β-Receptor activation can also cause cardiac metabolism to increase and require more oxygen.

β-Blockers decrease myocardial oxygen consumption by decreasing heart rate, contractility, blood pressure, and afterload, especially during exercise. They also decrease catecholamines in the ischemic heart. For these reasons, β-blockers given to myocardial infarction patients can limit infarct size and decrease the incidence of arrhythmias. β-Blockers are used for prophylaxis of angina to decrease the frequency and severity of attacks.

β-Blockers can cause bradycardia and exacerbation of chest pain on drug withdrawal unless a drug taper is scheduled. β-Blockers are contraindicated in patients with bronchial asthma or pulmonary disease that is due to induced bronchoconstriction. If a β-blocker is needed to treat angina in a patient with bronchial constriction, a selective β_1-agent is preferred. In addition to their β-receptor selectivity, β-blockers differ in their duration of action, pharmacokinetics, and price. See Table 9-3 for a comparison of β-blockers.

TABLE 9-3 Comparison of β-Blockers

Drug	Dosing Frequency	Relative β_1-Selectivity[a]	Lipid Solubility[b]
atenolol (Tenormin®)	Daily to b.i.d.	+ +	Low
acebutolol (Sectral®)	b.i.d.	+ +	Moderate
bisoprolol (Zebeta®)	Daily	+ +	Low
betaxolol (Kerlone®)	Daily	+ +	Low
carvedilol (Coreg®)	b.i.d.	0	High
labetalol (Trandate®)	b.i.d.	0	Moderate
metoprolol (Lopressor®, Toprol-XL®)	Daily to b.i.d.	+	Moderate to high
nadolol (Corgard®)	Daily	0	Low
propranolol (Inderal®)	Daily to b.i.d.	0	High

[a] *None are entirely β_1-specific. Use cautiously in patients with asthma, COPD, or peripheral vascular insufficiency.*

[b] *Highly lipid-soluble agents have shortest $T_{1/2}$, more hepatic metabolism, more variability in dose due to first-pass metabolism, and possibly more CNS side effect. Low–lipid solubility drugs have longer $T_{1/2}$, greater renal clearance, narrower dosage ranges, and possibly less CNS penetration.*

9.5d Calcium-Channel Blockers as Antianginals

Calcium-channel blockers inhibit the calcium influx into muscle that initiates contraction. They are also vasodilators, because they act directly on vascular smooth muscle. As noted in the section of this chapter on antiarrhythmics, they also decrease contractility, AV conduction, and automaticity.

Because calcium-channel blockers decrease myocardial oxygen demand by reducing afterload, contractility, and heart rate, you might expect this drug class to have the same benefits in an acute MI as β-blockers. Laboratory studies and animal data do show this, but clinical conditions do not, which is always the dilemma when evaluating medical literature. Within the calcium-channel blocker class, drugs differ in how much vasodilation and cardiac suppression individual agents cause. See Table 9-4 for a comparison of calcium-channel blockers.

TABLE 9-4 Comparison of Calcium-Channel Blockers

	diltiazem	nifedipine	verapamil
Coronary vasodilation	+ + +	+ + +	+ +
Peripheral vasodilation	+	+ + +	+ +
Contractility	↓	↑↓	↓

9.5e Nitroglycerin as an Antianginal

Nitroglycerin works like the naturally occurring vasodilator endothelium-derived relaxing factor (EDRF) to relax smooth muscle (vascular and nonvascular). It works to increase cGMP formation by the release of nitric oxide from nitrates. Relaxation is probably due to cGMP activation of protein kinase. Relaxation causes a decrease in heart wall tension and reduction of preload, with a lesser decrease in afterload. Nitroglycerin causes a reflex tachycardia, which can outweigh its beneficial effects. This is why combination use of nitrates and β-blockers, which slow the heart rate, can be beneficial.

Venodilation also causes orthostatic hypotension and headache. It affects nonvascular smooth muscle, so relaxation of the bronchi and other smooth muscles can occur. Heart pain and heartburn symptoms can be very similar, so a response to nitroglycerin may not allow you to distinguish cardiac from GI pain. Chronic administration of nitrates can lead to tolerance and lessened effects, as discussed in Chapter 1. This is prevented by a daily nitrate-free interval, such as removing a topical patch at night or not taking the last oral dose after 7:00 p.m. at night.

Nitroglycerin is available in the following formulations: intravenous, sublingual, buccal, spray, oral, ointment, and patch. For alleviation of anginal attacks, the sublingual, buccal, or spray are used. Prevention of angina is the goal of prophylactic oral or transdermal products. Other nitrate compounds include isosorbide dinitrate (ISDN), which is metabolized to isosorbide mononitrate (ISMN). These products have a longer half-life than nitroglycerin. See Table 9-5 for a comparison of antianginals.

TABLE 9-5 Comparison of Antianginals

	Contractility	Afterload	Preload	HR
Calcium-channel blockers	↓	↓		
β-Adrenergic blockers	↓	↓		↓
Nitrates		↓	↓	↑

9.5f Ranolazine

Ranolazine (Ranexa®) was approved in 2006 by the FDA for the treatment of chronic stable angina. It has a unique mechanism of action. It is thought to prevent calcium overload in the myocardial cell by inhibiting the late-phase sodium channel in ischemic cardiac myocytes. The decrease in calcium results in an increase in the relaxation of the heart muscle and a reduction in oxygen consumption by the heart. This hopefully decreases angina.

This effect on the sodium channel may lead to a prolonged ECG QT interval. Because of this, the FDA recommended reserving this medication for patients who have an inadequate response to other antianginal therapies. Other adverse effects of ranolazine include bradycardia, headache, dizziness, and confusion.

9.6 ACUTE CORONARY SYNDROMES

Acute coronary syndromes (ACS) include unstable angina and myocardial infarction. ACS is caused by rupture of an atherosclerotic plaque with resulting platelet adherence, activation, aggregation, and activation of the clotting cascade. Different treatment guidelines exist for ACS patients with ST-segment versus non–ST-segment findings on ECG. ST-segment-elevation ACS is treated with early reperfusion therapy with either primary percutaneous coronary intervention (PCI) or administration of a fibrinolytic agent. Concurrent intranasal oxygen, aspirin, sublingual nitroglycerin, intravenous nitroglycerin, intravenous β-blockers, and unfractionated heparin are used. Patients with non–ST-segment-elevation receive additional clopidogrel (Plavix®) or prasugrel (Effient®) and/or glycoprotein IIb/IIIa–receptor blocker.

Clinical pearl

Consensus guidelines indicate that clinicians cannot rule out an acute coronary syndrome in patients with typical ischemic chest pain symptoms on the basis of history, physical examination, risk-factor evaluation, and clinical judgment alone. A 6- to 12-hour observation period with repeat ECG and cardiac biomarkers is needed, often referred to as a "6-hour rule-out."

9.6a Myocardial Infarction

Treatment goals for acute MI are to save the myocardium, preserve left ventricular function, and reduce the risk of complications. Treatment strategies include reperfusion therapy and antithrombosis and anti-ischemic therapy. Some of the same drugs discussed in the section on angina are also used for MI. Reperfusion therapy and antithrombosis therapies are discussed in Chapter 10. Long-term therapy follow-up post–MI includes aspirin, a β-blocker, and an ACE inhibitor for prevention of stroke, recurrent myocardial infarction, and death. Most patients also receive a lipid-lowering agent called a statin to lower cholesterol.

9.6b Diabetes Mellitus

Diabetes has a very strong impact on the cardiovascular system. Diabetes mellitus is a group of metabolic disorders of fat, carbohydrate, and protein metabolism resulting from defects in insulin secretion, sensitivity, or both. There are two major classifications of diabetes mellitus (Type I and Type II) that differ in clinical presentation, onset, and etiology. Type I is a failure to produce insulin, whereas Type II is a failure of the cells to properly utilize insulin. Both Type I and Type II are associated with microvascular and macrovascular disease complications. The risk for coronary heart disease is 2–4 times greater in patients with diabetes than in nondiabetics. Aggressive management of cardiovascular disease risk factors includes smoking cessation, use of antiplatelet therapy, and lipid and hypertension management. More and more research suggests that these risk factors are not independent and may be related to a common factor of insulin resistance. See Table 9-6 for the ABCs of diabetes care. From this table you can see the importance of lab monitoring to check diabetes and lipid control.

Clinical pearl

Many cardiac problems are attributable to poor health habits or bad genes or a combination of both. It is easy for patients to think that medications for heart problems are magic bullets and will allow them to ignore diet and exercise. Diet and exercise are important treatment components of cardiovascular disease.

TABLE 9-6 The ABCs of Diabetes Care

- Hemoglobin A1c: less than 7% (ADA)[a] = average of 150 mg/dl glucose
- Blood pressure: <140/90 mm Hg
- Cholesterol
  - LDL-C: <100 mg/dl (70 mg/dl in very high-risk person)[a]
  - HDL-C: >40 mg/dl in men and >50 mg/dl in women[a]
  - TGs: <150 mg/dl[a]

[a]American Diabetes Association. *Diabetes Care* 2014;37(suppl 1):S1.

9.6c Classes of Diabetes Drugs

Insulin and oral agents are options for diabetes, with oral agents an option only for Type II diabetics and not Type I diabetics. See Table 9-7 for drug classes and their different mechanisms of action. See Table 9-8 for types of insulin. Because these drugs work differently, they may be used in combination. An inhaled insulin product was withdrawn from the market by the manufacturer in part due to slow sales. It was a dry-powder formulation of recombinant human insulin delivered systemically by a pulmonary inhaler. Another inhaled insulin product has recently been approved by the FDA and should become available for clinical use in 2015. Afrezza® is the brand name for the new inhaled insulin product. Since it is a rapid-acting insulin, it is meant to be used before meals to prevent the rise in blood sugar associated with food. Different doses may be delivered by picking either a 4- or 8-unit cartridge, which is loaded into an inhaler device for patient administration.

TABLE 9-7 Pharmacologic Agents for Diabetes

Drug Class/Example	Mechanism
Sulfonylureas/meglitinides/glipizide	↑ Insulin release
Biguanide/metformin	↓ Gluconeogenesis
Thiazolidinediones/pioglitazone	Insulin sensitizers
α-Glucosidase inhibitors/acarbose	Delay absorption of glucose
GLP-1 agonists/exenatide	↑ Insulin secretion
Insulin	Replace insulin deficiency
DPP-IV inhibitors/sitagliptin	Increase insulin synthesis and decrease glucagon secretion

TABLE 9-8 Types of Insulin

	Onset (hr)	Peak (hr)	Duration (hr)
Insulin lispro	0.25	0.5–1.5	4–5
Insulin aspart	5–10 min	1–3	3–5
Regular	0.5–1	2–4	5–7
Lente	1–3	6–14	24
NPH	1–2	6–14	24
Ultralente	4–6	18–24	36
Insulin glargine	1.5	None	24

9.6d Lipid-Lowering Agents

Cholesterol lowering with drug therapy is becoming so important to mortality and stroke prevention that one of the drug classes commonly referred to as "statins" may become available over-the-counter instead of as a prescription. Cholesterol-lowering guidelines are recommended by the National Cholesterol Education Program (NCEP) Adult Treatment Panel. Pharmacologic therapy is based on the specific lipoprotein disorder. A fasting lipoprotein profile includes total cholesterol, low-density lipoprotein (LDL), high-density lipoprotein (HDL), and triglyceride. Classification of numbers is then combined with major risk factors to determine individual patient goals for LDL and total cholesterol.

Therapeutic lifestyle change (TLC) is a part of hyperlipidemia treatment and is used in combination with lipid-lowering agents. Drugs used to treat hyperlipidemia include bile acid resins (BARs) or sequestrants (colestipol, cholestyramine, colesevelam), HMG-CoA reductase inhibitors (statins), niacin, gemfibrozil (Lopid®), fish oil, or ezetimibe (Zetia®). See Table 9-9 for lipid-lowering agents. Statins interrupt the biochemical rate-limiting step in cholesterol biosynthesis. The bile acid resins decrease cholesterol absorption, as does ezetimibe, though by a different mechanism. Niacin (nicotinic acid) reduces synthesis of LDL. Gemfibrozil lowers triglycerides but may increase LDL. Omega-three polyunsaturated fatty acids (fish oils) are found in fatty fish such as sardines, salmon, and mackerel. Diets high in these oils may reduce the risk of cardiovascular mortality in post–MI patients. Because the average American diet contains less than one-fifth of the recommended amount of these oils, supplements are available in the form of fish oil capsules. These may be used to lower triglycerides as well, if used in higher doses. Because these drugs all work differently, they are often used in combination.

Clinical pearl

In general, for every 1% reduction in LDL there is a 1% reduction in cardiovascular heart disease (CHD) event rates. Because HDL is the "good cholesterol," elevation of HDL of 1% reduces CHD events by approximately 2%.

Table 9-9 **Lipid-Lowering Agents**

Name	Adverse Effects
Bile acid resins (cholestyramine, colestipol, colesevelam)	Bloating, binds to other drugs
niacin	Cutaneous flushing, hepatitis, increased blood glucose
Statins (lovastatin, pravastatin, simvastatin, fluvastatin, atorvastatin, rosuvastatin)	Myopathy, elevated liver function tests
ezetimibe	Dizziness, headache, diarrhea
Fibric acids (gemfibrozil, fenofibrate)	Gallstones
Fish oil capsules	Fishy taste, gas, diarrhea

Controversy

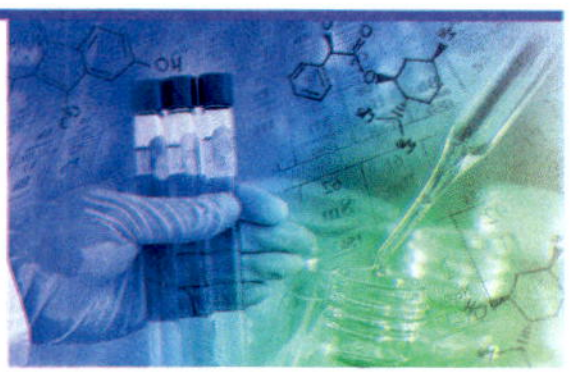

How low should we go? Some experts recommend a goal LDL of less than 70 mg/dl for all patients with known heart disease. Given the wide prevalence of hyperlipidemia and the cost of treatment, this change in aggressiveness of therapy is controversial.

Another controversy surrounds lowering cholesterol with ezetimibe. While ezetimibe lowers LDL cholesterol, there is no definitive evidence that it prevents cardiovascular disease when used alone, but it may have a small additional benefit in terms of reducing complications of ischemic cardiac disease when used with a statin.

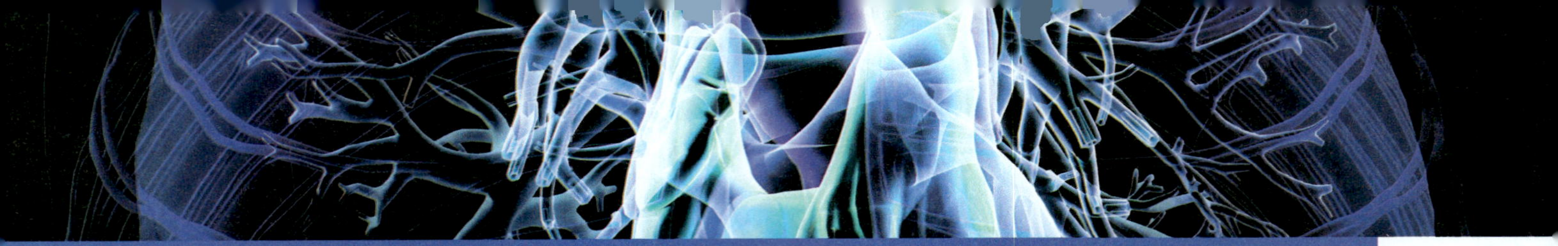

Summary

To facilitate a complete understanding of complex cardiopulmonary drug classifications, this chapter related cardiac and renal physiology to pharmacology and explored the interrelationships of the cardiovascular, respiratory, and renal systems. Various agents to treat various cardiac arrhythmias, heart failure, acute coronary syndromes, myocardial infarction, diabetes, hyperlipidemia, and angina were discussed, with emphasis on their mechanisms of action. Several of the medications have multiple indications and multiple mechanisms of action, with ACE inhibitors being a classic example. Cardiovascular agents demonstrate that drug selection is frequently controversial and always requires a balance between efficacy and toxicity. Keep this in mind as you continue on to yet more cardiovascular pharmacotherapy in the next chapter.

REVIEW QUESTIONS

1. A 68-year-old patient was started on digoxin for HF yesterday. Today he is complaining of swollen ankles and respiratory difficulty. Auscultation reveals diffuse crackles suggesting lung fluid. What could be possible causes?
   (a) positive inotropic effect
   (b) acute exacerbation of HF
   (c) new-onset asthma triggered by digoxin
   (d) diuresis

2. Match the diuretic drug name with its class:

thiazide	furosemide
loop	spironolactone
K-sparing	chlorothiazide

3. Match the term with its cardiac function:

chronotropic	rate
inotropic	rhythm
dromotropic	force of contraction

4. Arrhythmias can occur
   (a) in normal hearts
   (b) in abnormal hearts
   (c) with symptoms
   (d) without symptoms
   (e) all of the above

5. Vasodilators for HF may include
   (a) digoxin
   (b) propranolol
   (c) hydralazine
   (d) atropine
   (e) all of the above
6. What are some of the issues when considering whether or not to use an antiarrhythmic?
7. Explain the rationale for ACE inhibitors post–MI.
8. Describe different mechanisms of action for antianginals as they relate to mechanisms of cardiac ischemia.
9. Describe how antiarrhythmics differ from each other.
10. What is a proarrhythmia?

CASE STUDY 1

An elderly female

An elderly female presents to the emergency department with complaints of shortness of breath and pedal edema (swollen ankles). Breath sounds show diffuse crackles, suggesting pulmonary congestion. She is being treated with a diuretic and an ACE inhibitor. What potential medical problems may she have? What is the role and pharmacologic effect of a diuretic and ACE inhibitor for the medical condition you have hypothesized? What would be some side effects to watch for? What are other drug options if her current therapy isn't effective?

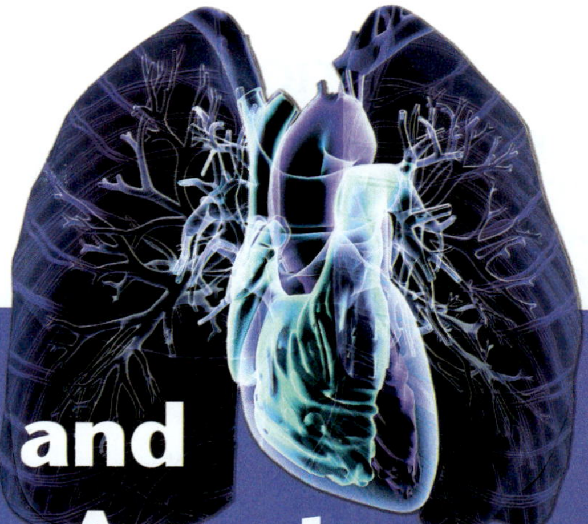

Chapter 10

Blood Pressure and Antithrombotic Agents

OBJECTIVES

Upon completion of this chapter you will be able to

- Understand the variables that affect blood pressure.
- Define key terms related to blood pressure and antithrombotic agents.
- Relate cardiovascular physiology to pharmacologic treatments.
- Describe indications and pharmacologic effects of various types of antihypertensive agents.
- Relate renal physiology to diuretic treatment.
- Describe indications and pharmacologic effects of anticoagulants, antiplatelet agents, and fibrinolytic agents.

KEY TERMS

afterload
anticoagulant
antiplatelet
baroreceptor
compliance
essential hypertension
fibrinolytic
hypertension
preload
thromboembolism

ABBREVIATIONS

ACEI angiotensin-converting enzyme inhibitor
ACT activated clotting time
ADH antidiuretic hormone
ADP adenosine diphosphate
aPTT activated partial thromboplastin time
ARB angiotensin II–receptor blocker
BP blood pressure
CCB calcium-channel blocker
CO cardiac output
DTI direct thrombin inhibitor
DVT deep-vein thrombosis
GP glycoprotein
ICP intracranial pressure
INR international normalized ratio
JNC Joint National Committee
LMWH low-molecular-weight heparin
PCI percutaneous coronary intervention
PT prothrombin time
TE thromboembolism
TOD target organ disease
tPA tissue plasminogen activator
TPR total peripheral resistance
UFH unfractionated heparin

Chapter 9 focused on drugs that affect the heart. This chapter focuses on regulating the pressure within the cardiovascular system. The drugs that regulate pressure in the cardiovascular system primarily affect sympathetic tone, the diameter of the blood vessels, or the actual blood volume. Diuretics work on the renal system and affect blood volume and therefore indirectly affect blood pressure. Although diuretics were mentioned in the previous chapter, they are discussed further in this chapter. In addition, this chapter discusses agents that ensure the blood itself flows freely through blood vessels and is not affected by intravascular blood clots. Anticoagulants prevent vascular clots from ever forming or extending and/or breaking off to form a clot to block vital blood flow to tissues and organs. In addition, this chapter discusses fibrinolytic agents that dissolve already-existing blood clots, as well as antiplatelet agents that prevent adhesion and aggregation of platelets.

10.1 BLOOD PRESSURE

10.1a The Basics

The cardiovascular system must be pressurized in order for blood to flow throughout it and to provide vital gas exchange, nutrients, immunologic defense, and other functions. Too much pressure can be disruptive and have serious consequences, whereas too little pressure will not allow enough perfusion to vital areas such as the brain or kidneys and can again have dire consequences.

The heart, as discussed in Chapter 9, is the pump that is connected to a roadway of blood vessels traveling throughout the body. Circulatory flow results as pressure differences are created in the system by the cardiac contraction. The vessels offer varying resistance to flow, depending on their diameter or level of dilation or constriction. Just as the heart can be broken down into a right- and left-sided pump with different purposes, the circulatory system can be divided between the pulmonary vascular and systemic vascular systems. The pulmonary vascular system represents the vessels that flow through the lungs for gas exchange. The systemic vascular system comprises all the other vessels that supply all the tissues and organs with blood flow (perfusion). Each system contains arteries, arterioles (small arteries), veins, venules (small veins), and capillaries.

10.1b The Blood Vessels

BVT *Lab*

Flashcards are available for this chapter at www.BVTLab.com.

A layer of endothelial cells lines each vessel in the vascular system. This layer is a passive barrier that keeps cells and proteins from going into tissues; it also contains substances that control the contraction of underlying smooth muscle, such as prostacyclin (vasodilator), nitric oxide (vasodilator), and endothelin (vasoconstrictor) (see Figure 10-1). Some of the proposed pathophysiology of the cardiac system may be related to endothelial dysfunction. In Figure 10-1, notice that the walls of arteries, arterioles, veins, and venules all contain smooth muscle but in different proportions. The capillaries contain no smooth muscle, because this would act as a diffusion barrier to the vital gas exchange that occurs in capillaries. It is important to remember that arteries carry blood away from the heart to the organs and tissues, and veins carry blood back to the heart.

FIGURE 10-1 Schematic Diagram of Various Blood Vessels

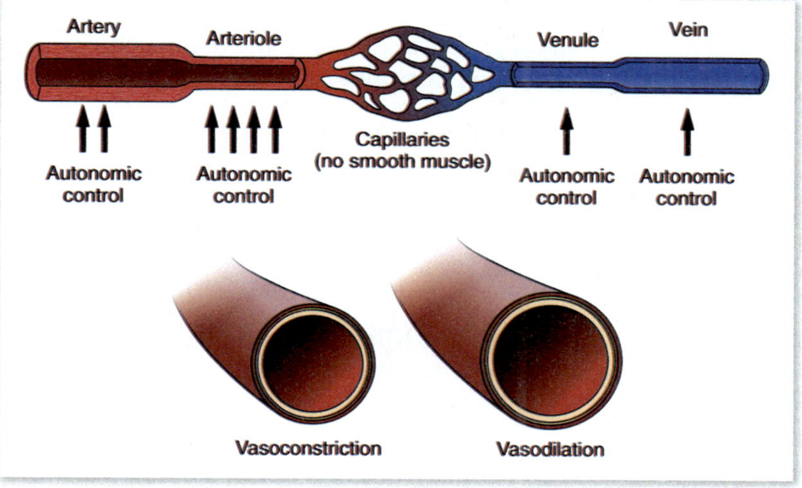

The sympathetic nervous system, discussed in Chapter 3, controls the activity of smooth muscle. Both neural and humoral (circulating within the blood) mechanisms control blood vessel contraction. Because the arterioles contain more smooth muscle and are under more nervous system control, they are the main *resistance vessels* and regulate the force against which the heart must pump, or the **afterload**. If the arterioles are vasoconstricted, this will narrow the circulatory highway, thereby increasing afterload and systemic vascular resistance. This leads to an increase in blood pressure. Conversely, vasodilation relaxes the smooth muscle layers in the vessels and thereby reduces afterload and lowers blood pressure. Arterioles branch into capillaries at the tissues, where vital gas exchange takes place, and the blood now delivers its oxygen and picks up waste carbon dioxide.

The systemic venules and veins then collect the deoxygenated blood from the tissue sites and return it to the right side of the heart to be pumped through the pulmonary vascular system to gain vital oxygen (inhalation) and rid the body of waste carbon dioxide (exhalation). The systemic veins and venules have a large capacity to hold blood and relatively little musculature compared to arteries and arterioles and therefore can distend much more easily without major pressure changes. The veins are therefore considered *capacitance vessels*; they regulate preload. **Preload** is the amount of blood returning to the heart and contained in the ventricles before a contraction.

Learning Hint

A balloon is a good way to understand these relationships. A new balloon is very noncompliant, so it takes more pressure to inflate. If you stretch the balloon (vasodilate it), it becomes more compliant and takes less pressure to inflate. A good disease analogy is an aneurysm, which is like a weak patch in a balloon. This section is too compliant, and high pressures (hypertension) could cause it to burst.

Compliance is the extent to which the pressure of the vascular system increases as volume increases. More work is needed to push blood through a constricted vessel, so compliance is decreased, resulting in a greater pressure. If the compliance increases and the vessels vasodilate, the pressure is reduced.

Thus far we have focused on the systemic vascular system; however it is important to note that pressure must also be regulated within the pulmonary vascular system, and this will be discussed in later chapters. Finally, the kidneys play a role in regulating blood pressure in addition to their other roles of ridding the body of waste products, excreting drugs or metabolites, and maintaining fluid, electrolyte, and acid–base balance. This role is discussed later in this chapter.

10.1c Regulation of Blood Pressure

Blood pressure is controlled by centers in the brain that respond to changes in the **baroreceptors** (pressure sensors) in the arterial system. Baroreceptor reflexes are the primary autonomic mechanism for blood pressure homeostasis. These reflexes react to input from the carotid sinus and output from parasympathetic and sympathetic nerves to maintain blood pressure control. If the baroreceptors are stretched too far, thus sensing high pressure, they send signals that decrease sympathetic tone and thus reduce blood pressure. If the receptors sense low pressure, they increase sympathetic tone to increase blood pressure and maintain perfusion.

A mathematical relationship describing blood pressure is helpful in understanding the various ways in which pharmacologic control of blood pressure can be exerted. The equation is

Blood pressure (BP) = cardiac output (CO) × total peripheral resistance (TPR)

From this equation, it is easy to see that anything that increases CO or TPR will increase blood pressure and vice versa. Cardiac output, as established in Chapter 9, is related directly to heart rate and stroke volume. Therefore anything that decreases heart rate, diminishes stroke volume, or decreases total peripheral resistance will lower blood pressure (see Figure 10-2).

FIGURE 10-2 Blood Pressure Homeostasis

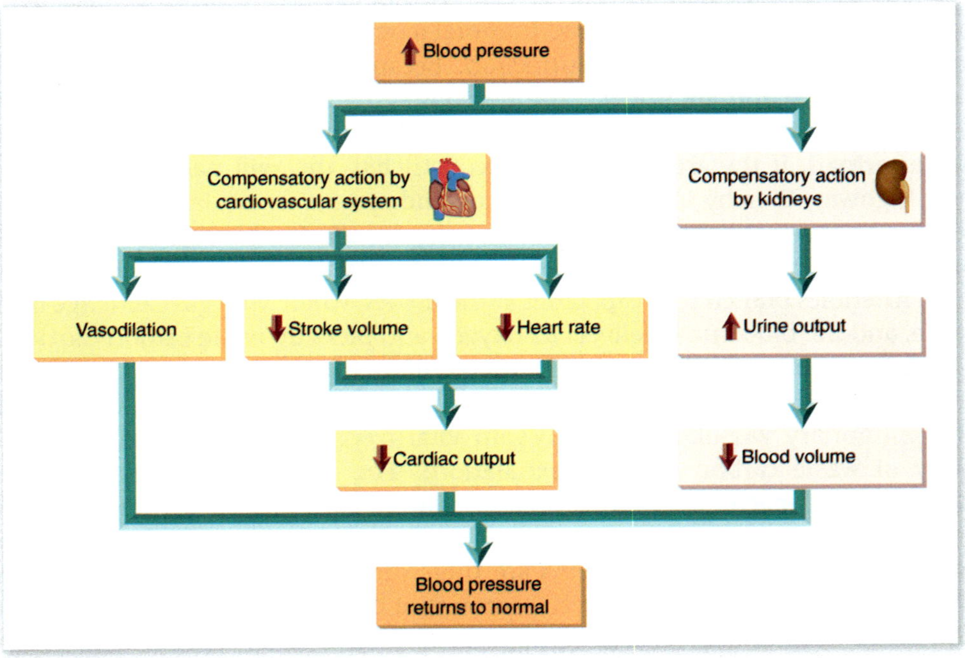

10.1d Hypertension

Hypertension can be characterized by an elevation in systolic blood pressure, diastolic blood pressure, or both. It is classified into stages as a guide to therapy. There are various causes of hypertension. If no specific cause can be found for the hypertension, it is termed **essential hypertension**; this is how we classify the majority of patients who have hypertension.

CONTROVERSY

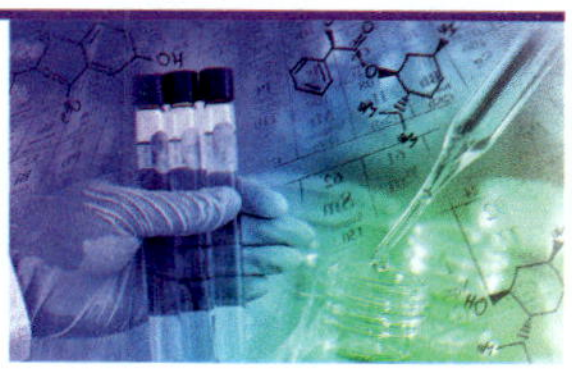

Some of the etiologic factors that may contribute to the pathophysiology of hypertension are subject to debate, including the following: abnormal renin–angiotensin–aldosterone system, defective baroreceptors, insulin resistance, defective kidney response to fluid and electrolytes, deficient nitric oxide release from the endothelium, excess sodium, potassium depletion, and even too little calcium in the diet.

Because the disease is usually asymptomatic, hypertension is frequently called the "silent killer." Hypertension, even without symptoms, is one of the leading causes of stroke, blindness, congestive heart failure, and renal disease. The Eighth Report of the Joint National Committee (JNC) on the Detection, Evaluation, and Treatment of High Blood Pressure was developed as national clinical guidelines to aid clinicians in managing hypertension (please see Table 10-1). If hypertension is not treated, target organ disease (TOD) can result. Target organ disease may include, for example, left ventricular hypertrophy, transient ischemic attacks, peripheral vascular disease, retinopathy, or protein in the urine. If TOD is present at the time of diagnosis, it suggests that hypertension has been present long term but not treated adequately.

Clinical pearl

Many people with hypertension are asymptomatic, yet other people with hypertension complain of a pounding in their heads. If pressure increases in your arms or legs, there is a certain "give" because the tissues are not rigid, allowing some of the pressure increase to dissipate. However, the skull does not allow this flexibility, and small increases in cerebral blood flow or pressure can increase the intracranial pressure (ICP) dramatically.

TABLE 10-1 **Management of Hypertension (JNC 8)**

Population Age	Systolic (mmHg) Goal	Diastolic (mmHg) Goal	Initial Drug Therapy
>60	<150	<90	thiazide, ACEI, ARB, or CCB
<60	<140	<90	thiazide, ACEI, ARB, or CCB
Any age with diabetes	<140	<90	thiazide, ACEI, ARB, or CCB
Any age with chronic kidney disease	≤140	≤90	ACEI or ARB

ACEI = angiotensin-converting enzyme (ACE) inhibitor
CCB = calcium-channel blocker
ARB = angiotensin II–receptor blocker

Source: The Eighth Report of the Joint National Committee on Prevention, Detection, Evaluation, and Treatment of High Blood Pressure, http://jama.jamanetwork.com/article.aspx?articleid=1791497

Antihypertensives work on different parts of the blood pressure equation to either decrease cardiac output or decrease total peripheral resistance. See Figure 10-3, which shows the relationship between antihypertensive agents and the blood pressure equation. Looking at Figure 10-3, you can clearly see the potential role for combination antihypertensive therapy, which includes two drugs that work on different parts of the equation.

FIGURE 10-3 Relationship Between Antihypertensive Agents and Blood Pressure Equation

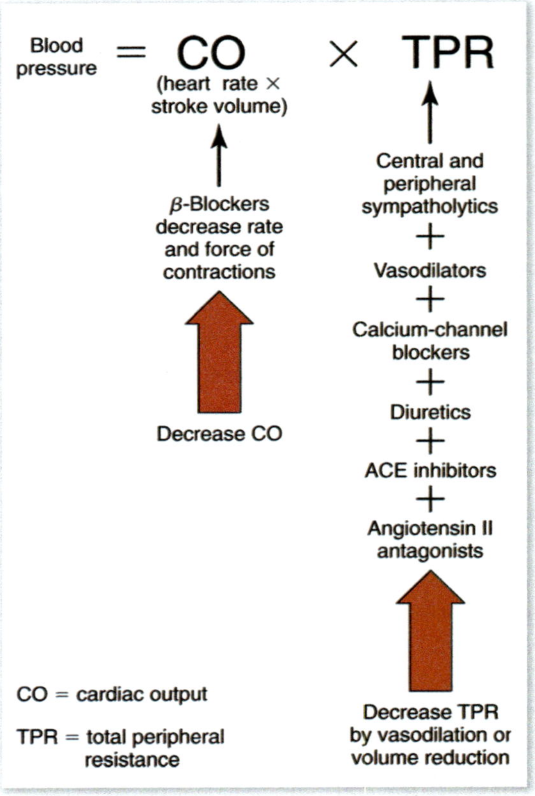

Patient & Family Education

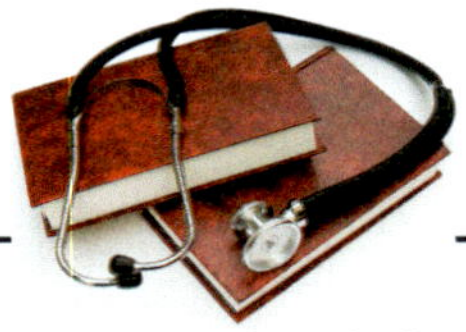

Because most patients with high blood pressure are not aware that their pressure is high, it is important to emphasize the long-term benefits of medicines they take for high blood pressure. This is especially important since the blood pressure medicines may make them feel worse until their body gets used to them. Remind patients and their families that the benefits of lowering blood pressure to normal levels include reductions in strokes, heart attacks, and heart and kidney failures.

Before discussing the various pharmacologic agents to treat hypertension, it should be noted that nonpharmacologic lifestyle modification treatment is preferred if possible. By using lifestyle changes such as exercise, weight loss, alcohol restriction, smoking cessation, and salt restriction, patients may be able to control high blood pressure or decrease the amount of drug needed to control the disease. Some individuals are more sensitive than others to dietary salt intake, and they are referred to as salt sensitive. Salt-sensitive patients achieve greater degrees of blood pressure lowering by restricting dietary sodium intake. Numerous genes are probably responsible for salt excretion by the kidney. The different mechanisms for the pathophysiology of hypertension may explain why patients respond differently to nonpharmacologic treatment as well as different antihypertensives. If the hypertension cannot be treated effectively nonpharmacologically, then initial drug therapy is individualized according to concurrent compelling medical indications (see Table 10-2). In general the goal blood pressure should be less than 140/90 mmHg if the patient is less than 60 years old or has diabetes or chronic kidney disease. For patients 60 years of age and older, a target blood pressure of 150/90 mmHg is the goal.

TABLE 10-2 Compelling Indications

Systolic heart failure	Diuretic, ACE inhibitor, β-blocker, ARB, aldosterone antagonist
Post–myocardial infarction	β-Blocker, ACE inhibitor, aldosterone antagonist
Diabetes mellitus	ACE inhibitor or ARB, diuretic, CCB
Chronic kidney disease	ACE inhibitor or ARB
Recurrent stroke	Diuretic or ACE inhibitor

An example of a treatment choice based on concurrent compelling medical condition is a hypertensive patient with systolic heart failure. This patient will most likely be started on an angiotensin-converting enzyme (ACE) inhibitor, because these drugs can treat both medical conditions. If single-drug therapy is not successful, then additional drugs from a different class or a new drug from a different class are given until the right combination works. The various types of antihypertensive agents include (1) diuretics, (2) central- and (3) peripheral-acting sympatholytics, (4) β-blockers, (5) ACE inhibitors, (6) angiotensin II–receptor blockers (ARBs) or antagonist, (7) calcium-channel blockers (CCBs), and (8) vasodilators. Again, please refer to Table 10-1 for the classification and management of blood pressure in adults and Table 10-2 for compelling indications for the various drug classes.

CONTROVERSY

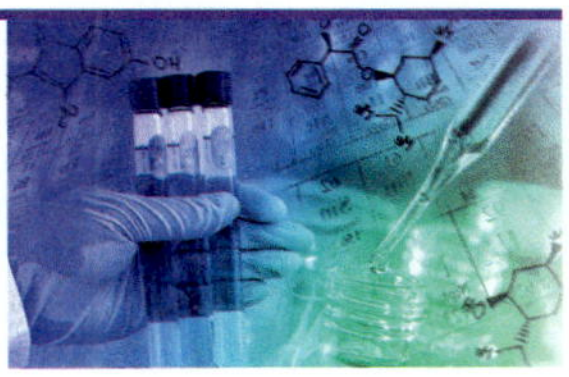

There is no agreement as to which antihypertensive medicine should be used first. Unless there is an underlying condition that would benefit from a beta-blocker, this class of high blood pressure medicines is not used as a first-line treatment option. Another controversial area is the choice of a thiazide. Most of the research using a thiazide diuretic was done using chlorthalidone, which is approximately twice as potent and much longer acting than hydrochlorothiazide, the most frequently prescribed diuretic. Whether hydrochlorothiazide is interchangeable for chlorthalidone in not only reducing blood pressure but also preventing clinically important outcomes is questionable.

10.2 CATEGORIES OF DRUGS TO TREAT HYPERTENSION

In Chapter 3 you learned that any agent that inhibits sympathetic nerve function results in decreased venous tone, decreased heart rate, decreased contractility of the heart, decreased cardiac output, and decreased total peripheral resistance. On this basis, it makes sense that sympatholytics are used as antihypertensives. Sympatholytic antihypertensives are classified by their central (the brain) or peripheral (circulating vessels) site or mechanism of action. These antihypertensive agents affect the α- or β-receptors.

10.2a Direct-Acting α_2-Agonists or Central-Acting Sympatholytics

Central-acting agents work directly on the α_2-receptors in the central nervous system (CNS) to decrease sympathetic outflow of activity from the CNS. When they are stimulated, α_2-receptors block the release of norepinephrine. Remember that norepinephrine is an endogenous vasoconstrictor, and thus its blockage causes vasodilation and reduces blood pressure. α_2-Selective agonists such as clonidine therefore decrease centrally controlled sympathetic outflow from the brain, thus resulting in decreased cardiac output and decreased vascular resistance.

Rebound hypertension may occur when a central α_2-agonist is discontinued. This means that the blood pressure can overshoot and become higher than it was before treatment. Another side effect to be aware of with this class and all antihypertensives is orthostatic hypotension. *Orthostatic hypotension* occurs when blood pressure drops as the patient moves from a sitting to a standing position. Patients should always rise slowly from a horizontal or sitting position to minimize dizziness that may accompany the orthostasis and lead to falls. The use of this class of drugs is limited due to a high incidence of common adverse effects such as sexual dysfunction, dry mouth, and sedation. Common types of central-acting or α_2-agonists are

- clonidine (Catapres®)
- guanfacine (Tenex®)

Clinical Pearl

Clonidine can also be used to treat withdrawal symptoms in patients who are giving up smoking or going through opiate withdrawal. It is proposed that it works by decreasing the noradrenergic hyperactivity that is common in these situations.

10.2b α_1-Blockers or Peripheral-Acting Sympatholytics

α_1-Receptors are found mainly in the blood vessels themselves, and their stimulation causes vasoconstriction. However α_1-blockers or antagonists block receptors in both arterioles and veins, thus causing vasodilation. α_1-Blockers such as prazosin therefore decrease vascular resistance. α-Blockers are well known for their ability to cause orthostatic hypotension, especially with the first dose. Other common adverse effects include headache and weakness. Patients should always be counseled to take their first dose at bedtime as a way to lessen first-dose hypotension. These drugs are generally not used as first-line therapy except possibly for older men with symptomatic benign prostatic hyperplasia for which these medications help improve symptoms. Some common α_1-blockers or peripheral-acting sympatholytics are

- prazosin (Minipress®)
- terazosin (Hytrin®)
- doxazosin (Cardura®)

Clinical Pearl

α-Blockers that are prescribed for hypertension are also effective for benign prostatic hyperplasia. They work because the prostate has α-receptors whose blockade results in decreased smooth muscle tone and less obstruction. For many patients, not only is their blood pressure lowered, but they also experience decreased frequency of urination, which is problematic in benign prostatic hyperplasia. Treating two diseases with one drug is like killing two birds with one stone (but what a terrible saying)!

10.2c β-Blockers

β_1-Receptors are found primarily in the heart, and their stimulation leads to an increase in the rate and force of contraction. β-Blockers therefore inhibit sympathetic activity and decrease the rate and force of contraction, thus lowering blood pressure. As discussed in Chapter 9, β-blockers differ in their selectivity for β_1- and β_2-receptors.

β-Blockers need to be used cautiously in patients with severe peripheral vascular disease and insulin-dependent diabetics. This is because β-blockers can exacerbate symptoms of arterial insufficiency and mask warning signs of hypoglycemia. β-blockers can also cause bradycardia or atrioventricular conduction abnormalities. β-Blockers that are *not* selective for β_1-receptors can exacerbate chronic obstructive pulmonary disease by blocking the β_2-receptors in the lung. β-Blockers can decrease HDL cholesterol, raise triglycerides, and elevate plasma glucose. Some common β-blockers include

- metoprolol (Lopressor®)
- propranolol (Inderal®)
- atenolol (Tenormin®)

See Figure 10-4, which illustrates the sites of action of sympatholytic antihypertensive agents.

FIGURE 10-4 Sites of Action of Sympatholytic Antihypertensive Agents

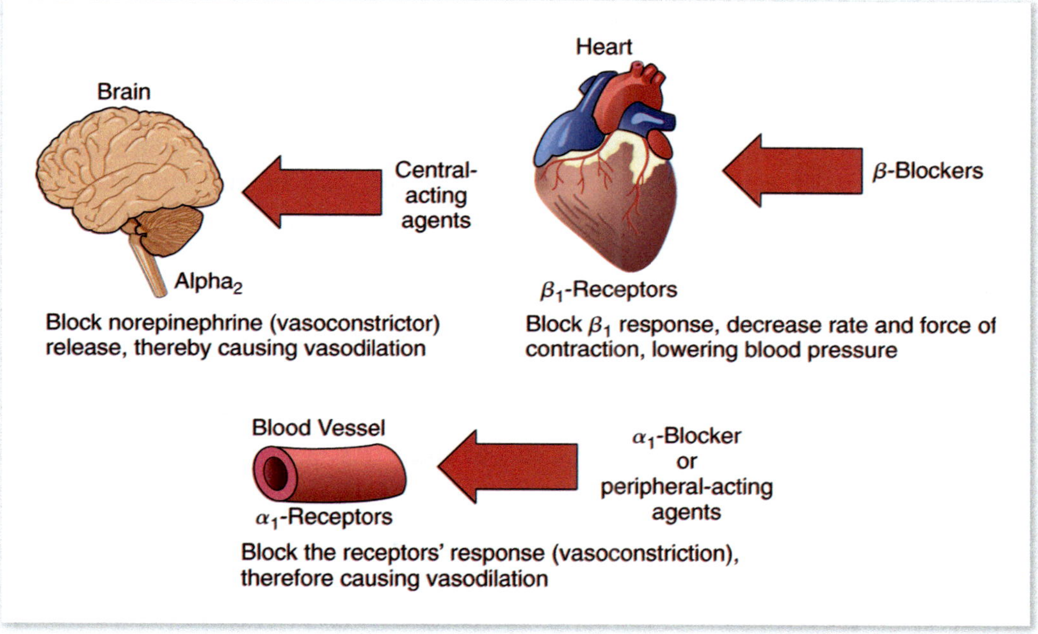

10.2d Diuretics

As discussed in Chapter 9, diuretics are used to treat edema associated with heart failure as well as to treat hypertension. To understand renal pharmacology, it is important to review the basics of renal physiology. Kidneys rid the body of waste products by filtering the blood. In addition the kidneys maintain fluid, electrolyte, and acid–base balance. The kidney is thought of primarily as an excretory organ; it also plays an important role in drug elimination.

The functional unit of the kidney is the *nephron,* which is comprised of the glomerulus, proximal convoluted tubule, the loop of Henle, the distal convoluted tubule, and the collecting duct. As blood is filtered in the glomerulus, it drains into the tubular systems, where parts of the filtrate can be reabsorbed back into the blood via the peritubular capillary system. The filtrate remaining in the tubular system is excreted via the urine.

Electrolytes or salts that are filtered are usually reabsorbed at a certain site along the kidney. Electrolytes regulate acid–base balance and affect neuromuscular activity. Blood volume is regulated by sodium and water reabsorption,

Learning Hint

To get a visual picture, imagine the tubular system as PVC piping—you know, the white plastic kind used for sink drains and such. Now wrap red yarn all around it to represent the peritubular capillary system. What stays in the pipe is excreted from the body via urination or goes down the drain. What is "reabsorbed" (via capillary diffusion) goes into the red yarn to be recirculated in the bloodstream.

which are affected by osmosis and concentration gradients and are also influenced by antidiuretic hormone (ADH) and aldosterone. Renal secretion of electrolytes is important in helping to control the acid–base balance of the body.

Diuretics basically do not allow sodium to be reabsorbed back into the peritubular capillary system (bloodstream). If sodium stays in the tubular system, it draws water via osmosis into the tubular system, which is then excreted as increased urine output.

All diuretics increase salt and water excretion, but the effect that diuretics have on other ions depends on the diuretic. Different diuretics work on different sites in the kidney, and they are classified according to the site in the nephron where they work. Because the mechanisms of reabsorption of sodium and water and of chloride and potassium are different in each segment of the kidney, diuretics acting on different segments have different mechanisms. In general thiazide diuretics are preferred as antihypertensives unless the patient has severe kidney disease. Initially thiazide diuretics lower blood volume by increasing sodium and water excretion and therefore lower blood pressure. Over the longer term blood volume returns to normal while systemic vascular resistance falls.

Three different classes of diuretics are used to treat hypertension: thiazides, loop, and potassium-sparing. Blood pressure–lowering effects are not necessarily dose-related. There can be a *ceiling effect* for drugs, as with the thiazide class of diuretics, in which increased doses just cause more side effects and do not lower blood pressure. Side effects of diuretics differ depending on the class and may include hypokalemia, hypomagnesemia, hyperuricemia, and hyperglycemia. Loop diuretics cause less hyperglycemia and differ from thiazides in that they cause hypocalcemia, whereas thiazides can be calcium-sparing. See Figure 10-5, which shows the mechanisms of action of diuretics.

FIGURE 10-5 Mechanisms of Action of Diuretics

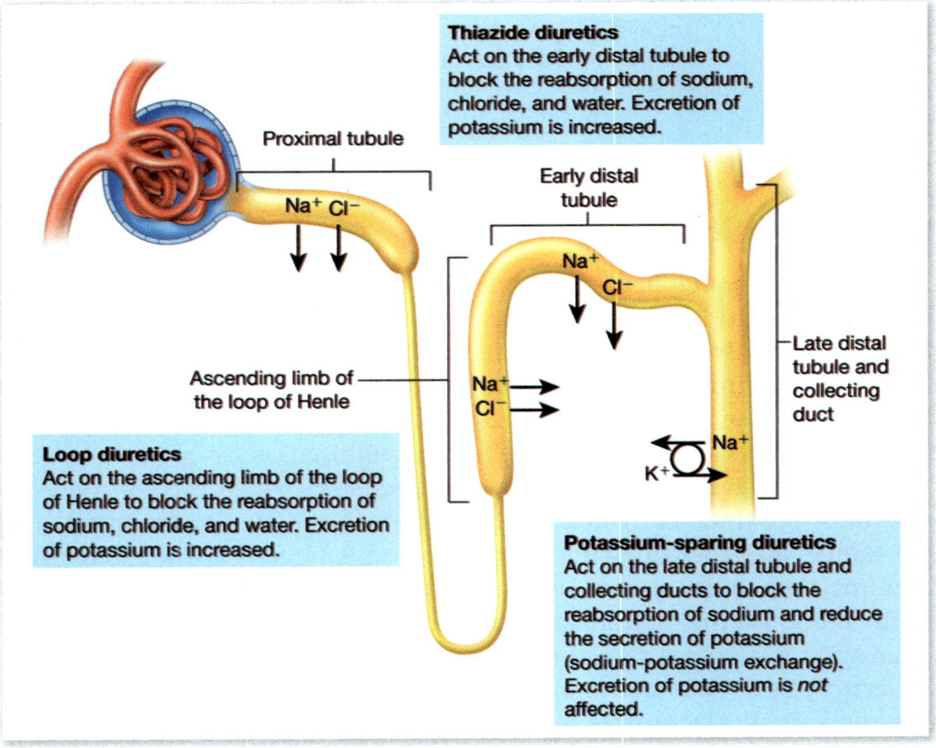

Specific Diuretics

The thiazide diuretics block the sodium and chloride reabsorption in the distal convoluted tubule resulting in excretion of about 6% of the filtered sodium. Water follows this salt, but salt is excreted in excess of water. Examples of thiazide diuretics include

- chlorthalidone (Thalitone®)
- hydrochlorothiazide (Microzide®)

Loop diuretics decrease sodium, chloride, and water absorption at the loop of Henle by blocking absorption of chloride into the bloodstream. Since sodium is cotransported with chloride, it follows the chloride and water out of the kidney. Water is excreted in excess of salt. These are the most potent diuretics. Examples of loop diuretics include

- bumetanide
- furosemide (Lasix®)

Loop diuretics such as furosemide (Lasix®) can be used for hypertension, but they have a shorter duration of action than thiazide diuretics; as mentioned previously, loop diuretics are generally reserved for patients with severe, chronic kidney failure. They are also useful in the treatment of edema and acute pulmonary edema. In that situation, in addition to diuresing, they act as venodilators via their effect on enhancing prostaglandin secretion. This is why patients report alleviation of their pulmonary edema symptoms before the medicine has caused an increase in urine production. Loop diuretics are also used in the treatment of hypercalcemia of malignancy to lower calcium levels.

Potassium-sparing diuretics do not allow potassium to be excreted along with the sodium as thiazides or loop diuretics do. The excessive loss of potassium leading to hypokalemia can have serious cardiac effects. Potassium-sparing diuretics include

- amiloride (Midamor®)
- spironolactone (Aldactone®)
- triamterene (Dyrenium®)
- eplerenone (Inspra®)

Potassium-sparing diuretics such as spironolactone (Aldactone®) may be administered in combination with other diuretics to prevent potassium depletion. They have a weak antihypertensive effect when used alone but can be additive with thiazide or loop diuretics. If the hypertension is aldosterone-mediated, an aldosterone-antagonist diuretic, such as spironolactone, is especially effective. Thiazide and loop diuretics both cause potassium loss and are not potassium-sparing. Thiazides are frequently used in combination with a potassium-sparing diuretic such as triamterene (Dyrenium®). This is conveniently available as a combination product called Maxzide®.

BVT Lab

Visit www.BVTLab.com to explore the student resources available for this chapter.

Life Span Considerations

Whether a person with high blood pressure is young or old, restricting salt in the diet is extremely important. This is difficult to do because 80% of our salt intake comes from foods we buy at the grocery store and not from the salt shakers on our dinner tables. Helping patients learn how to read food labels and to choose lower-sodium foods is one way of helping patients lower their dietary salt intake.

10.2e Angiotensin-Converting Enzyme (ACE) Inhibitors

The kidneys are involved in blood pressure regulation through the renin–angiotensin system. They release renin into the bloodstream when renal blood flow decreases. Renin acts on angiotensinogen (also known as angiotensin precursor) in the bloodstream to form angiotensin I. It is then converted to angiotensin II as it circulates through the lungs; angiotensin II is a powerful vasoconstrictor. Angiotensin II also causes the release of the hormone aldosterone, which increases sodium and water reabsorption into the bloodstream. The increased blood volume, along with the vasoconstriction, increases the blood pressure (see Figure 10-6). ACE inhibitors decrease blood levels of angiotensin II and aldosterone by interrupting the renin–angiotensin–aldosterone system and thereby lower blood pressure. They reduce peripheral arterial resistance without affecting heart rate and cardiac output.

These drugs have up to a 20% incidence of cough as a side effect. Cough can occur after anywhere from 1 week to 6 months of therapy and is more common in women than in men. Another side effect of ACE inhibitors is hyperkalemia, especially in patients with decreased renal function. ACE inhibitors may also cause a decline in renal function that could be severe, even though they are also used to protect renal function (renal-sparing) and they decrease protein loss in the urine in patients with diabetes. Acute kidney failure or a decline in kidney function is unusual unless the patient has bilateral renal artery stenosis or is volume depleted. Hypertension and diabetes frequently coexist in patients, making ACE inhibitors common drugs used. Common ACE inhibitors include

- benazepril (Lotensin®)
- captopril
- enalapril (Vasotec®)

FIGURE 10-6 The Renin–Angiotensin–Aldosterone Pathway

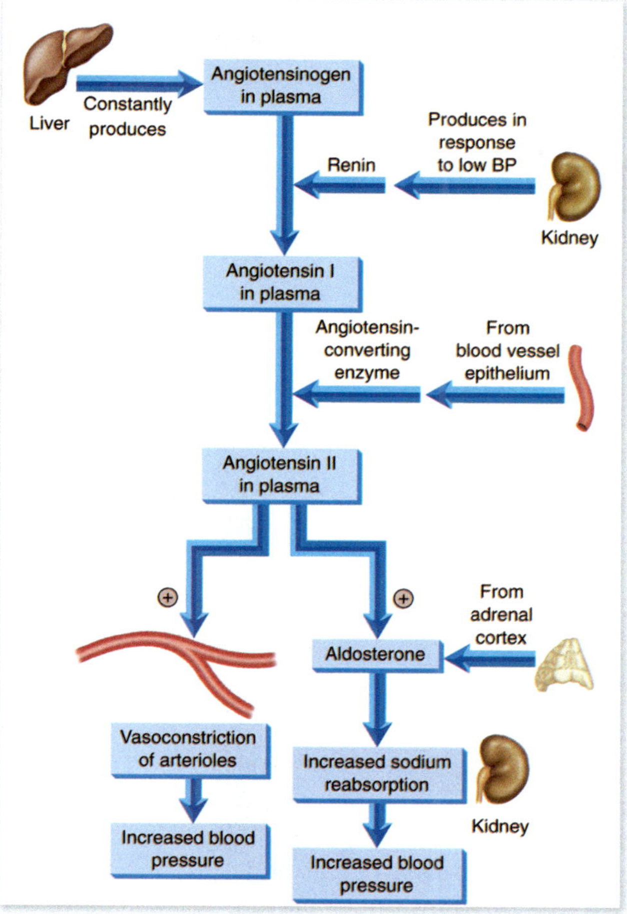

10.2f Angiotensin II–Receptor Blockers (ARBs)

Angiotensin II antagonists inhibit angiotensin II at receptor sites on the blood vessels and therefore act differently than ACE inhibitors. They are an alternative for patients with a cough side effect from an ACE inhibitor. They can also cause hyperkalemia and acute kidney failure as discussed previously for ACE inhibitors. Representative drugs in this category include

- losartan (Cozaar®)
- valsartan (Diovan®)

See Figure 10-7, which shows the site and mechanism of action of diuretics, ACE inhibitors, and angiotensin II–receptor blockers.

10.2g Calcium-Channel Blockers

Calcium-channel blockers (CCBs) produce arteriole relaxation by the same mechanisms they use to relieve angina. By blocking calcium needed for vascular smooth muscle contraction, they relax vascular smooth muscle, so vasodilation results. Any effects related to the drug's action on calcium in smooth muscle are unrelated to dietary calcium.

FIGURE 10-7 Mechanisms of Action of Diuretics, ACE Inhibitors, and Angiotension II–Receptor Blockers

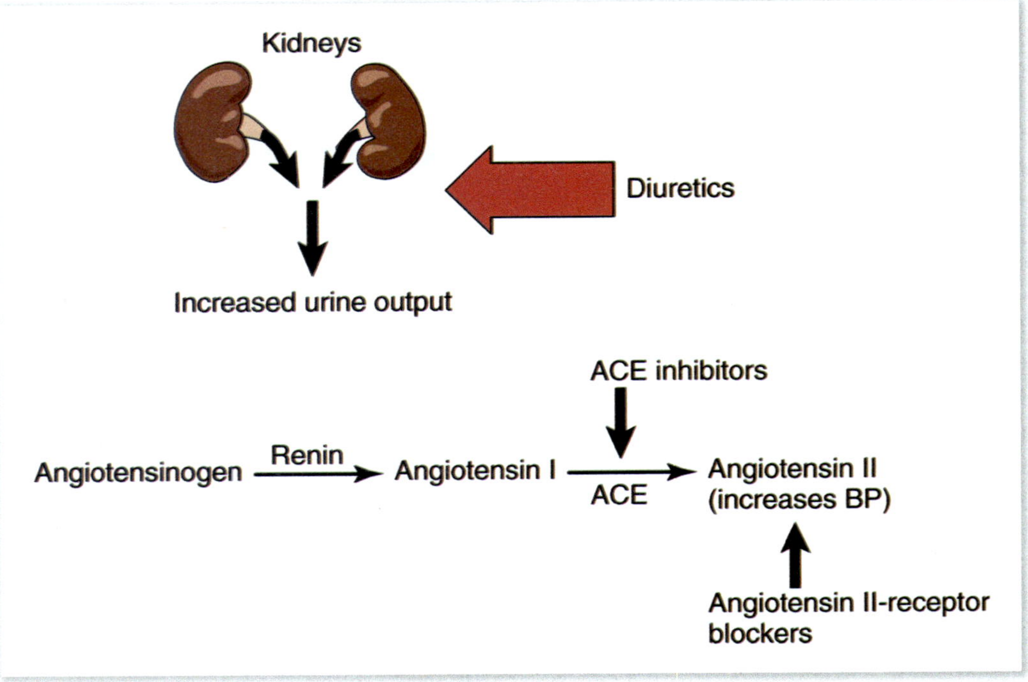

Learning Hint

Calcium-channel blockers are also known as calcium entry blockers (CEBs).

The most common side effects of CCBs are peripheral edema and dizziness. As explained in the section on arrhythmia in Chapter 9, CCBs have different effects on heart rate and atrioventricular nodal conduction. This may cause side effects when used for hypertension. Common CCBs include

- amlodipine (Norvasc®)
- diltiazem (Cardizem®)
- verapamil (Calan®)

10.2h Vasodilators

Vasodilators such as hydralazine are more effective at relaxing the smooth muscle in arteries than that in veins. Vasodilators are usually considered last-line therapy for nonacute hypertension treatment. Vasodilators can cause a reflex tachycardia and peripheral edema. For those reasons, they are frequently used in combination with a β-blocker and a diuretic. One vasodilator you may recognize by name is minoxidil (Loniten®). One of the side effects of minoxidil is hypertrichosis, or increased hair growth. Drug manufacturers capitalize on this side effect and market minoxidil (Rogaine®) for male-pattern baldness. The vasodilator action of Rogaine® reestablishes blood flow to the hair follicles of some individuals when it is applied topically. Common vasodilators include

- hydralazine
- minoxidil

time for review

After reading about all the side effects of blood pressure medications and reading about hypertension being a silent killer, how do you explain the importance of treatment compliance with antihypertensives?

10.2i Agents for Hypertensive Emergencies/Urgencies

Although hypertensive emergency and urgency may sound like the same condition, they are different medical conditions and are treated differently. The two conditions differ not so much by absolute blood pressure value as by the absence or presence of end-organ damage (e.g., retinal hemorrhages or acute kidney failure) along with the elevated blood pressure. Physicians must do a physical exam and order lab work to detect end-organ damage that may be present due to the elevated blood pressure. This can guide treatment aggressiveness and drug therapy selection.

Systolic blood pressure ≥180 mmHg or diastolic blood pressure ≥120 mmHg can be immediately life-threatening, requiring fast-acting treatment, or some patients can be relatively asymptomatic, presenting with just a headache. The optimal management in patients with minimal symptoms is unknown. In either case too rapid a reduction in blood pressure can be dangerous. Both oral and parenteral antihypertensive drugs are options. Oral drugs are usually used for hypertensive urgencies, while intravenous medications are reserved for hypertensive emergencies. The oral antihypertensives clonidine (Catapres®) and captopril (Capoten®) have been given in loading doses in the past to achieve a fast response, but now they are generally given as a single dose for hypertensive urgencies along with allowing the patient to rest quietly in a dark room for 20 minutes.

Nitroprusside sodium (Nitropress®) is a potent agent that is used for minute-to-minute control of hypertensive emergencies. Nitroprusside is a potent vasodilator that dilates both venous and arterial vessels and has an immediate onset of action, within 30 to 60 seconds. Its most common side effect is too rapid a reduction in blood pressure, which, as previously mentioned, can be dangerous. Another problem with nitroprusside is the potential for cyanide toxicity. This problem is uncommon when nitroprusside is used at low doses or for brief periods. Cyanide toxicity can be fatal, so this medicine is usually only used in patients refractory to other antihypertensives and is stopped as soon as possible.

Clinical pearl

Excessive doses of nitroprusside can cause cyanide toxicity, as it is metabolized to cyanide.

Intravenous nitroglycerin dilates both arterioles and veins, reducing both preload and afterload. It is especially useful when hypertension occurs concurrently with myocardial ischemia.

Fenoldopam (Corlopam®) is a dopamine-1 antagonist with a quick onset of action. It is titrated by intravenous infusion and is commonly used for perioperative hypertension. Because it improves renal blood flow, it is useful for patients with renal insufficiency. Coronary, renal, mesenteric, and peripheral arteries are vasodilated and renal blood flow increases with this drug. Fenoldopam is more expensive than nitroprusside and is used primarily in patients at high risk for cyanide toxicity.

Nicardipine (Cardene®) and clevidipine (Cleviprex®) are intravenous calcium-channel blockers useful in most hypertensive emergencies except acute heart failure. Adverse effects include tachycardia and flushing. Clevidipine is formulated within a 20% fat emulsion, which may result in hypertriglyceridemia, especially when used in high doses for extended periods of time.

Labetelol (Normodyne®, Trandate®) is a combination α- and β-blocker for intravenous infusion in most hypertensive emergencies except acute heart failure. Adverse effects include bronchoconstriction and heart block.

See Table 10-3, which lists the various categories of antihypertensive agents, along with representative drugs. See Figure 10-8, which shows the mechanism of action of antihypertensive drugs.

TABLE 10-3 Categories of Antihypertensive Agents with Representative Drugs

Class	Action Name	Generic Name	Brand Name
Sympatholytics (central)	Decrease in sympathetic outflow from brain	guanfacine	Tenex®
		clonidine	Catapres®
Sympatholytics (peripheral) α-blockers	Peripheral vasodilation	doxazosin	Cardura®
		prazosin	Minipress®
		terazosin	Hytrin®
β-Blockers	Decrease in CO	acebutolol	Sectral®
		atenolol	Tenormin®
		metoprolol	Lopressor®
		propranolol	Inderal® LA
Diuretics	Decrease in blood volume	chlorthalidone	Thalitone®
		furosemide	Lasix®
		spironolactone	Aldactone®
ACE inhibitors	Vasodilation	benazepril	Lotensin®
		captopril	
		enalapril	Vasotec®
Angiotensin II antagonists	Vasodilation	losartan	Cozaar®
		valsartan	Diovan®
Calcium-channel blockers	Vasodilation	amlodipine	Norvasc®
		verapamil	Calan®
		diltiazem	Cardizem®
Vasodilators	Direct relaxation of smooth muscle	hydralazine	
		minoxidil	
Emergency/urgency antihypertensives	Acute vasodilation	nitroprusside	Nipride®
		nicardipine IV	Cardene®
		clevidipine IV	Cleviprex®
		nitroglycerin IV	

FIGURE 10-8 Mechanism of Action of Antihypertensive Drugs

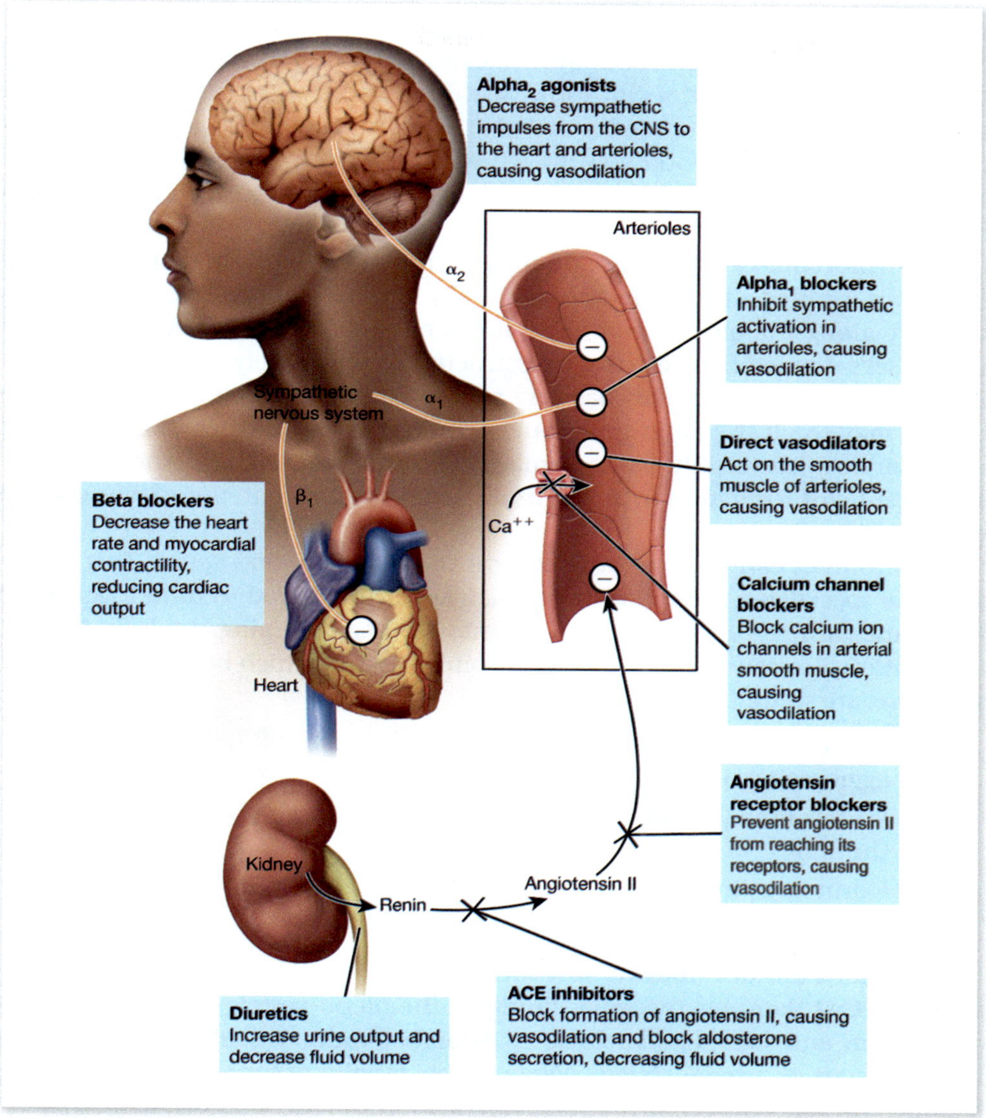

10.2j Treating Hypotension

The treatment of hypotension and shock will be covered in Chapter 15 as part of the discussion of Advanced Cardiac Life Support (ACLS). These drugs are primarily vasopressor and cardiotonic agents. Vasopressor drugs increase smooth muscle tone and thus cause vasoconstriction. Cardiotonic agents stimulate the heart to increase the rate and/or force of contraction of the heart to increase blood pressure and perfusion.

10.3 THE HEMOSTATIC SYSTEM

10.3a The Clotting Process

One of the amazing things about blood is its normal ability to flow freely through blood vessels and yet clot when the need arises. The hemostatic system's job is to

Clinical pearl

An *embolism* is a general term for an obstruction of a blood vessel by a foreign substance. This may be fat or even a gas bubble. A *thromboembolism* refers specifically to a blood clot.

maintain fluidity of blood within the vasculature and minimize blood loss when blood leaks outside the vessels by clotting. Without the clotting mechanism, a minor cut would cause us to literally bleed to death. However, the clotting mechanism, like all physiologic mechanisms, can get out of balance owing to disease states or other factors. If a clot forms within a blood vessel or an organ cavity such as the heart, it is termed a *thrombus*. This intravascular clot can partially or totally occlude the blood flow, which will diminish or stop the supply to the local tissue being fed by this vessel. Lack of blood flow leads to infarction and subsequent tissue necrosis.

The thrombus can dislodge and travel through the bloodstream. A traveling thrombus is called a **thromboembolism** (TE). The thromboembolism continues to move along the bloodstream until it reaches a vessel where its size matches the vessel's diameter; eventually it obstructs and completely blocks blood flow beyond the obstruction. This has very serious consequences, especially because emboli may reach the lungs (pulmonary emboli) or brain (cerebral emboli) and cause serious, irreversible tissue damage. The goal of anticoagulant therapy is to prevent clot formation in patients at risk and to prevent clot extension and embolization.

A thrombus can form because of local trauma to a blood vessel. This stimulates the specialized thrombocytes or platelets in the blood to bind together or aggregate, forming a sticky gelatinous mass to begin to plug the leak. Platelet aggregation also causes the release of thromboplastin, which begins a cascade of steps that are simplified as follows:

1. Thromboplastin forms in the presence of vitamin K (released from aggregating platelets).
2. Prothrombin, in the presence of thromboplastin and calcium, forms thrombin.
3. Fibrinogen, in the presence of thrombin, forms fibrin, which causes the clot.

Vascular stasis or turbulent flow such as occurs in atherosclerotic disease and anything that damages the inner lining of the blood vessels can cause platelet aggregation and subsequent release of thromboplastin. Vascular clots can form in the venous or arterial system. Venous clots usually occur as a result of stasis, because the venous system is a relatively low-pressure/low-flow system. Platelet aggregation usually occurs in the higher flow/higher pressure of the arterial system.

Drugs are used to treat or prevent the formation of thrombi. **Anticoagulants** prevent the formation of the fibrin clot by interfering with one of the steps leading to fibrin formation. **Antiplatelet** drugs inhibit the aggregation and release of thromboplastin to begin the process. Finally **fibrinolytics** (thrombolytics) actually dissolve and liquefy the fibrin of the existing clot. Thrombolytics enhance the conversion of plasminogen to plasmin, which degrades the fibrin.

10.3b Anticoagulants

Anticoagulants are distinguished as either indirect or direct thrombin inhibitors. Indirect thrombin inhibitors include warfarin, unfractionated heparin, and low-molecular-weight heparin. Direct thrombin inhibitors include dabigatran (Pradaxa®), argatroban, and bivalirudin (Angiomax®). Anticoagulants inhibit steps in the clotting cascade leading to fibrin formation and *do not* dissolve existing clots. They do prevent new clots, as well as the extension of existing clots, from forming. They prevent mostly venous thrombosis formation. Anticoagulants are used primarily prophylactically to prevent deep-vein thrombosis (DVT) after surgery and to decrease the risk of stroke in patients with atrial fibrillation or artificial heart valves. Candidates for anticoagulants may have any of the following:

- A history of embolus formation
- Prolonged bedrest
- Coronary artery disease
- Venous thrombosis
- Phlebitis
- Surgery with previous history of thrombosis (especially orthopedic surgery)

Heparin

Standard (unfractionated) heparin (UFH) is a parenteral anticoagulant that binds with antithrombin to inhibit the conversion by thrombin of fibrinogen to fibrin. See Figure 10-9 for an illustration of its mechanism of action.

FIGURE 10-9 Mechanism of Action of Heparin

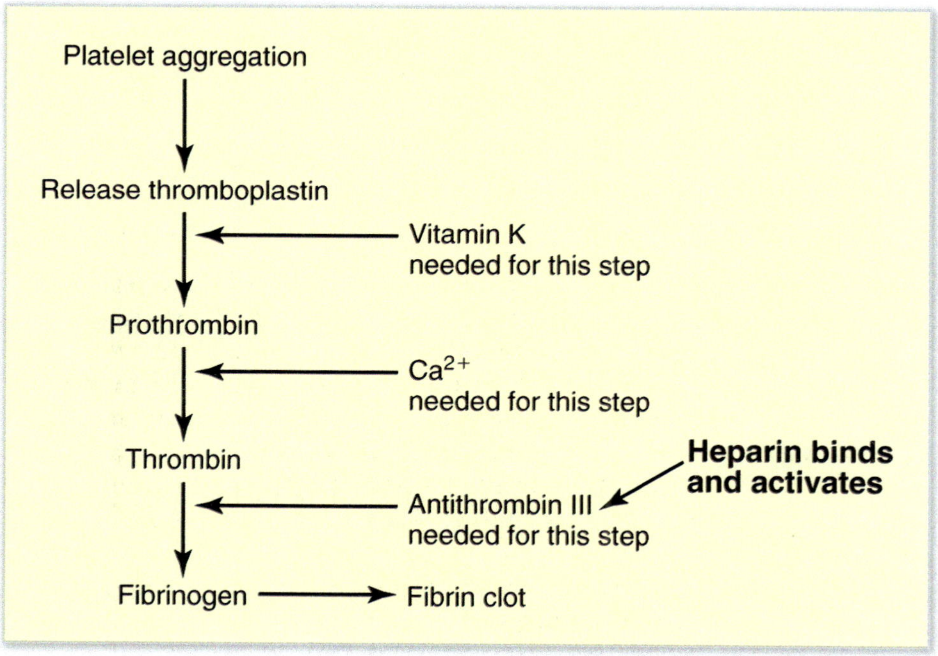

Heparin is a naturally occurring substance in mast cells and is broken down in the stomach, so it is effective only as an injectable medication. Low-dose subcutaneous heparin is used to prevent venous thromboembolism in immobile, bedridden patients postoperatively. Weight-based IV boluses and infusions of heparin are used to treat pulmonary emboli. Heparin is also used to prevent clots in cannulas or may be included in an IV or in procedures such as hemodialysis.

In arterial blood sampling kits, needles and syringes are heparinized to prevent clotting from occurring and blocking the return of blood into the syringe.

The therapeutic goals, depending on the heparin indication, are aimed at increasing the activated partial thromboplastin time to a certain laboratory-defined range. The *activated partial thromboplastin time* (aPTT) lab test is used to make dosage adjustments for heparin. The aPTT time should be maintained within a specific therapeutic range depending on the indication. These ranges should be published by a hospital's laboratory and will vary depending on the type of thromboplastin used. The aPTT lab test is different from the prothrombin time (PT) lab test, which is used to make dosage adjustments for warfarin. The PT measures the vitamin K–dependent factors. It has been largely replaced by the more reliable international normalized ratio (INR), which will be discussed later in connection with warfarin.

Side Effects of Heparin

Standard heparin does not cross the placental barrier, has a rapid action, and is readily metabolized (because the body recognizes it). However, bleeding is the most important side effect of heparin. Watch for bleeding in the mucosa (petechiae) and gums and for hematuria and GI bleeding. An antidote for excess bleeding is protamine sulfate, which complexes with heparin to antagonize its action.

Clinical pearl

Protamine, which is derived from salmon sperm, is an anticoagulant alone, but given with heparin neutralizes its effects. This reversal agent acts instantaneously and is long acting.

Heparin can cause thrombocytopenia and even osteoporosis with long-term use. Heparin is contraindicated with any serious active bleeding or thrombocytopenia. Use of heparin with brain, eye, or spinal cord surgery can be very risky, because the slightest bleed could increase intracranial pressure (brain bleed), cause paralysis (spinal cord bleed), or blindness.

Low-molecular-weight heparins (LMWHs) are the more modern version of heparin. They can be conveniently administered by the subcutaneous route, and since their absorption is more predictable than standard heparin, they are dosed based on body weight and rarely require monitoring with special coagulation tests. These agents differ in their antithrombotic properties, pharmacokinetics, side effects, and monitoring. As suggested by the name, LMWH is smaller in weight than standard heparin. This allows LMWH to have a different antithrombotic effect that is as effective as standard heparin but may have fewer side effects and less need for monitoring. A representative drug is the low-molecular-weight heparin enoxaparin (Lovenox®).

Fondaparinux

Fondaparinux is a pentasaccharide that binds specifically but reversibly to antithrombin. It selectively inhibits factor Xa activity and prevents thrombus generation and clot formation by directly inhibiting factor Xa activity through its interaction with anithrombin. It is different from UFH and LMWH in that it has no direct effect on thrombin activity, but it is similar in that it is administered parenterally by subcutaneous injection. Apixaban (Eliquis®) and rivaroxaban (Xarelto®) are oral factor-Xa inhibitors. These medications, along with dabigatran discussed previously, are replacing warfarin in a number of clinical situations because they do not require routine blood monitoring and they appear to be as good as, or better than, warfarin in preventing strokes in patients with atrial fibrillation. They also have no effect on platelet function and, as previously mentioned, routine coagulation testing is not needed, other than a periodic blood count to detect occult bleeding. They are eliminated by the kidneys, and their use in patients with kidney disease is either contraindicated or they must be used at a reduced dose depending on the severity of the kidney disease.

time for review

What precautions would you take if you were obtaining an arterial blood gas from someone on heparin?

Warfarin

Warfarin is an orally administered anticoagulant that has been around for more than 50 years. Warfarin acts differently than heparin and works on vitamin K–dependent liver synthesis of certain clotting factors by inhibiting vitamin K, which is vital to the clotting process (see Figure 10-10 for this mechanism).

Clinical pearl

Warfarin is an oral anticoagulant that is sometimes referred to by patients as "rat poison," because the active components are similar. This drug was discovered when cattle died mysteriously after eating sweet clover. It turned out that the sweet clover was spoiled. This led to the isolation of the chemical components of the spoiled sweet clover and development of oral anticoagulants.

FIGURE 10-10 Mechanism of Action of Warfarin

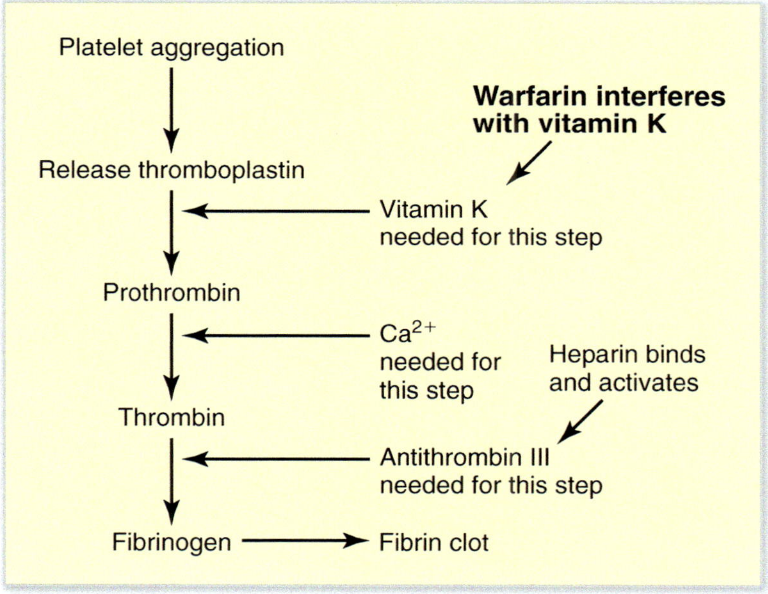

Warfarin is used to prevent blood clots in patients with various medical conditions, such as atrial fibrillation, a prosthetic mechanical heart valve, or stroke. Depending on the indication, the goal international normalized ratio (INR) may be 2 to 3 or higher. Chronic warfarin therapy requires monthly lab monitoring and frequent dosage manipulations, because the anticoagulant effect of warfarin is affected by many things such as dietary vitamin K intake, drug interactions, and other disease states.

Clinical pearl

Dabigatran, rivaroxaban, and apixaban cannot be used to prevent stroke in patients with mechanical heart valves. A study comparing warfarin to dabigatran was halted when the number of strokes in the dabigatran group far exceeded the number of strokes in the warfarin group.

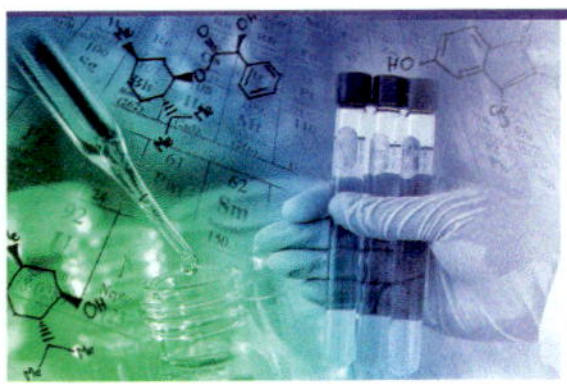

CONTROVERSY

A person's genetic makeup may influence how he or she responds to warfarin. Patients with variations in two genes may need lower doses of warfarin than people without these variations. The two genes are called VKORC1 and CYP2C9. The VKORC1 gene helps regulate warfarin's ability to prevent blood from clotting, and the CYP2C9 gene is involved with the metabolism of warfarin. Tests are commercially available to test for these gene variations, but testing is controversial until there is more information about how the results will inform patient care.

Interactions and Side Effects of Warfarin

Diet drug interactions with warfarin are important. Anything that increases vitamin K, such as yellow or green leafy vegetables, can also affect warfarin response. This can be used advantageously in cases of over anticoagulation by administering pharmacologic doses of vitamin K. Patients on anticoagulants need to be monitored for bleeding gums, nose bleeds, petechiae, or blood in the urine or stool. Before surgery or certain dental procedures, warfarin patients may need to withhold doses. Any drug has the potential to interact with warfarin on the basis of the mechanistic principles described in Chapter 1. Most, but not all, patients on warfarin are instructed not to take aspirin concurrently, because it may increase bleeding potential.

A representative drug is

- warfarin (Coumadin®)

Clinical pearl

Hirudin is an anticoagulant protein found in leeches that was one of the first direct thrombin inhibitors. Leeches are dispensed from some hospital pharmacies to be used as an anticoagulant.

10.3c Direct Thrombin Inhibitors

Direct thrombin inhibitors (DTIs) do not require antithrombin to have antithrombotic activity and are able to inhibit both circulating and clot-bound thrombin. The prototype of this class came from the medical leech (hirudin). Others include desirudin, bivalirudin, and argatroban available parenterally. Dabigatran is a new oral DTI that is used as an alternative to warfarin in a number of clinical situations.

Argatroban

The direct thrombin inhibitor argatroban has distinct pharmacologic properties relating to how it interacts with thrombin. This drug may be used in conjunction with aspirin in patients with unstable angina who are undergoing percutaneous transluminal coronary intervention (PCI) or as an alternative to heparin in patients with heparin-induced thrombocytopenia. Argatroban is monitored using the aPTT test, and bivalirudin by the activated clotting time (ACT). ACT is a point-of-care test done bedside, such as in the cardiac catheterization suite.

A representative drug is

- bivalirudin (Angiomax®)

time for review

What is the difference between the PT, aPTT, ACT, and INR lab tests, and why are they important to pharmacotherapy?

10.3d Antiplatelet Drugs

Antiplatelet agents inhibit the platelet phase of clotting (see Figure 10-11). Antiplatelet drugs are also called antithrombotic drugs and include aspirin. Aspirin irreversibly inhibits the enzyme prostaglandin synthetase, which is required for the formation of prostaglandin precursors. This means that once aspirin is taken, a platelet will be affected by aspirin's antiplatelet effects for the lifetime of that platelet. The cardioprotective effects of an aspirin a day warrant that most patients, with few exceptions, take daily low-dose aspirin. One of the controversies addressed in the consensus guidelines on the Web is whether a baby aspirin is enough or whether a full dose of aspirin is needed.

FIGURE 10-11 Mechanism of Action of Antiplatelet Drugs

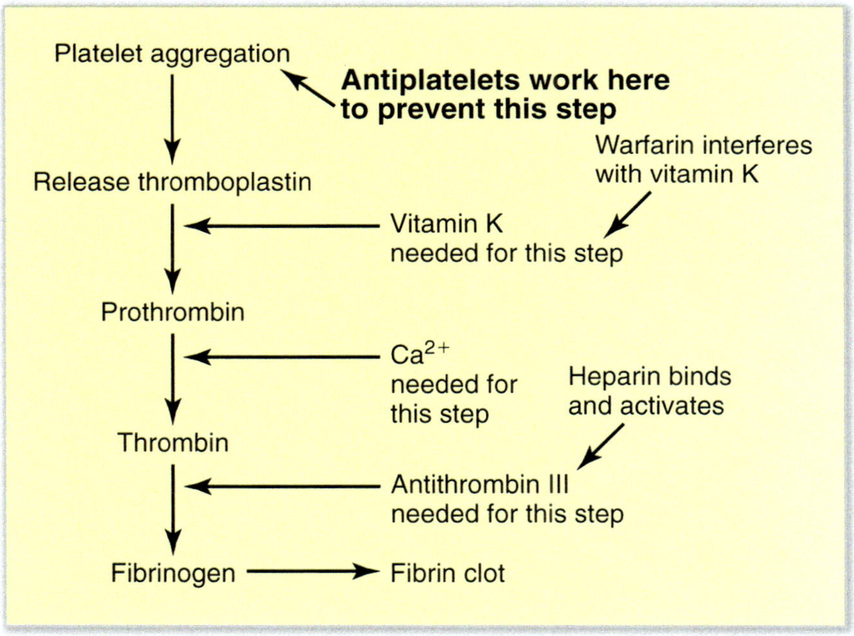

Besides aspirin, representative antiplatelet drugs include

- dipyridamole (Persantine®)
- ticlopidine (Ticlid®)
- clopidogrel (Plavix®)
- prasugrel (Effient®)
- ticagrelor (Brillinta®)

These drugs are usually used if patients "fail" or still have symptoms on aspirin or don't tolerate aspirin, although their use is becoming more widespread. They are also used in combination with aspirin to prevent clot formation in bare-metal and drug-eluting stents. These stents are placed by interventional cardiologists in the coronary arteries of patients with coronary artery disease. Clopidogrel, prasugrel, and ticlopidine are thienopyridines that block adenosine diphosphate (ADP) receptors on platelets.

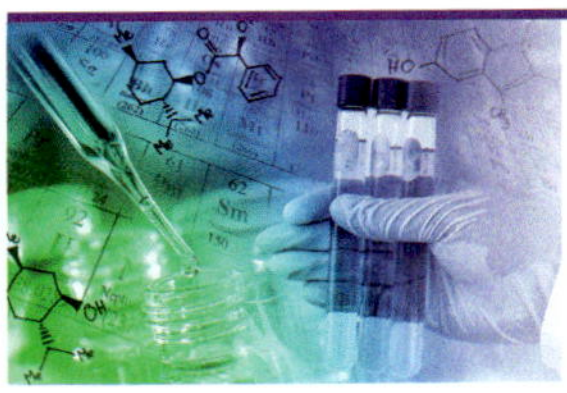

CONTROVERSY

Clopidogrel is a prodrug. This means it must be metabolized by the liver to its active metabolite before it can do its job of blocking platelets. The liver enzyme CYP2C9 is responsible for this metabolism. Depending on the genetic profile of the patient, some patients may not be able to convert clopidogrel to its active form as efficiently as others and therefore may have a reduced benefit from this medicine. A test is commercially available to see how well a patient is likely to metabolize clopidogrel. In patients found to be poor metabolizers, it isn't clear whether the dose of clopidogrel should be increased or whether the patient should switch to a different medicine.

10.3e Platelet Glycoprotein IIB/IIIA–Receptor Inhibitors

Clinical pearl

Abciximab (ReoPro®) is often used in patients undergoing primary PCI who have not received fibrinolytics.

Platelet glycoprotein (GP) IIb/IIIa–receptor inhibitors are a newer class of drugs that are administered parenterally. They bind with and block GP IIb/IIIa receptors, which initiate platelet aggregation. They are used for unstable angina and myocardial infarction, and they have been used concurrently with heparin. Representative platelet GP IIb/IIIa–receptor inhibitors include

- tirofiban (Aggrastat®)
- eptifibatide (Integrilin®)
- abciximab (ReoPro®)

10.3f Fibrinolytics

Fibrinolytics stimulate fibrinolytic mechanisms to dissolve existing clots. Pharmacologic thrombolysis occurs when plasminogen is converted to plasmin, an enzyme that digests fibrin strands. In essence thrombolytics promote the lysis of the fibrin to a gel or liquid, thereby dissolving the existing clot. Thrombolytics are used for patients with acute myocardial infarction, because these drugs lyse the thrombus that caused the infarction and can reduce mortality and salvage heart tissue by reperfusion. These drugs dissolve existing clots but do not affect the underlying cause of the occlusion.

There are different generations of thrombolytics, each generation striving to be better than the previous. Improvements include things such as longer half-life, bolus IV administration, and fewer side effects. This is important because the goal is to treat myocardial infarction or stroke patients as early as possible after the onset of chest pain or within 4.5 hours of the onset of stroke symptoms.

There are two main types of thrombolytics: enzymes and tissue plasminogen activators (tPAs). The enzyme thrombolytic streptokinase (no longer commercially available) is derived from *Streptococcus* and can cause antigenicity, making repeat administration not safe. The tPAs are produced commercially by DNA technology. Clinical studies influence which thrombolytic is used most often. Because fibrinolytics can't differentiate between pathologic clots and hemostatic plugs, the biggest complication of fibrinolytics is bleeding. Representative thrombolytics include

- alteplase (Activase®) (rtPA) (FDA approved to treat both heart attacks and strokes)
- reteplase (Retavase®) (rPA)
- tenecteplase (TNKase®) (TNK-tPA)

See Table 10-4 for a summary of the classes of antithrombotic agents.

Learning Hint

Notice that all the thrombolytic drugs end in "ase," which is a formal suffix denoting an enzyme.

TABLE 10-4 Classes and Representative Drugs Used for Antithrombotic Therapy

Class	Generic Name	Brand Name
Unfractionated heparin	heparin sodium	Calciparine®
Low-molecular-weight heparin	enoxaparin	Lovenox®
Vitamin K antagonist	warfarin sodium	Coumadin®
Direct thrombin inhibitor	lepirudin	Refludan®
	bivalirudin	Angiomax®
	dabigatran	Pradaxa®
Antiplatelet agents	aspirin	
	dipyridamole	Persantine®
	ticlopidine	Ticlid®
	clopidogrel	Plavix®
	prasugrel	Effient®
Factor- Xa inhibitors	fondaparinux	Arixtra®
	rivaroxaban	Xarelto®
	apixaban	Eliquis®
Fibrinolytic agents	alteplase	Activase®
	tenecteplase	TNKase®
	reteplase	Retavase®
Platelet glycoprotein IIb/IIIa–receptor inhibitors	tirofiban	Aggrastat®
	eptifibatide	Integrilin®
	abciximab	ReoPro®

CONTROVERSY

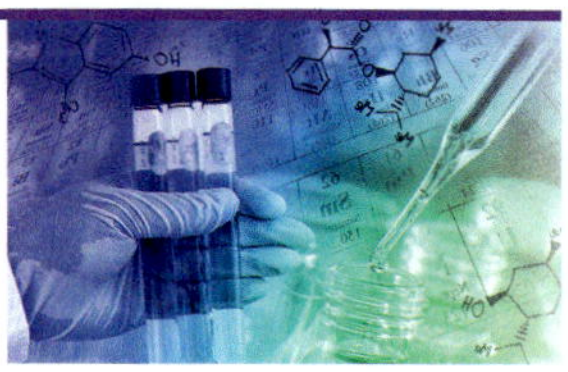

In patients older than age 75, fibrinolytic therapy is controversial. A benefit–risk decision between risk of intracranial hemorrhage, risk of stroke, and the fact that 60% of all MI deaths occur in this age group makes the decision to use the drug different in individual situations. Because of these bleeding risks and the possible failure of the drug to open the occluded coronary artery, most heart attack patients today are taken to a cardiac catheterization laboratory to have their artery opened by specially trained cardiologists. Unfortunately not all parts of the United States have this type of health-care service available in the community.

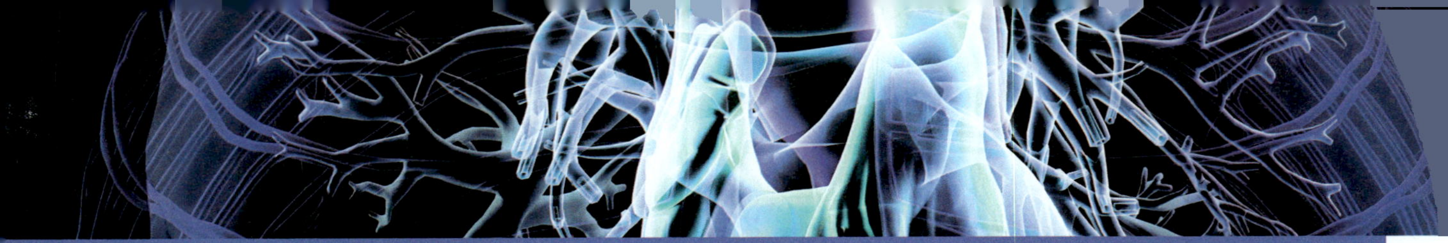

Summary

This chapter concluded a two-chapter sequence on cardiac pharmacotherapy. Antihypertensives, anticoagulants, antiplatelet agents, and thrombolytic agents have greatly influenced cardiac morbidity and mortality. The high prevalence of the conditions these drugs are used to treat indicates that you will encounter these drugs frequently in your professional practice and even in your personal life.

REVIEW QUESTIONS

1. Nonpharmacologic approaches to hypertensive treatment include
   (a) fluid restriction
   (b) salt supplementation
   (c) exercise
   (d) folic acid
   (e) vitamin C

2. Which of the following is not an antihypertensive drug class?
   (a) β-agonist
   (b) β-blocker
   (c) α-agonist
   (d) α-blocker
   (e) diuretic

3. Sympatholytics
   (a) decrease venous tone
   (b) increase heart rate
   (c) increase cardiac contractility
   (d) increase total peripheral resistance
   (e) increase cerebral blood flow

4. Diuretics
   (a) can cause bleeding
   (b) have dose-related antihypertensive effects
   (c) are classified by where they work in the kidney
   (d) should not be used with other antihypertensives
   (e) (b) and (c)

5. ACE inhibitors
   (a) may cause a cough
   (b) may cause hypokalemia
   (c) increase aldosterone
   (d) work the same as angiotensin II–receptor blockers
   (e) may cause heart failure
6. Explain the mathematical equation that describes blood pressure and how it relates to antihypertensive therapy.
7. Discuss the factors that influence which antihypertensive is used in an individual patient.
8. Explain the steps involved in platelet aggregation and clot formation.
9. Describe three categories of drugs used to treat or prevent thrombus formation.
10. A 47-year-old man presents with prehypertension (BP 136/86 mmHg) without target organ disease (TOD). Is pharmacotherapy indicated at this point? If not, what suggestions would you make?
11. A 53-year-old woman with a medical history of pulmonary emboli is admitted for pelvic surgery. What prophylactic pharmacotherapy may be indicated presurgery? What would be the therapeutic goal? What tests would help to confirm the effectiveness of the presurgical medications?

CASE STUDY 1

An obese 75-year-old woman

An obese 75-year-old woman was admitted to the hospital for hypertensive emergency and chest pain 2 days ago. She now complains of shortness of breath, swelling, and soreness of her left calf. What potential medical problem might she have? What are her risk factors for this? What additional information do you need? What are some of the drug options available? What kind of adverse effects of drug therapy would you be concerned about? If this patient is discharged to home, what medications might be prescribed and what precautions emphasized?

Chapter **11**

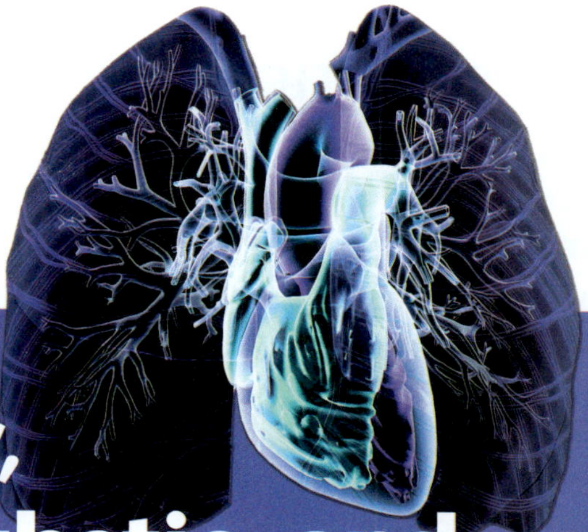

Neuromuscular, Sedative, Anesthetic, and Analgesic Agents

OBJECTIVES

Upon completion of this chapter you will be able to

- Apply the principles of nerve transmission to pharmacology of neuromuscular blocking drugs.
- Describe the clinical applications of neuromuscular blocking drugs.
- Discuss the mechanisms of action of medications that are hypnotic, sedative, or anxiolytic and their importance in cardiorespiratory practice.
- Describe the mechanism and role of ventilatory stimulants.
- Explain the pain pathway (nociceptive pathway) and the role of medications that are used as analgesics.
- Discuss the role of medications used for general anesthesia and distinguish them from those used for local anesthesia.
- Describe pharmacologic prevention therapies for postoperative nausea and vomiting.

KEY TERMS

action potential
analeptic
analgesic
anxiolytic
depolarizing agent
general anesthesia
hypnotic
local anesthesia
malignant hyperthermia
nondepolarizing agent
opioid
sedative
train-of-four
ventilatory stimulant

ABBREVIATIONS

ACh	acetylcholine
AChE	acetylcholinesterase
APAP	acetaminophen
ASA	aspirin
CDC	Centers for Disease Control and Prevention
CNS	central nervous system
COD	codeine
COX	cyclo-oxygenase
CSF	cerebrospinal fluid
DEA	Drug Enforcement Agency
DTs	delirium tremens
EMS	emergency medical services
FDA	Food and Drug Administration
GABA	γ-aminobutyric acid
MAC	minimum alveolar concentration
NMBA	neuromuscular blocking agent
NSAID	nonsteroidal anti-inflammatory drug
PCA	patient-controlled analgesia
PONV	postoperative nausea and vomiting
REM	rapid eye movement
SSRI	selective serotonin reuptake inhibitor
TCA	tricyclic antidepressant
TOF	train-of-four

Health-care professionals are responsible for the safe administration of all medications utilized in the provision of patient care. There is no better example of the complete control that health-care providers have than the case of general anesthesia, or when medications are administered to cause paralysis of respiratory muscles. If a patient were not on ventilatory support in either of these circumstances, rapid death would ensue. To appreciate and understand the pharmacologic activities of these medications, it is imperative to have a thorough understanding of nervous system transmission, explained previously in Chapter 3 but reviewed briefly in this chapter.

Many medications covered in this chapter somehow influence muscle contraction or patient sensorium. Drug classes in this chapter are commonly used to facilitate ventilation. In some situations, in order to achieve effective ventilation, the muscles around the airway must be relaxed. Sometimes relaxation and sedation of the individual alone is enough to provide sufficient muscle relaxation for the situation, although at other times complete and total respiratory paralysis is the desired outcome, to reduce the work of breathing and decrease oxygen consumption. Once the patient and/or respiratory muscles are relaxed and ventilation is appropriately controlled, there is frequently a need to decrease the pain associated with invasive cardiorespiratory procedures. This is accomplished by using analgesics or local anesthesia. If the need is broader, general or surgical anesthesia is used, and the practitioner must make decisions about using intravenous or inhalational routes. There may also be a need for sedation, so sedatives, anxiolytics, and hypnotics are discussed in this chapter. Postoperative nausea and vomiting are common complications that are discussed. The consequences of drugs from each of these classes for blood pressure and heart rate must be considered, not just the isolated respiratory effects. In each situation a different drug and dose must be indicated.

This chapter also discusses the role of opioid and nonopioid pain medications and their corresponding relationships to the cardiorespiratory system. For completeness and balance to the discussion of all these drugs, which potentially cause respiratory depression, this chapter also discusses the role of ventilatory pharmacologic stimulants.

11.1 NERVE TRANSMISSION

11.1a Physiology of Muscle Contraction

Agents that affect skeletal muscle contraction affect the somatic part of the peripheral nervous system. As you will recall from Chapter 3, the somatic nervous system originates in the central nervous system (CNS) and is the portion of the nervous system that is responsible for skeletal and respiratory muscle activity.

Nerve conduction occurs when ions move across cells, and electrical energy moving along the fiber results in eventual interaction at the target organ. That target organ may be another nerve junction, as in the case of the ganglia, or it may be a target organ such as muscle in the eye, arms, legs, or diaphragm. When a nerve impulse reaches the end of the fiber, it is converted into a chemical that facilitates propagation of the impulse. There are a variety of types of nerve fibers as well as chemicals that help to continue the impulse. These nervous system chemicals are called neurotransmitters.

Nerve conduction occurs only when there is a precise transfer of electrolytes such as potassium and sodium, which results in cellular depolarization. Cells have a particular electrical charge at which a cell is most likely to depolarize; this is called the *threshold level*. When electrical energy moves along the fiber and is depolarized, there is a time period during which that nerve cannot accept any more electrolyte transfer. This time period is called the *refractory period*. Once depolarization and muscle contraction occur, *repolarization* must take place. All of this occurs at incredible speed. The traveling of the impulse down the fiber is referred to as an **action potential.**

The nerve junction with skeletal muscles is referred to as the *motor endplate*. This is where the binding sites for acetylcholine are located. When these receptors are stimulated, they become activated, and acetylcholine is released into the synapse and allows calcium influx. Depolarization of the muscle fiber occurs when calcium is released. Calcium is required for the contractile proteins actin and myosin to interact, resulting in muscle contraction (see Figure 11-1, which illustrates this process).

FIGURE 11-1 Nerve Transmission and Muscle Contraction

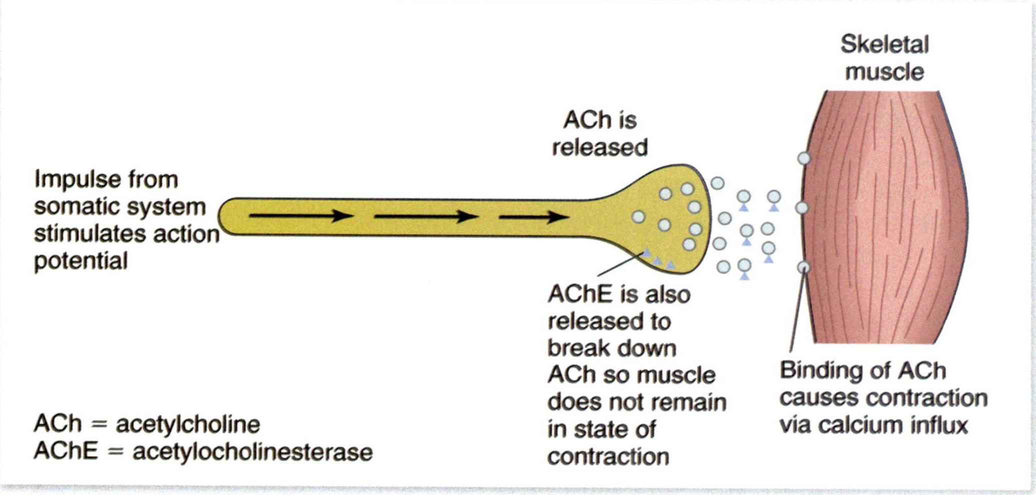

Different tissues specialize in conduction of different impulses. In Chapter 9 we talked about cardiac muscle and its action potential and refractory periods. In that case the different action potential and refractory period were what maintained a proper balance between the stimulation of the cardiac muscle and the contraction of the heart as an effective pump. In this case the same can be said about the proper balance of skeletal muscle contraction and relaxation.

From this discussion you can see that several things can happen at the neuromuscular junction. Cholinergic agonists can stimulate more acetylcholine (ACh) and thus facilitate muscle contraction. Conversely, agents can be given to decrease levels of ACh or block its action and thus result in neuromuscular blockade, which inhibits muscle contraction.

Learning Hint

All this talk of ACh and AChE can be confusing. Remember that *-ase* is the suffix for an enzyme. Think of ACh as the army that causes the muscle contraction and AChE as the opposing army, which causes muscle relaxation. Anything that inhibits ACh function or stimulates AChE function therefore tips the battle in favor of muscle relaxation.

11.1b Acetylcholinesterase

Acetylcholinesterase (AChE) breaks down acetylcholine, ending the contraction, or else we would be in a constant state of contraction. AChE is the enzyme that inactivates acetylcholine to relax the muscle, end the contraction, and result in a resting state. When AChE is inhibited, more acetylcholine is available at the muscle endplate. Drugs can stimulate muscles by stopping the breakdown of ACh by the enzyme AChE. This makes impulse transmission easier and makes the duration of action of acetylcholine longer. For this reason cholinesterase inhibitors are considered cholinergic stimulants.

11.1c Neuromuscular Blocking Agents

Neuromuscular blocking agents (NMBAs) have several indications pre- and postoperatively and in the emergency and critical-care departments. One of the factors that has influenced neuromuscular blockade use over the years has been the method of ventilation available. In the past, the more the patient "fought the ventilator," the more likely pharmacologic paralysis was to be needed. Today, however, pharmacologic paralysis of mechanically ventilated patients is avoided due to serious complications such as prolonged muscle weakness. It is better to try and match ventilator settings to patient demand and use sedation and analgesia to make this experience tolerable for the patient.

With the correct application of sedation and analgesia protocols, practitioners can generally alleviate problems associated with the patient being out of "sync" with the ventilator. If pharmacologic paralysis is necessary, bolus doses may be tried first to allow for patient recovery of muscle function in between doses, or continuous infusions may be necessary for patients requiring sustained paralysis. It's unusual to need these drugs for longer than 72 hours. Neuromuscular blocking agents may be beneficial for use with mechanical ventilation therapy because they (1) reduce spontaneous breathing, (2) prevent movement that can dislodge chest tubes, (3) reduce oxygen consumption in patients with poor cardiopulmonary function, and (4) improve patient ventilator synchrony, thereby reducing the pressure needed for mechanical ventilation. NMBAs may also be used to facilitate endotracheal intubation as a one-time dose.

Clinical pearl

Neuromuscular blockers do not have CNS effects, because they cannot cross the blood–brain barrier. This is important to keep in mind, because patients are alert, feel pain, and frequently need concurrent analgesia and sedative medications with neuromuscular blockers. Think of being paralyzed but having your full senses about you and being able to feel but not react to pain.

Now that we have talked in generalities about NMBA uses, let's get specific about the pharmacology of various types of neuromuscular blockers. We will then pick up again with some clinical applications. Neuromuscular blockers can be classified as nondepolarizing or depolarizing agents, and we discuss them according to this classification.

11.1d Nondepolarizing Agents

Nondepolarizing agents are competitive antagonists and bind to the receptor sites that acetylcholine would occupy. If a binding site is occupied by a nondepolarizing neuromuscular blocking agent, acetylcholine cannot stimulate the muscle, and muscle paralysis results. The drugs are called nondepolarizing because they prevent the motor endplate from depolarizing. These drugs are competitive antagonists, which means that their effect can be reversed if more acetylcholine is available to compete at the receptor site.

Nondepolarizing agents are nonselective in cholinergic receptor stimulation, which means they will bind with other cholinergic sites that stimulate parasympathetic responses, as in the heart. This is what causes side effects such as hypotension and tachycardia and is one factor that influences selection of NMBAs.

Nondepolarizing agents can be reversed. This is useful in situations of toxicity or side effects. The antidote for a nondepolarizer's neuromuscular blockade is to increase ACh levels at receptor sites. Neuromuscular blocking action ceases when the drug's plasma concentrations decline via metabolism or the effect is reversed by cholinesterase inhibitors. These inhibitors inhibit the enzyme acetylcholinesterase, which breaks down acetylcholine. More acetylcholine is then available to compete with the neuromuscular blocker. During the reversal situation, it's important to recover spontaneous ventilation and neuromuscular transmission before the artificial ventilation is discontinued. Examples of nondepolarizing agents include pancuronium, rocuronium, and rapacuronium, to name a few. Examples of agents that reverse neuromuscular blockade, or cholinesterase inhibitors, include neostigmine and pyridostigmine.

BVT Lab

Flashcards are available for this chapter at www.BVTLab.com.

time for review

What respiratory intervention is needed for patients on a nondepolarizing agent?

11.1e Depolarizing Agents

Depolarizing agents are agonists that actually bind to the ACh receptor sites and initiate a massive depolarization of the muscle, which then sends it into a prolonged refractory period. Muscle twitching (fasciculation) takes place, followed by complete muscle paralysis. This is different from nondepolarizing agents, which do not cause the initial muscle fasciculations and go straight to muscle paralysis.

Depolarizing neuromuscular blocking agents such as succinylcholine bind with cholinergic receptors and start depolarization by causing total body muscle contraction, followed by muscle paralysis. This lasts until the binding of the receptor by the depolarizing agent ends, or the drug is inactivated by the enzyme pseudocholinesterase. Cholinesterase inhibitors cannot reverse the effects of depolarizing neuromuscular blocking agents the way they can nondepolarizing agents. Because depolarizing agents have a short duration of action, this is not a

Clinical pearl

To fasciculate or not to fasciculate? Fasciculations may increase gastric pressure and put a patient at risk for gastric reflux, which could lead to aspiration.

Clinical pearl

Even anesthesia in the dentist's office requires strict monitoring. A 17-year-old undergoing dental surgery was given succinylcholine and had to be resuscitated and ventilated after finding out the hard way that she had a genetic deficiency of the enzyme pseudocholinesterase. There is a lab test available to identify whether this deficiency is present and may therefore result in this adverse effect of succinylcholine.

problem clinically, except in those rare patients who have a genetic deficiency of pseudocholinesterase. In those cases paralysis can last for hours.

Neuromuscular blockers may have drug interactions with inhalation anesthetics, antibiotics, and other drugs, so they require close monitoring and dosing. Neuromuscular blockade is monitored clinically and subjectively by patient movement (or lack thereof) and objectively by nerve stimulation with a peripheral nerve stimulator. There are also new devices that measure hypnotic effects of anesthetics and sedatives. These devices may decrease the amount of anesthetic that needs to be administered and facilitate recovery.

Neuromuscular blocking agents are classified not only by the type of block produced (either depolarizing or nondepolarizing), but also by chemical structure, side effects, duration of action, and onset of action. See Table 11-1 for some representative neuromuscular blocking agents.

TABLE 11-1 Neuromuscular Blocking Agents

Generic Name	Trade Name
Depolarizing neuromuscular blocking agents	
succinylcholine	Anectine®
Nondepolarizing neuromuscular blocking agents	
pancuronium	
vecuronium	
atracurium	
rocuronium	Zemuron®
cisatracurium	Nimbex®

11.1f NMBA Selection Factors

Clinical pearl

Patients actually hear better when they are on NMBAs, because the drugs make muscles in the ear relax. Be careful what you say when you are providing patient care to someone who can't communicate with you verbally. Patients on an NMBA should be treated as if they are completely awake and should always be treated with sedatives with or without analgesics.

Before administering a drug, it's important to know which patients should or should not receive a drug and which patients might be at risk. The ideal NMBA is one that is not influenced by the liver or renal dysfunction common in acutely ill patients and one that does not have the vagolytic activity that increases heart rate or releases histamine to cause hypotension or reflex tachycardia. It's also important to know what other drugs the patient is on to avoid drug interactions. Neuromuscular blocking drugs may have drug interactions with inhalation anesthetics such as isoflurane, antibiotics such as aminoglycosides, and other drugs such as furosemide and theophylline.

It is important to keep in mind that neuromuscular blocking agents do not affect pain or consciousness. All patients who receive NMBAs should receive sedatives or anxiolytics and analgesics first, to decrease awareness and anxiety and to relieve pain. Patients on NMBAs and mechanical ventilation frequently also require blood thinning to decrease their risk of developing a blood clot secondary to immobility. Because concurrent use of these drugs with NMBAs is necessary, drug interactions are always a potential and need to be monitored for.

time for review

Resistance has been reported with nondepolarizing NMBAs. How would you know whether this were occurring?

Usually, once paralysis is no longer needed, patients regain muscle function spontaneously upon discontinuation of NMBAs. This is assessed clinically by patient ability to open the eyes wide, protrude the tongue, grip a hand, lift the head, or cough on demand. If reversal needs to be done, acetylcholinesterase inhibitors are used.

As mentioned previously, NMBAs differ in some of their pharmacologic properties. See Table 11-2 for a comparison of neuromuscular blocking agents. The U.S. Food and Drug Administration (FDA) defines NMBAs by their onset and duration of action. Ultrashort-onset NMBAs respond in a minute or less, intermediate ones in 2 to 4 minutes, and long or slow ones in 4 minutes or longer. The duration of ultrashort NMBAs is less than 8 minutes; intermediate, from 20 to 50 minutes; and long, more than 50 minutes.

TABLE 11-2 Comparison of Neuromuscular Blocking Agents

Category	Drug	Onset (min)	Duration (min)	Cardiovascular Effects
Ultrashort duration	succinylcholine	1–1.5	7–12	+ +
Intermediate duration	atracurium	3–4	35–45	+ +
	cisatracurium	4–6	40–50	0
	rocuronium	1.5–3	30–40	+
	vecuronium	3–4	35–45	0
Long duration	pancuronium	3–5	90–120	+++

The onset and duration information is approximate and may vary depending on patient characteristics.

LIFE SPAN CONSIDERATIONS

Even though we mentioned it previously, it is important to remember that muscle relaxant medications do not provide sedation or analgesia to patients of any age requiring their use. Therefore please make sure your patients are properly sedated and pain is addressed prior to using this class of medications. Otherwise they will be paralyzed without the ability to communicate their fear, anxiety, and need for pain relief.

Following is a brief summary of available NMBAs.

Succinylcholine (Anectine®)

With various neuromuscular blocking drugs on the market, there is a need to compare and contrast them and to define their roles. We start with a review of succinylcholine, the single depolarizing agent and long the "gold standard" drug for quick action for intubation. This drug has been used for more than 50 years. Its rapid onset and short duration of action make it a popular drug, especially in rapid-sequence intubation.

Succinylcholine can be used as a bolus or infusion, and it works quickly at the vocal cords, which makes for good intubating conditions and rapid recovery. Unfortunately it has cardiovascular effects such as dysrhythmias and pulmonary edema; increases intraocular, intragastric, and intracranial pressure; and has been associated with hyperkalemia and myoglobinemia.

Patients with genetic muscle weakness disorders are prone to hyperkalemia when they are given succinylcholine, inhalation anesthetics, or a combination of the two. Patients with burns, polio, or Guillain-Barré syndrome are also at higher risk for hyperkalemia with succinylcholine, so it should not be used for such patients.

Succinylcholine has also been associated with malignant hyperthermia. This is a life-threatening, autosomal-dominant inherited, pharmacogenetic disorder. Triggering events can include volatile anesthetics and depolarizing muscle relaxants. It is characterized by spasm of the jaw muscles, skeletal muscle damage, hyperthermia, rapid breathing, and death if not treated properly. Metabolic and respiratory acidosis are commonly associated with it. In addition succinylcholine has been shown to cause rhabdomyolysis (rapid breakdown of skeletal muscles) in some patients.

Pancuronium

Pancuronium has a higher incidence of residual neuromuscular blockade postoperatively than other agents, probably owing to its duration of action. This might put a patient at risk for pulmonary complications. Patients with renal failure have longer recovery times with pancuronium.

Rocuronium (Zemuron®)

Rocuronium has a faster onset of action and controllable duration of action relative to other intermediate-duration drugs. It has neutral cardiac side effects and is available in a liquid dosage form, which may allow for faster administration. It rarely causes histamine release.

Cisatracurium (Nimbex®)

This drug is a chemical isomer of atracurium that is less likely to cause histamine release. It has a longer duration of action than atracurium and does not depend on liver or renal elimination but rather is broken down in the bloodstream.

Atracurium

Atracurium requires no dosage change for patients with renal or liver impairment. It has a metabolite that can cause seizures in dogs at very high doses but not in humans. It produces histamine release and probably should not be used in unstable ICU patients.

Vecuronium

Vecuronium is very similar to rocuronium. It has a neutral cardiac side-effect profile with no histamine release. It requires reconstitution before administration.

When neuromuscular blocking agents are used in critically ill patients, it is recommended that the depth of paralysis be monitored using a peripheral nerve stimulator. The **train-of-four** (TOF) method involves placing electrode pads on the skin several centimeters from the muscle that will be stimulated. The ulnar nerve at the wrist is usually used. The muscle that is stimulated by this nerve is the adductor pollicis nerve, which, when stimulated, causes the thumb to twitch. The peripheral nerve stimulator delivers four stimuli over a 2-second period. Patients treated with NMBAs have a progressive reduction in the response to each stimuli. For most patients the goal would be 2 twitches out of 4 when the nerve stimulator is activated.

11.2 SKELETAL MUSCLE RELAXANTS

In many situations mild relaxation rather than paralysis of the muscle is needed. For example someone experiencing painful back spasms or the typical "pulled muscle" will benefit from a muscle relaxant but will certainly not require paralysis. Skeletal muscle relaxants relieve musculoskeletal pain or spasm. They are used to treat spasticity in patients with multiple sclerosis, spinal cord injuries, and stroke patients. These medications are used occasionally as an adjunct to pain control, which will be discussed later.

Skeletal muscle relaxants can be divided into two classes: central-acting and peripheral-acting. Unlike the neuromuscular blocking agents, central-acting relaxants do not block the motor endplate junction but are thought to act directly on the CNS to decrease muscular tone by interfering with overstimulated reflex nerve pathways in the spinal cord. These drugs are frequently used for acute and chronic back pain.

Peripheral muscle relaxants work on the muscles themselves. Peripheral muscle relaxants such as dantrolene (Dantrium®) decrease the force of skeletal muscle contraction by stopping the release of calcium. This results in less actin and myosin linkage and decreased force of contraction, because calcium is a necessary part of that mechanism. Its major effect is directly on muscle rather than on the brain, so dantrolene causes fewer CNS side effects than centrally acting agents. It is used for treatment of malignant hyperthermia. Examples of common muscle relaxants are listed in Table 11-3.

Clinical Pearl

All of the muscle relaxants can cause drowsiness. When used in combination with other centrally acting agents, the effect may be enhanced. This is important to keep in mind when combination treatment for pain, injuries, and chronic diseases is needed. This is why the CNS depressant alcohol should not be taken in conjunction with these medications.

TABLE 11-3 Common Muscle Relaxants

Generic Name	Trade Name (and Type)
methocarbamol	Robaxin® (central)
cyclobenzaprine	Flexeril® (central)
orphenadrine	Norflex® (central)
chlorzoxazone	Parafon Forte® (central)
carisoprodol	Soma® (central)
dantrolene	Dantrium® (peripheral or direct-acting)

11.3 SEDATIVES, HYPNOTICS, AND ANXIOLYTICS

11.3a Terminology

A drug that reduces CNS arousal is a **sedative.** Any medication that induces sleep is a **hypnotic.** Any medication that reduces the symptoms of anxiety is an **anxiolytic.** Some drug classes, such as benzodiazepines, may have all of these characteristics and be categorized as all three. Differences among sedatives, hypnotics, and anxiolytics are in reality minor and may be dose-related.

Sedatives are often needed with analgesics to improve tolerance of endotracheal tubes, facilitate acceptance of mechanical ventilation, suppress spontaneous ventilation, and prevent self-extubation. It's preferable to adjust the ventilator to patient tolerance rather than to sedate the patient to match the ventilator, but this may not always be possible. One of the biggest challenges is to measure the level of sedation in patients. Different modes of ventilation require different amounts of sedation. Sometimes sedation allows avoidance of neuromuscular blocking agents.

Clinical pearl

Use of long-acting sedatives can present a risk of delay in weaning a patient from mechanical ventilation, because of drug accumulation and decreased spontaneous respirations.

Tolerance and dependence are real possibilities with these drug classes. These concepts are defined later in this chapter in the discussion of opioids. Depending on the drug indication, some of these drugs are used only for the short term to avoid this potential. With indications such as chronic anxiety, long-term use is the reality. Duration of use of what we refer to as sleeping pills or hypnotics, regardless of the drug class to which they belong, needs to be assessed periodically. Some of these pharmacologic agents are intended to be used for a maximum of only 1 or 2 consecutive weeks at a time. With longer-term use, some hypnotics can change the characteristics of a normal sleep cycle and alter rapid eye movement (REM), sleep quality, and sleep quantity.

11.3b Benzodiazepines

Benzodiazepines are by far the most common drug class with sedative, hypnotic, and anxiolytic pharmacologic effects. Benzodiazepines work by enhancing the inhibitory effect on the receptor for the neurotransmitter γ-aminobutyric acid (GABA) within the brain. Benzodiazepines can cause respiratory effects such as loss of airway reflexes at high doses and decreased tidal volume at lower doses. The duration of action influences the extent of hypnotic hangover felt in the morning. One of the common short-acting sedative benzodiazepines is midazolam (Versed®). See Table 11-4 for more examples of the benzodiazepines.

TABLE 11-4 Common Benzodiazepines

Generic Name	Trade Name
alprazolam	Xanax®
chlordiazepoxide	No U.S. trade name
diazepam	Valium®
midazolam	Versed®
lorazepam	Ativan®

Clinical pearl

Benzodiazepines are also used for effects other than sedative, hypnotic, and anxiolytic. Status epilepticus is treated with intravenous lorazepam. Symptoms of alcohol withdrawal and delirium tremens (DTs) are prevented by giving benzodiazepines. One of the short-acting agents, midazolam (Versed®) is used as an adjunct to anesthesia. There is a drug available that is an antagonist to GABA receptors and that can be used in benzodiazepine overdoses; it is called flumazenil (Romazicon®).

time for review

It's 3 o'clock in the morning and you can't get back to sleep. Should you take another dose of the same sleeping pill that you took right before bedtime? Why or why not?

11.3c α_2-Adrenergic Agonist (Sedative)

Dexmedetomidine (Precedex®) is used in the intensive care unit for sedation of mechanically ventilated patients and for sedation prior to and/or during surgical procedures in patients without intubation. It works by stimulating central α_2-receptors resulting in anesthetic and sedative properties. When compared to sedation with benzodiazepines, dexmedetomidine has a lower incidence of delirium. However the acquisition cost of dexmedetomidine is high and a significant proportion of patients develop hypotension and bradycardia (similar to clonidine, which is another central α_2-adrenergic agonist).

11.3d Nonbenzodiazepines

Nonbenzodiazepine sedative hypnotics have pharmacokinetic differences from benzodiazepines that may cause fewer side effects. They are sometimes referred to as the "Z" compounds: zolpidem (Ambien®), eszopiclone (Lunesta®), and zaleplon (Sonata®). Ramelteon (Rozerem®) is a melatonin-receptor agonist that is a new class of hypnotic. These drugs have a shorter half-life and are more selective for GABA, so fewer daytime residual effects occur. They also have less effect on respiratory and cardiac function. They are being promoted as being safer for long-term use.

11.3e Barbiturates

Barbiturates are some of the oldest drugs around; they have been used for many years to treat seizure, sleep, and anxiety disorders. Barbiturates work differently than benzodiazepines to block the excitatory impulse and decrease the level of arousal in the CNS. Like benzodiazepines, the barbiturates differ in their onset of action and duration of action. The primary side effect—drowsiness—is a natural extension of their desired actions. Patients who use these drugs for seizure treatment fortunately become tolerant of this side effect. In overdose situations, barbiturates cause respiratory depression, CNS depression, cardiovascular collapse, coma, and death. For this reason, barbiturates, even though they are a time-honored drug class, are not used as frequently as benzodiazepines. Phenobarbital is generally not used for sedation in the ICU since its long half-life prevents rapid awakening of the patient when he or she is ready for extubation. Another disadvantage is the drug interactions that may occur, because phenobarbital is an enzyme inducer.

Clinical pearl

Usually, daily attempts at withholding all sedative medicines and/or dose reduction are effective at decreasing the duration of unneeded drug administration. Respiratory therapy–driven ventilator protocols along with sedation and analgesia protocols have been shown to decrease patient-days on the ventilator.

11.3f Cocktails

A variety of drugs are used in surgical and office procedure arenas to decrease the patient's level of consciousness and produce a retrograde amnesia so the patient won't remember the negative aspects of the procedure. Sometimes these drug combinations are referred to as "cocktails." Individual prescribers frequently develop their own combination or recipe of drugs they feel comfortable with to decrease patient consciousness. Two such examples are midazolam given in combination with fentanyl or morphine given with lorazepam. The desired endpoint is to make a patient comfortable yet still able to respond to commands such as "lift your arm" or "open your eyes."

11.4 ANESTHETICS

11.4a General Versus Local

The term *anesthesia* refers to the inability to perceive sensations. The route and the type of agent administered depend on the individual patient situation. **Local anesthesia** refers to the administration of an agent that acts locally to stop the transmission of sensations from that area. **General anesthesia** refers to the induction of a total anesthetic state in which the patient does not respond to any stimuli. General anesthesia is reserved for surgical procedures in which the normal stresses placed on the patient are substantial.

11.4b General Anesthesia

Important anesthesia terms are induction, maintenance, and termination. *Induction* relates to the time it takes to create the appropriate level of anesthesia. *Maintenance* relates to continuation of the anesthetized state. *Termination* refers to the time it takes for a patient to recover from the anesthesia. Pharmacologic and patient characteristics of each agent determine and influence each of these components of anesthesia.

One of the most influential factors in determining which anesthetic medication a patient receives, or whether the person is even a candidate for anesthesia, is the medical condition of the patient. Age, organ function, and the disease being treated all influence the selection process. Elderly people tend to have decreased liver, kidney, lung, and immune function, as well as a lower serum albumin concentration. All of these contribute to altered efficacy, elimination, accumulation, and potential toxicities of the anesthetic agents. Likewise neonatal patients may have a reduced ability to clear medications, and this may result in drug accumulation and toxicity.

Drug allergy or sensitivity may also affect which route and type of anesthetic medication is administered. Patients who have experienced an adverse effect from a particular type of anesthetic or analgesic in the past are more likely to have that same adverse event the next time they receive the medication. These adverse reactions may range from mild gastrointestinal discomfort after receiving an opioid analgesic or a dysphoric reaction (unpleasant CNS sensations) with inhaled nitrous oxide all the way to severe cardiovascular collapse following the administration of inhaled general anesthetic medications.

BVT Lab

Visit www.BVTLab.com to explore the student resources available for this chapter.

Drug factors also influence the type of anesthetic used. The characteristics of the drug molecule determine whether it may be administered by an enteral, parenteral, or inhaled route. Onset of action is critical for each of these routes, as is the duration of medication action. Termination of the effect of an inhaled anesthetic is termed *decrement time*. It can be quantified as the time required for the concentration of the anesthetic to decrease by 90% or "90% decrement time." Decrement time is influenced by the duration of time the anesthetic is administered.

11.4c Stages of Anesthesia

The depth of anesthesia can be categorized as stages 1 through 4. Stage 1 is analgesia, with the patient retaining consciousness without experiencing pain. Stage 1 anesthesia is sometimes called "conscious sedation" and is frequently used for outpatient endoscopies, colonoscopies, and minor procedures. Stage 2 anesthesia is the level representing a loss of consciousness. During stage 2, the patient may have a number of reflexes activated that result in coughing, increased salivation, increase in cardiovascular output, and increase in blood pressure. Stage 3 anesthesia is surgical anesthesia and progresses to a state of complete respiratory depression. During stage 3, there is a loss of the blink reflex and loss of eye movement, and respiratory depression soon ensues. Stage 4 is complete loss of respiratory drive, and there may be a loss of cardiovascular tone. As you can see, there is a fine line between the desired level of anesthesia and the level that produces adverse effects.

time for review

As the level of anesthesia progresses, some characteristic responses can be anticipated. Can you think of any medication that can be administered as a "preanesthetic" to decrease the complications of general anesthesia?

11.4d Specific General Anesthetics

You can administer medications to create a state of surgical anesthesia. These medications are administered by the inhaled route or by the intravenous route. General anesthesia has four characteristics: unconsciousness, analgesia, muscle relaxation, and depression of reflexes. Undesirable characteristics that can occur with anesthesia relate to cardiovascular hemodynamics.

Inhaled general anesthetics work by binding to a protein-binding site in the neurons of the CNS. The interaction of the anesthetics and the neurons results in a decrease in the neuronal firing rate. Inhaled anesthetics are a diverse group of compounds that exist in a gaseous state. The medications must pass through the alveoli, diffuse through the bloodstream, cross the blood–brain barrier, and then diffuse into the CNS. Characteristics of the individual compounds determine the ease with which they pass through membranes. It is nearly impossible to determine the actual concentration of the medication in the CNS, so inhaled anesthetic medications are discussed and compared by using a concept called *minimum alveolar concentration* (MAC). MAC is a number that correlates to the minimum inhaled drug concentration that results in 50% of patients failing to move in response to surgical incision. You have to feel bad for the other 50%, who do move, but remember that they usually have no memory of this event.

The desired CNS actions of inhaled anesthetics are useful for surgery. However, as the chemicals are distributing throughout the body, they come in contact with all organ systems. Side effects of inhaled anesthetics include cardiovascular complications such as reduction in blood pressure, increase in peripheral tissue blood flow, decrease in vessel and cardiac response to sympathetic nervous system activity, and alteration of cardiac conduction. Respiratory complications include reduction in the ventilatory response to falling O_2 levels, decrease in depth of respiration, increase or decrease in rate of respiration, and alteration of the ventilatory response to rising CO_2 levels.

Muscle complications may include increased sensitivity of motor endplate to the actions of neuromuscular blocking agents, relaxation of skeletal muscles, or, rarely, development of **malignant hyperthermia.** Malignant hyperthermia is a condition in which there is sustained skeletal muscle contraction that if untreated results in muscle breakdown and potential renal impairment. See Table 11-5, which lists common inhaled anesthetics.

Clinical pearl

Agitation in ICU patients affects 50%–70% of patients and can be associated with interference with mechanical ventilation, among other things. Agitated ICU patients may develop propylene glycol toxicity with high doses of lorazepam or hypertriglyceridemia with propofol. Patients tend to associate the actual surgery with high risk; however, when there are problems, anesthesia may be a contributing factor. Neuromuscular blocking agents have been implicated in anesthesia-related anaphylaxis more than any other drug. Other drugs or surgical materials that may cause anaphylaxis are latex, preoperative antibiotics, contrast, or induction agents/hypnotics such as thiopental, propofol, or midazolam. Because the surgical patient is unconscious, sedated, and under drapes, early signs of anaphylaxis may not be obvious. Early signs to watch for include hypotension, bronchospasm, and cutaneous signs such as urticaria or flushing.

TABLE 11-5 Inhaled Anesthetics

Generic Name	Trade Name
nitrous oxide	
enflurane	Ethrane®
isoflurane	Forane®
sevoflurane	Ultane®
desflurane	Suprane®

Intravenous anesthetics are commonly used as adjuncts to inhaled anesthesia or as the primary agent for maintaining a state of anesthesia. IV induction agents rapidly induce unconsciousness in a predictable way. These medications are generally classified as rapid-acting barbiturates (thiopental), rapid-acting benzodiazepines (midazolam), or as miscellaneous agents. These medications when administered by the intravenous route cross into the CNS and cause a global reduction in neuronal activity. This may be done by the inhibition of pre- and postsynaptic neuronal interactions (barbiturates), by alterations of electrolyte channels (barbiturates and benzodiazepines), or by an unknown global cerebral suppression (propofol). Importantly they blunt the stress response to laryngoscopy and intubation.

They also induce a short-lived global amnesia. Complications of barbiturates have included respiratory depression, suppression of cardiac conduction, and severe reductions in arterial blood pressure. Because of these complications, the short-acting benzodiazepines have become the preferred agents in the acute setting. Midazolam (Versed®) is an ultrashort-acting benzodiazepine.

This medication is used to induce an amnesia state in major and minor surgical procedures.

Propofol (Diprivan®) is a lipid-soluble medication that can be administered intravenously to induce and maintain general anesthesia. Propofol is chemically unrelated to barbiturates, benzodiazepines, and inhaled anesthetics, and its exact mechanism of action is unknown, but it is thought to be an agonist at GABA receptors in the brain. Propofol comes in a lipid emulsion containing soybean oil, which can occasionally cause an elevation of serum triglycerides. This intravenous anesthetic is used frequently in the ICU setting to assist with sedation of the mechanically ventilated patient. Since it is a phenolic compound, propofol may cause a green discoloration of urine, hair, or nailbeds. It can be discontinued with a rapid taper and allows for earlier extubation. Some of these drugs can be used for maintenance of general anesthesia alone or in combination with inhalational anesthetics.

Ketamine (Ketalar®) is used clinically intravenously as an analgesic and sedative at lower doses and an anesthetic at high doses. It can be used in nonintubated patients but has been reported to be associated with aspiration and ventilatory compromise. Ketamine is also a bronchodilator, but it can increase respiratory secretions.

See Table 11-6 for a list of common IV anesthetics.

TABLE 11-6 IV Anesthetics

Type	Generic Name	Trade Name
Barbiturate	methohexital	Brevital®
Miscellaneous	propofol	Diprivan®
	etomidate	Amidate®
	ketamine	Ketalar®
Benzodiazepine	midazolam	Versed®

11.4e Local Anesthetics

Many circumstances in medicine do not require administration of general anesthesia. Local anesthesia relates to the administration of a medication that will make a specific region of the body insensitive to pain without loss of consciousness. The most common situation for local anesthesia is when a potentially painful procedure is required. Suturing, removing moles, and taking skin biopsies are examples of times when administration of a topical local anesthetic is appropriate.

For certain procedures, such as a bronchoscopy or an intubation, local anesthetics help deaden the gag reflex that can cause the patient discomfort or, worse yet, aspiration of vomitus into the lungs. Another situation in which local anesthetics may be administered is in joint injuries that may require a joint-space injection. Among athletes, torn rotator cuffs and sprained fingers are frequently injected with local anesthetics. They can also be used topically on mucous membranes for surface anesthesia to decrease pain and discomfort. Local anesthetics are found in hemorrhoidal cream preparations and in topical sprays that may be used for sunburn or even sore throats. The most commonly known drug with local anesthetic properties is cocaine. It also has therapeutic pharmacologic applications for ophthalmic anesthesia when used topically.

Clinical pearl

Another instance in which local anesthetics may be administered is when a local block is desired in a particular anatomic site. Regional spinal anesthesia is frequently used in surgical situations. Epidural anesthesia refers to the injection of the analgesic medication into the dural tissue, as in the case of obstetrical cesarean section birth. Intrathecal anesthesia results with the direct injection of the medication into the CSF. These local blocks can be accomplished with narcotic analgesics or with local anesthetic medications.

time for review

The last time you went to the dentist and had a cavity fixed, or perhaps a root canal, what types of local anesthetics did you receive?

Clinical pearl

A common application of local anesthetics is subcutaneous lidocaine injected before inserting an arterial line.

Local anesthetics work by binding to a membrane site that when stimulated results in an inability of the neuron to depolarize. This action is related to the closing of the sodium channels that propagate the action potential. Adverse effects of local anesthetics are related primarily to a skin sensitivity to the structure of the medications. "Caine" anesthetic medications can be divided chemically into amide and ester types. If a patient has had an adverse reaction to an amide-type anesthetic, there is a high probability of a cross-reaction to any other structurally related products. Examples of the amide-type anesthetics include lidocaine (Xylocaine®), bupivacaine (Marcaine®), and mepivacaine (Carbocaine®). The second type of local anesthetic is known as esters. These medications include cocaine, benzocaine (Anbesol®), and chloroprocaine (Nesacaine®). See Table 11-7, which describes local anesthetics.

Clinical pearl

A lidocaine spray is often used before a bronchoscopy procedure to reduce the gag reflex and aid patient comfort. Once the area is numb (no gag reflex or sensation with tongue depressor), adding more lidocaine will not numb it further. Rather the additional drug will just be absorbed systemically and might cause a seizure.

Table 11-7 **Common Local Anesthetics**

Type	Generic Name	Trade Name	Duration of Action (hrs)
Ester	chloroprocaine	Nesacaine®	0.5–1.5
	benzocaine	Anbesol®	0.5–1.5
	tetracaine	Pontocaine®	1.25–3
Amide	lidocaine	Xylocaine®	0.5–1
	mepivacaine	Carbocaine®	0.5–1.5
	bupivacaine	Marcaine®	2–4
	ropivacaine	Naropin®	3–15

11.4f Postoperative Nausea and Vomiting

Postoperative nausea and vomiting (PONV) can occur in 25%–30% of surgical experiences and may be related to the anesthesia. Prevention is important to avoid not only patient discomfort but also complications such as dehydration and aspiration pneumonitis. Risk factors for PONV may be patient-specific, such as females and nonsmokers, or related to the type and duration of surgery. Strategies to reduce risk for PONV are based on risk factors (Table 11-8). Antiemetic drugs can be used for both prevention and treatment. Antiemetic drugs include antimuscarinics, serotonin antagonists, and dopamine antagonists. See Table 11-9 for examples.

Table 11-8 Strategies Recommended to Decrease PONV Risk

- Use regional anesthesia.
- Use propofol for induction and maintenance of anesthesia.
- Avoid nitrous oxide.
- Avoid volatile anesthetics.
- Use supplemental oxygen.
- Maintain hydration.
- Minimize use of opioids and neostigmine.

Table 11-9 Antiemetic Drug Classes

Dopamine antagonists	droperidol
	prochlorperazine
	metoclopromide (Reglan®)
Serotonin antagonists	odansetron (Zofran®)
	granisetron (Kytril®)
Antimuscarinics	promethazine (Phenergan®)
	dimenhydrinate (Dramamine®)

11.5 VENTILATORY STIMULANTS

So far, we have talked mostly about depressing the respiratory system. However there are times when we need to stimulate the ventilatory drive with **ventilatory stimulants**. A drug that causes nervous system arousal and increases the rate and depth of ventilation is technically classified as an **analeptic** but is more commonly referred to as a ventilatory stimulant. These drugs possibly act on the respiratory center in the medulla to increase the rate and depth of ventilation, but their true mechanism of action is unknown. Drugs that are useful as ventilatory stimulants also stimulate the CNS, although not all CNS stimulants are useful as ventilatory stimulants.

Drugs used clinically for these effects include doxapram (Dopram®), caffeine, theophylline, protriptyline (Vivactyl®), and medroxyprogesterone (Depo-Provera®). In reality these drugs are used infrequently for this indication and are not practical for reversing CNS depression. It makes sense that by stimulating respiration, breathing becomes more work and requires more oxygen, which may exacerbate tissue hypoxia.

Ventilatory stimulants are used to treat sleep apnea, postanesthesia respiratory depression, acute hypercapnea in chronic pulmonary patients, patients who need to be weaned from ventilators, and apnea of prematurity.

Caffeine is well known as a CNS stimulant but less well known as a xanthine that can increase the ventilatory drive, similar to theophylline. One of the differences between caffeine and theophylline for this indication is the potency and duration of action. Side effects of the stimulants include nausea, vomiting, nervousness, insomnia, tremors, and even convulsions but are lower with caffeine than theophylline.

Medroxyprogesterone is a progesterone hormone that stimulates alveolar ventilation and increases the body's ventilatory response to hypercapnea and hypoxia. Because it increases the sensitivity of the medullary respiratory centers to respond to hypercapnea and hypoxia, it was used to treat patients with obstructive sleep apnea (now referred to as obesity hypoventilation syndrome). However, due to significant side effects such as venous thromboembolism, nervousness, nausea, male impotence, and alopecia, it is rarely used today.

Protriptyline is an antidepressant used for sleep apnea, although its mechanism is not that of a ventilatory stimulant. Rather it suppresses REM sleep, which is the sleep period most associated with loss of upper-airway muscle tone. It also increases muscle tone of the upper airways. It does not affect arterial carbon dioxide tension directly. Due to a lack of evidence supporting improved clinical outcomes and significant side effects, it is rarely used today. See Table 11-10 for a list of ventilatory stimulants.

TABLE 11-10 Ventilatory Stimulants

Drug	Indication
medroxyprogesterone	Obesity hypoventilation syndrome
protriptyline	Daytime symptoms of obstructive sleep apnea
doxapram	Postanesthesia for drug-induced respiratory depression
caffeine	Apnea of prematurity

11.6 ANALGESIA

11.6a Principles of Analgesia

Analgesia refers to the reduction in the sensation of pain. Anything that decreases the patient's perception of pain or pain intensity is an **analgesic**. The physiologic consequence of stress response caused by pain may include tachycardia, increased oxygen consumption, and immunosuppression. One of the roles of analgesics is to minimize physiologic results of pain by decreasing pulmonary complications. Almost all ICU patients are in pain, whether because of an endotracheal tube, postoperative discomfort, trauma, or inability to position themselves comfortably.

Pain can certainly impair ventilatory function if the pain is located in the abdominal thoracic region. If you have ever damaged your ribs, you became "painfully aware" of your breathing process and even more aware of your cough reflex. Postoperative abdominal and/or thoracic patients must be encouraged to breathe deeply or the pain may lead to hypoventilation and poor cough effort. This in turn can lead to atelectasis (lung collapse), pneumonia, or even the need for mechanical ventilation.

Analgesics include drugs that relax a patient or decrease patient pain perception, as well as drugs or devices that interrupt nerve transmission. This section focuses on pharmacologic analgesic treatment. The principles that guide the use of analgesic medications are similar to those that guide other medications and include medication class, mechanism of action, side effects, patient tolerability, cost, and route of administration. Frequently medications from different classes are combined for synergistic effects.

Analgesics work on neurotransmitters and different locations in the pain pathway. Morphine-like drugs target opioid-binding sites. Steroidal and nonsteroidal anti-inflammatory agents inhibit the formation of pain-producing cytokines that start the pain impulse. Other drugs, such as some of the antidepressants, increase levels of the regulatory neurotransmitters norepinephrine and serotonin. And still other drugs, such as some of those used for seizures, slow the nerve impulses for pain.

11.6b The Pain Response

The specialty organ system that is responsible for dealing with painful noxious stimuli is the *nociceptive nervous system*. It is also worthwhile to consider that pain is a normal protective response that helps to warn the organ system (you!) of any potential or real damage. Acute pain is a normal response after tissue injury and subsides with healing. Chronic pain persists for longer than the expected time frame for healing.

Clinical pearl

The word *nociception* is related to the word *noxious*, which refers to any type of stimulus that may be damaging or a threat. Everyone is familiar with noxious smells, which elicit the normal response of backing away or plugging your nose!

Pain receptors are referred to as *nociceptors*. There are four different types of receptors that we will discuss briefly, although in reality there are probably dozens of different types and subtypes of nociceptors that can start an impulse. These four are stretch, temperature, pressure, and chemical receptors. Types of receptors differ in location and tissue density.

The stretch receptors—located in joints, for example—fire before there is damage and serve in a protective role. The temperature receptors have their highest density in the hands, lips, and mouth. They help warn us if we grab or try to eat something outside of our temperature tolerance. The deep pressure receptors have no pharmacologic interventions yet, but stay tuned as developments occur. The chemical receptors regulate the inflammatory and healing responses. When tissue damage has taken place, chemicals such as prostaglandins are released as a natural response to damaged tissue by the arachidonic acid cascade.

Once impulses from pain receptors reach the brain, there are hundreds, if not millions, of innervations in the cerebral cortex that allow for the psychological, behavioral, and physical responses to the impulse. Psychological activity in response to pain is usually an increase in arousal and awareness. Behavioral and physical responses include increased heart rate and blood pressure, increased motor activity (attempts to get away from the painful stimuli), and vocalization (usually cursing in acute pain and moaning and groaning in chronic pain).

The World Health Organization is in the process of developing three treatment guidelines that will cover chronic pain in children, chronic pain in adults, and acute pain. It is important to treat patients' pain, but it is also important to understand what medicines and nonpharmacologic therapies are the most effective for different types of pain. The Centers for Disease Control and Prevention (CDC) has published data indicating that deaths from drug overdoses have risen steadily, more than doubling over the last two decades. In 2013 in the United States, there were 16,235 deaths involving opioid analgesics. Health-care providers must work together to make sure pain is treated effectively and safely.

time for review

What are some physical symptoms to look for in a patient who may not be able to verbalize his or her level of pain (e.g., a ventilated patient in the ICU)?

11.6c Analgesics

This section focuses on pharmacologic modalities that have analgesic properties. The principles that govern the use of analgesic medications include medication type, mechanisms of action, side effects, patient tolerability, and cost. Routes of administration become important and may include oral, transdermal, intravenous, intramuscular, or direct infusion of medications into the cerebrospinal fluid space (intrathecal administration).

Also important is whether a local analgesic can be administered, contrasting with a major surgical procedure that may require a general anesthetic. Frequently multiple medications from different classes are used for synergistic analgesia. All patient factors and medication factors need to be taken into account to determine the ideal analgesic regimen.

11.6d Outcomes Assessment Analgesic Therapy

No two people report pain in the same way. It is therefore very difficult to quantify such a subjective perception. The best way to quantify the pain response is to let patients rate their pain on a visual analog scale or a verbal number scale. If time allows a more thorough discussion with the patient, a few simple questions may start to reveal contributing factors to the patient's pain response. Occasionally, the acronym PQRST is used to help with the pain assessment. **P**alliative information relates to what relieves the pain. **Q**uality relates to a description of the pain (such as sharp, acute, penetrating versus dull, aching, or sickening pain qualities). **R**adiation helps to identify where the pain starts and where it goes—internal pain often presents with a characteristic radiating pattern; the heart-attack patient who presents with neck, shoulder, and jaw pain illustrates this example. **S**everity relates to the perceived intensity of the pain; the analog scales help to quantify the severity assessment. "T" translates into the **t**ime course of pain. This may be time of day, time of month, time of year, or any relationship to an event that may exacerbate the pain response. The Joint Commission on Accreditation of Healthcare Organizations (JCAHO) recognizes pain as the fifth vital sign.

11.6e Pain-Related Terminology

Misunderstandings among health-care providers, patients, the public, and regulators can occur as a result of inconsistent use of terms. The end result may be patients who are not adequately treated with pain medications. Health-care professionals must be able to treat real pain and not risk undertreating because of concerns about inappropriate use. Physical dependence, tolerance, cross-tolerance, addiction, and pseudoaddiction are all terms with different definitions.

Physical dependence is a state of adaptation manifested by a drug class– specific withdrawal syndrome precipitated by abrupt cessation, rapid dose reduction, decreasing blood level of the drug, or administration of an antagonist. Physical dependence is common in patients receiving daily opioid therapy for longer than 3 weeks.

Tolerance is a state of adaptation in which repeated exposure to a drug induces changes that result in a decrease of one or more of the drug's effects over time. Tolerance is common, which explains why patients may require higher-than-normal doses to achieve the same level of analgesic effect. It is important to distinguish tolerance from increase in pain as the reason for needing higher doses. The good news is that tolerance can also develop to reduce some side effects.

Cross-tolerance is the ability of one drug to suppress the manifestations of physical withdrawal produced by another drug and to maintain the physically dependent state. Some patients rotate opioids, and caution must be used because tolerance to opioid analgesic and nonanalgesic effects do not fully transfer to the new drug. This is the basis for recommending a decrease in dosage of the new opioid by 30%–50% when initiating a different opioid.

Addiction is a maladaptive pattern of substance abuse leading to clinically significant impairment or distress.

Pseudoaddiction occurs when patients with severe unrelieved pain become preoccupied with finding opioids. Behavior usually resolves with adequate pain control. The CDC reports that each day 46 people die from overdoses of prescription pain medications in the United States. More must be done to prevent overprescribing while ensuring patients' access to effective and safe pain therapy.

11.6f Classes of Analgesics

Analgesics exert their mechanisms of action by targeting a number of different locations and neurotransmitters in the nociceptive pathway. These medications may target opioid-binding sites, causing the opioid receptors' inhibition of the pain impulse (morphine-like drugs), or they may inhibit the formation of the pain-production cytokines that start the pain impulse (steroids and nonsteroidal anti-inflammatory agents). Other medications that are used in pain situations may act to increase the regulatory neurotransmitters norepinephrine and serotonin or slow the propagation of nerve impulses.

11.6g Opioids

One of the first analgesic medications to be used was heroin, obtained from the poppy seed. The juice of the poppy seed contains a number of opiate congeners that have been shown to have analgesic properties as well as many unwanted CNS side effects. Morphine sulfate is the best known of this class of medications. The term **opioid** refers to any natural or synthetic chemical that can bind to an opioid receptor and exert an action. Opioids differ in their potency, onset of action, duration of action, chemical structure, available routes of administration, side effects, abuse potential, and cost. See Table 11-11 for a list of the opioid analgesics.

Clinical pearl

Remember from Chapter 9 that the opioid morphine is also beneficial for its ability to decrease preload, which may help patients with pulmonary edema, heart failure, and myocardial infarction when indicated to relieve pain.

TABLE 11-11 Opioid Analgesics

Generic Name	Trade Name	Parenteral Dose (mg)	Oral Dose (mg)	Onset (min)	Duration (hr)
morphine	Many	10	30	IV, 5; PO, 30	3–6
hydromorphone	Dilaudid®	1.5	7.5	See morphine	3–6
levorphanol	Levo-Dromoran®	2	4	30–90	4–6
oxymorphone	Opana®	1.5	N/A	10–90	3–6
fentanyl		0.1	N/A	IV, almost immediate	0.5–2
sufentanil	Sufenta®	10 mcg	N/A	IV, 1–3; epidural, 10	2–4
methadone	Dolophine®	5	10	sc, IM = 10–20	6–8
codeine	Many	36	60	See morphine	3–6
hydrocodone	Many	N/A	30	10–20	4–8
oxycodone	Many	N/A	20	10–15	4–6
meperidine	Demerol®	100	400	PO, 10–15; IV, 5	1–3
buprenorphine	Buprenex®	0.3	N/A	10–30	6–8
butorphanol		2	N/A	IV, <10; Nasal ,<15	3–4
nalbuphine	Nubain®	10	N/A	IV, 2–3; SC, < 15	4–6

The opioids that cross more quickly into the CNS and produce rapid analgesia and euphoric effects are the agents more likely to be abused by patients with addictive personalities. It should be noted that in acute pain situations, when the source of the pain is very well defined, there is a very low probability of patients demonstrating drug-seeking behavior or progressing to opioid addiction. However in chronic pain situations, when the source of pain is not well defined, patients frequently present with drug-seeking behavior and chemical dependency.

The FDA, in conjunction with the Drug Enforcement Agency (DEA), heavily regulates the manufacture, distribution, and sale of opioid analgesics. The scheduling of controlled drugs is based on the potency and potential for abuse of the various chemicals. See Table 11-12 for drug schedules and their regulations.

TABLE 11-12 Drug Schedules

Schedule	Criteria	Examples
I	No medical use; high addiction potential	heroin
II	Medical use; high addiction potential	cocaine, opioids, amphetamines
III	Medical use; moderate potential for dependence	codeine, hydrocodone
IV	Medical use; low abuse potential	benzodiazepines

The route of administration of opioid analgesics depends on the severity of the pain. If a patient is in mild to moderate pain, oral administration of opioids is appropriate. If the patient is not controlled on oral regimens, intramuscular, subcutaneous, or intravenous medications may be administered. A self-administration technique is patient-controlled analgesia (PCA). This allows the prescriber to determine the medication, continuous infusion rates, and bolus doses. However, the patient can self-dose the medication to an appropriate level of analgesia by pressing a button that is connected to the PCA infusion device. PCA infusion devices have decreased patients' pain and suffering while minimizing nursing and prescriber time in acute pain settings.

An additional option for the management of pain is to infuse opioids directly into the CNS. This may be done in the acute situation, such as delivering a baby, with epidural administration. Epidural anesthesia is a type of regional anesthesia in which drugs are injected into the epidural space of the spinal cord. In a more prolonged surgery, a drug may be infused directly into the intrathecal space to produce local analgesia. In the circumstance of malignant pain, catheters placed intrathecally or epidurally may be connected to continuous-infusion pumps. In each of these situations, the goal is to provide optimal analgesia while minimizing the central side effects.

Opioid analgesics exert similar side effects. They differ slightly in their ability to cause side effects such as respiratory depression or constipation. It is important to note that patients who have not had opioids in their systems (opioid-naive patients) are more likely to have serious side effects such as respiratory depression. Patients who are not opioid-naive are much more tolerant to larger doses and side effects. Administration of opioid analgesics causes a central depression of the brainstem's ability to sense CO_2. This can result in a decrease in respiratory rate, tidal volume, minute ventilation, and the CO_2 response-curve slope. The peak respiratory depression effect corresponds to the route of administration and the peak in CNS concentration of the opioids. For example the peak actions following IV morphine are in 8–10 minutes. See Table 11-13 for a list of opioid analgesic side effects. Predisposing factors to respiratory depression include being overweight, sleep apnea, and asthma.

Clinical pearl

Ziconotide (Prialt®) is a unique analgesic that blocks calcium influx into the cells through voltage-gated or N-type calcium channels. These channels are present in the afferent neuron and in the dorsal horn ganglion. Blockage prevents subsequent neuronal depolarization. The drug is derived synthetically from a toxin produced by a snail. It is administered intrathecally for severe chronic pain in patients who are intolerant to or refractory to other treatments.

TABLE 11-13 Side Effects of Opioid Analgesics

System or Area of Concern	Side Effect
Major concerns	Respiratory depression, apnea, circulatory depression, shock, respiratory arrest, cardiac arrest
CNS	Light-headedness, dizziness, syncope, seizures, dysphoria, hallucinations
Respiratory	Depression, decreased rate and depth of breathing
Cardiovascular	Reduction in venous and arterial pressures
Skin	Histamine release resulting in blood vessel dilation, flushing, sweating, pruritus
GI	Nausea, inhibition of peristaltic waves leading to constipation

11.6h Opioid Antagonists

Opioid antagonists such as naloxone (Narcan®) reverse the CNS and ventilatory depression that can be caused by opioids. The antagonism they cause at the opioid receptor can be as soon as 5 minutes after administration. Because naloxone administration in the absence of opioids is not harmful, naloxone administration is frequently used in cases in which narcotic overdose is suspected but unknown. It does not reverse CNS and ventilatory depression from other causes. Recently the FDA approved a form of naloxone (Evzio®) available in an auto-injector delivery device intended for "buddy" administration to a person who either accidentally or purposefully overdosed on opioids while

Clinical pearl

All opiates produce equivalent respiratory depression in equipotent doses. Regular use of opiates can cause tolerance to respiratory depression.

awaiting emergency medical services (EMS) arrival (see Figure 11-2). There are printed instructions on the device as well as electronic voice instructions that can be heard through a speaker on the device instructing the lay person on proper administration. The auto-injector administers the dose either IM or SC. Immediate medical attention should be sought after administration because the duration of action of most opioids exceeds that of naloxone.

FIGURE 11-2 Evzio(®) Auto-injector Delivery Device

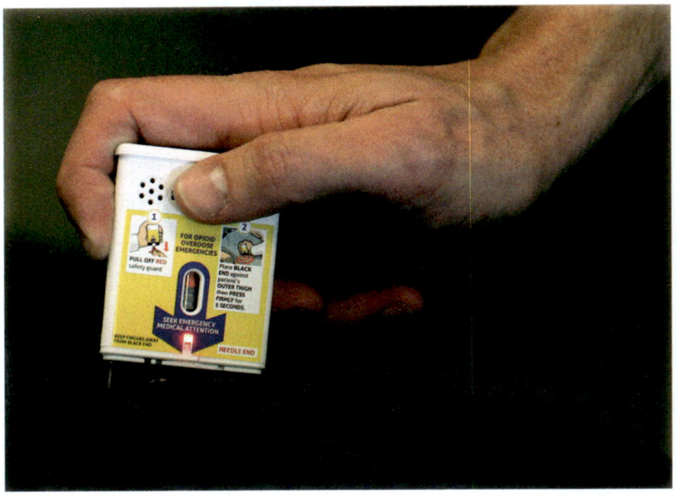

Source: AP Images

11.6i Steroid Anti-Inflammatory Agents

Whenever tissue is destroyed, the arachidonic acid cascade is activated. The end products of this cascade include leukotrienes, which act as inflammatory mediators, as well as prostaglandins, which are potent stimulators of the chemical nociceptors. Corticosteroid anti-inflammatory medications act to inhibit the arachidonic acid cascade, resulting in decreased production of leukotrienes and prostaglandins.

Corticosteroids for pain may be administered by a number of routes. Systemic routes include enteral administration of oral tablets or solutions, or parenteral administration of intravenous or intramuscular injections. Short-term systemic administration of corticosteroids is occasionally very helpful in controlling the pain response. However, long-term side effects of systemic corticosteroids—including peptic ulcer disease, bone demineralization, alteration of blood glucose, and muscle atrophy—limit their use.

Corticosteroids are utilized by local injections into painful joints for analgesic/ anti-inflammatory action. Corticosteroid joint injections are limited by the amount of fluid that can be injected into the space. Naturally, a large shoulder joint will require a larger volume than a small finger joint. One of the complications of joint injections is that they mask the damage at the joint. If injured athletes do not want to take time off from the sport to allow the injury to heal, they may receive a joint injection that will mask the pain, which may result in further injury to the joint.

PATIENT & FAMILY EDUCATION

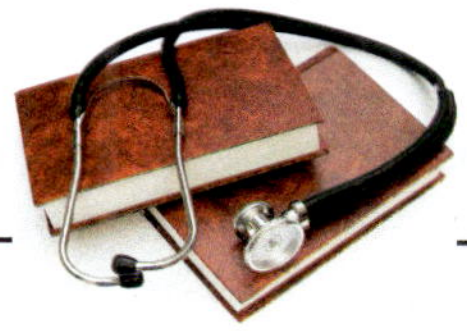

It is important to provide detailed instructions for patients who are in need of pain medications. These instructions should include the purpose of each analgesic prescribed if more than one (e.g., "MS Contin® is your background medication, meaning it keeps a constant level of medicine in your blood"), how to take them (e.g., "around the clock" versus "as needed"), how much to take, side effects to expect, and what to do if pain is not well controlled.

11.6j Nonsteroidal Anti-Inflammatory Agents

One of the most commonly used classes of analgesic medications is the nonsteroidal anti-inflammatory drugs (NSAIDs). NSAIDs are considered the drugs of choice in situations of tissue-destruction pain. Any circumstance that has caused a disruption of the tissues will respond to NSAID therapy. NSAIDs have antipyretic, anti-inflammatory, and analgesic properties. NSAIDs exert their mechanism of action by inhibiting the enzyme system known as *cyclo-oxygenase*. This enzyme system causes the production of thromboxanes, prostacyclins, and prostaglandins. NSAIDs can be used for acute pain, chronic pain, malignant pain, osteoarthritis pain, arthritis pain, migraine headache, regular headache, and gout pain. Side effects of bleeding can be related to cyclo-oxygenase (COX) inhibition. This has resulted in the development of COX-2–specific NSAIDs or COX-2 inhibitors. Examples of COX-2 inhibitors include celecoxib (Celebrex®). Recent controversies with this drug class relate to the increased cardiovascular risk of myocardial infarction that prompted lawsuits and withdrawal of rofecoxib (Vioxx®) from the market. See Table 11-14 for a list of nonsteroidal anti-inflammatory medications.

TABLE 11-14 Common Nonsteroidal Anti-Inflammatory Medications

Generic Name	Brand Name
aspirin	Bayer®, etc.
ibuprofen	Motrin®, etc.
ketoprofen	
naproxen HCl	Naprosyn®, etc.
naproxen sodium	Anaprox®, etc.
indomethacin	Indocin®, etc.
sulindac	Clinoril®
piroxicam	Feldene®
ketorolac	
celecoxib	Celebrex®

Side effects of NSAIDs are primarily an extension of the desired action. Inhibition of prostaglandin production can result in a decrease in the protective effects of prostaglandins on the GI tract. This may present acutely with gastritis, irritation, and intestinal discomfort; chronically, it may contribute to peptic ulcer disease. CNS effects include dizziness and drowsiness—but to a much lesser degree than with the opioid-type medications. NSAIDs may also alter renal function and can contribute to renal dysfunction in patients with underlying tenuous renal perfusion, such as patients with heart failure, diabetes, or kidney disease. NSAIDs are also metabolized extensively in the liver, and these medications can occasionally cause toxicities to the liver cells.

11.6k Analgesic Synergy

It should be apparent that there is a pharmacologic rationale for the administration of analgesics from different classes to better control the pain. Remember from Chapter 1 that the concept of synergy relates to the phenomenon best illustrated with a numeric example: 1 + 1 = 3. When you use two medications, the analgesia is better than the sum of the two agents separately. A significant number of combination products are commercially available. Acetaminophen (an analgesic but not an anti-inflammatory) is combined with codeine to create the product line known as Tylenol® with codeine. It is also combined with a number of different strengths of hydrocodone to form the product lines Vicodin®, Anexia®, and Lortab®. Aspirin plus the potent opioid oxycodone is known as Percodan®. Not to be outdone, ibuprofen has been added to hydrocodone to form the product Vicoprofen®. All of these medications have been shown to be more effective than either medication by itself in improving pain scores. See Table 11-15 for suggested pain-severity dosing regimens.

TABLE 11-15 Suggested Pain Dosing Regimens

Mild Pain	Moderate Pain	Severe Pain
APAP 650 mg q 4 hr ASA 650 mg q 6 hr ibuprofen 600 mg q 6 hr tramadol (Ultram®) 50 mg t.i.d. hydrocodone 2.5/500 1–2 q 4–6 hr APAP 300/COD 15 mg 1–2 q 4–6 hr	tramadol (Ultram®) 50 mg q 6 hr ketorolac 10 mg q 6 hr hydrocodone 5/500 1–2 q 4–6 hr APAP 325/oxycodone 5 mg q 4 hr APAP-325/COD 60 mg 1–2 q 4–6 hr hydrocodone 7.5/500 1–2 q 4–6 hr	ketorolac (Toradol®) 30–60 mg IM, 15–30 mg IV hydrocodone/APAP (Lorcet®) 10/650 1–2 q 4–6 hr hydrocodone/APAP (Norco®) 10/325 1–2 q 4–6 hr oxycodone/APAP (Tylox®) 5/500 1–2 q 3–4 hr oxycodone/ASA (Percodan®) 5/ 325 1–2 q 4–6 hr morphine 15 mg q 4 hr levorphanol (Levo-Dromoran®) 2 mg 1–2 q 6–8 hr methadone (Dolophine®) 20 mg q 12 hr meperidine (Demerol®) 50 mg 4–6 tabs q 6 hr hydromorphone (Dilaudid®) 4 mg q 4 hr morphine controlled-release 60 mg q 8 hr

Abbreviations: APAP, acetaminophen; ASA, aspirin; COD, codeine.

11.6l Adjuncts to Analgesics

A number of other medications have been utilized as adjunctive analgesics. Phenothiazine antiemetic medications have been administered to decrease the nausea and vomiting associated with the pain response. These medications include prochlorperazine (Compazine®) and promethazine (Phenergan®). They were previously mentioned in this chapter as treatments for PONV.

Patients with chronic pain are known to have a functional decrease in circulating levels of the neurotransmitters serotonin and norepinephrine. Tricyclic antidepressant (TCA) medications have been shown to be effective in improving pain-response scores. These medications act by blocking the presynaptic uptake of catecholamines released into the synaptic cleft. This results in an increase in serotonin and norepinephrine that then decreases the release of the pain-propagating neurotransmitter called substance P. See Table 11-16 for common antidepressant medications.

In the treatment of depression, there has been a recent emphasis on putting patients on selective serotonin reuptake inhibitors (SSRIs). This has happened largely because of their lower side-effect profiles and greater safety in an overdose setting. However, in pain situations, the selective SSRIs are *not* more effective than the older TCA types of medications. This is probably because the TCAs also block the reuptake of norepinephrine, which also regulates the pain transmission process. SSRIs, however, affect only the serotonin-related aspects of pain transmission.

TABLE 11-16 Common Antidepressant Medications

Category	Generic Name	Trade Name
Tricyclic antidepressants (TCAs)	amitriptyline	
	imipramine	Tofranil®
	doxepin	
	nortriptyline	Pamelor®
	desipramine	Norpramin®
Selective serotonin reuptake inhibitors (SSRIs)	fluoxetine	Prozac®
	paroxetine	Paxil®
	sertraline	Zoloft®
	citalopram	Celexa®

Tricyclic antidepressants have a characteristic side-effect profile that may affect a patient's tolerance. Drowsiness and confusion are the first side effects. These go away if the dose is started low and titrated upward on a weekly basis. Dry mouth, urinary retention, hot dry skin, and constipation are the other anticipated side effects of this class of medications.

Neuropathic pain is characterized by well-defined nerve pathway involvement. This pain is generally described as sharp and piercing, or a constant burning along a specific nerve root. A good example of neuropathic pain is post-herpetic neuralgia, which may become quite debilitating in patients following a herpes zoster infection (shingles). Neuropathic pain also presents in diabetic patients and HIV patients, and occasionally following injuries. The medications that work well in this circumstance are some of the antiseizure medications. These medications act by decreasing the membrane depolarization and somehow decreasing the intensity of pain. Carbamazepine (Tegretol®), divalproex sodium (Depakote®), topiramate (Topamax®), and gabapentin (Neurontin®) have all been shown to be helpful in select nerve-pain situations.

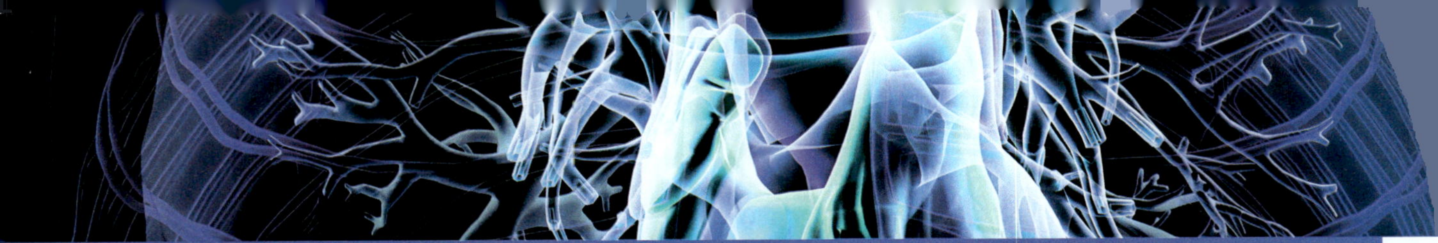

Summary

In this chapter we have learned about the role of neuromuscular function–blocking agents before surgery, in intubations, with mechanical ventilation, and in specialized cases postoperatively. We have learned that these drugs can have consequences on blood pressure and heart rate and not just isolated respiratory effects. Because analgesia must accompany neuromuscular relaxation, and pain can impair ventilation, other broad classifications of drugs were also reviewed. In addition anesthesia agents were reviewed, with special attention to the effect on the respiratory system.

REVIEW QUESTIONS

1. Neuromuscular blocking agents are classified by
   (a) duration of action
   (b) the type of block produced
   (c) the route by which they are administered
   (d) all of the above
2. The terms *induction*, *maintenance*, and *termination* are relevant to
   (a) local anesthesia
   (b) sedative/hypnotics
   (c) general anesthesia
   (d) anxiolytics
3. Inhaled anesthetics may adversely affect
   (a) cardiovascular function
   (b) respiratory function
   (c) muscular function
   (d) all of the above
4. Match the NMBA to its duration of action:

pancuronium	long
succinylcholine	intermediate
vecuronium	ultrashort

5. Match the drug with its pharmacologic class

ibuprofen	anxiolytic
morphine	NSAID
Valium®	opioid

6. Explain some of the principles that guide the use of analgesics.

7. Describe some of the different neurotransmitters involved in the pain pathway and why they are important to cardiorespiratory pharmacotherapy.
8. What are some of the side effects of opioid analgesics?
9. What is the role of concurrent analgesic use with NMBAs?
10. Describe the characteristics of an ideal drug used to facilitate endotracheal intubation.
11. What are some methods of monitoring the efficacy of neuromuscular blocking agents?
12. What pharmacologic effects do the benzodiazepines have?
13. A vehicular accident patient with massive chest injuries requires emergency intubation. What pharmacologic agent is indicated? Once intubated, the patient is difficult to ventilate because he is combative; in addition the physician wants to depress spontaneous ventilation to assist in healing the chest trauma. What pharmacologic agents are indicated?

Chapter 12

Therapeutic Medical Gases

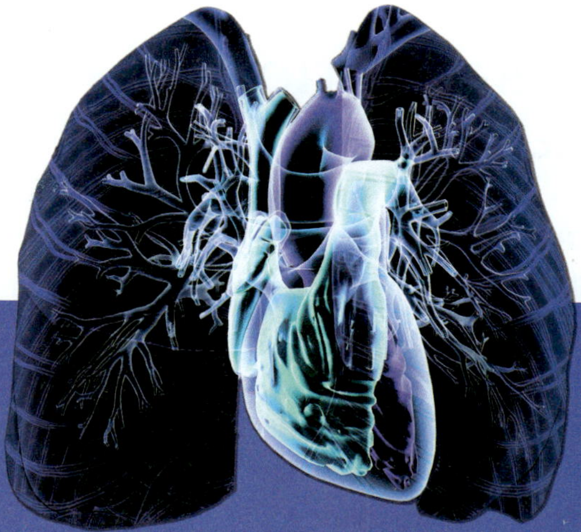

OBJECTIVES

Upon completion of this chapter you will be able to

- Identify the indications for oxygen, helium, and nitric oxide therapy.
- List and describe the function of oxygen delivery devices.
- Describe the effects of oxygen, helium, and nitric oxide therapy.
- List the hazards of oxygen, helium, and nitric oxide therapy.
- Describe the monitoring and assessment of oxygen, helium, and nitric oxide therapy.

KEY TERMS

absorptive atelectasis
anemic hypoxia
bland aerosol therapy
cyanosis
demand hypoxia
free radicals
heated humidified high-flow therapy
heliox
hemoglobin
high-flow oxygen system
high-flow therapy
histotoxic hypoxia
hypoxemia
hypoxemic hypoxia
hypoxia
hypoxic drive
inhaled nitric oxide
jet mixing mask
large-volume nebulizer
low-flow oxygen system
nasal cannula
nonrebreathing mask
oxygen therapy
oxygen toxicity
peripheral chemoreceptor
polycythemia
respiration
simple mask
stagnant hypoxia
ventilation

ABBREVIATIONS

ABG arterial blood gas
CO carbon monoxide
CPAP continuous positive airway pressure
EDRF endothelium-derived relaxing factor
FIO_2 fraction of inspired oxygen
He helium
HFT high-flow therapy
HHHF heated humidified high-flow therapy
INO inhaled nitric oxide
IRDS infant respiratory distress syndrome
MI myocardial infarction
NO nitric oxide
NO_2 nitrogen dioxide
$PaCO_2$ blood gas measurement of the pressure of carbon dioxide in the arterial system
PaO_2 blood gas measurement of the pressure of oxygen in the arterial system
PEEP positive end-expiratory pressure
PPHN persistent pulmonary hypertension of the neonate
ppm parts per million
ROP retinopathy of prematurity
SaO_2 arterial blood gas measurement of the saturation of oxygen on the hemoglobin molecule
SpO_2 measure of hemoglobin saturation via pulse oximetry
USP United States Pharmacopoeia
V/Q relationship of alveolar ventilation (V) to capillary perfusion (Q)

Learning Hint

Think of hemoglobin as a bus and the oxygen molecules as kids who can get on and off the bus. Hemoglobin (the bus) has an affinity for (wants to pick up) oxygen (kids) at the lungs. When oxygen-rich hemoglobin reaches the tissues, the oxygen molecules are released to the tissues and carbon dioxide is picked up to return to the lungs for exhalation. This bus analogy will be used throughout this chapter.

Therapeutic gases are indeed drugs because they exert physiologic effects on the body. *Oxygen* is listed in the United States Pharmacopeia (USP), and **oxygen therapy** is used extensively in both hospital and home settings. The transport and delivery of oxygen to the body's tissues is vital for life. Without adequate oxygen delivery to tissues, we suffer irreversible brain damage in 4 to 6 minutes. However too much oxygen can also be dangerous and have serious consequences by disrupting normal tissue function, possibly leading to oxygen toxicity.

Oxygen therapy can be administered with relative ease. However, many misconceptions, and the fact that it is easy to administer, can lead to situations in which oxygen therapy is taken for granted and is not used rationally or properly. Working through this chapter will give you the knowledge to decide when and how to properly administer oxygen therapy to your patients. In addition this chapter focuses on gases mixed with oxygen to achieve certain desired physiologic effects. These gases include helium and nitric oxide.

12.1 OXYGEN THERAPY

12.1a Physiologic Background

One of the most basic human functions in maintaining life is the extraction of oxygen from the atmosphere and its delivery via the bloodstream to cells and tissues to be used for such functions as energy, growth, and repair. We obtain oxygen from the atmosphere and deliver it to our bloodstream by the processes of **ventilation** and **respiration.** Ventilation is simply the process of breathing in and out or carrying the oxygen-rich atmosphere from outside the body to the millions of thin-walled alveoli in the lungs. Respiration is the process of gas exchange at the alveolar capillary membrane, where oxygen is transferred from the alveoli into the bloodstream and the waste product carbon dioxide is transferred to the alveoli to be exhaled. External respiration occurs via diffusion of gases from areas of high concentration to areas of low concentration in the lungs. In essence the fundamental purpose of the respiratory system is to supply oxygen to the individual tissue cells and to remove their gaseous waste product, carbon dioxide. Disruption or impairment of either the ventilation or the respiration process impairs oxygenation of the blood. See Figure 12-1 for the process of respiration at the alveolar–capillary membrane.

FIGURE 12-1 Respiration at the Alveolar–Capillary Membrane

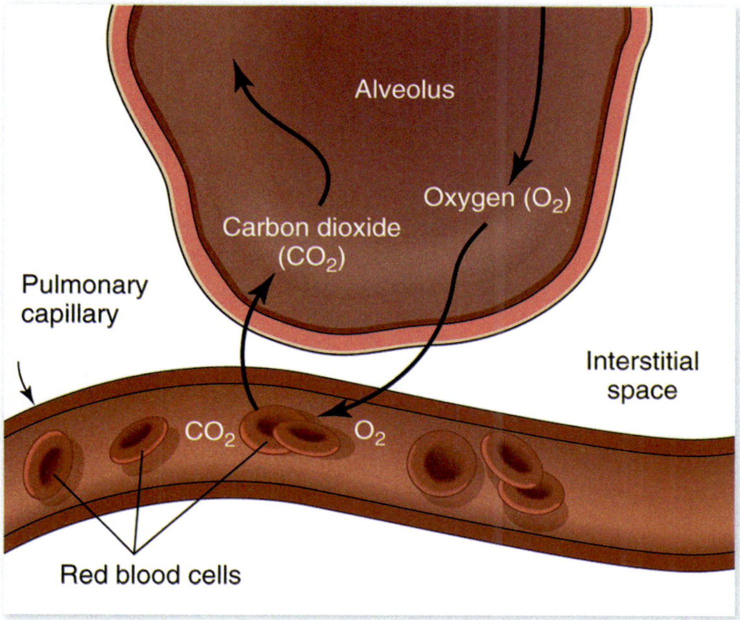

Once oxygen is transported across the alveoli into the bloodstream, it must be carried to the tissues via hemoglobin molecules, found in red blood. **Hemoglobin** has an affinity to bind with oxygen in a reversible manner and thus can combine with oxygen at the alveoli and then release it to the tissues (internal respiration).

This basic background can now be used as a foundation to explain the indications for oxygen therapy.

12.1b Hypoxemia

Although **hypoxemia** and **hypoxia** sound similar, they are related but different clinical terms. First we will discuss hypoxemia. Hypoxemia is defined as low levels of oxygen in the blood that can be verified by measuring arterial blood gas (ABG), which shows the partial pressure of oxygen dissolved in the blood (PaO_2). Normal PaO_2 values range between 80 and 100 mmHg. A PaO_2 of less than 80 mmHg indicates hypoxemia. See Table 12-1 for a classification of the types of hypoxemia according to the PaO_2 value.

Learning Hint

Whenever health-care workers draw and analyze arterial blood gas for oxygen levels, they are measuring the amount of oxygen dissolved in the blood—*not* the amount on the hemoglobin molecule. The amount of oxygen dissolved in the blood is called the partial pressure of arterial oxygen or PaO_2 value. You can think of this value as representing kids running around outside the bus waiting to get in. If a lot of kids are running around outside the bus (high PaO_2), then the bus is probably too full to fit any more (saturated); if there aren't many kids around (low PaO_2), then the bus is probably not very full.

BVT Lab

Flashcards are available for this chapter at www.BVTLab.com.

TABLE 12-1 Classification of Hypoxemia

Type	PaO_2
Hyperoxemia	>100 mmHg
No hypoxemia (normoxemia)	80–100 mmHg
Mild hypoxemia	60–79 mmHg
Moderate hypoxemia	40–59 mmHg
Severe hypoxemia	<40 mmHg

LIFE SPAN CONSIDERATIONS

PaO_2 normally decreases with age, and this fact must be considered. There are different ways to adjust for age and decreasing PaO_2. One method used is for every year of age over 60, subtract 1 mmHg from the normal range limits. For example, a 75-year-old patient would have 65 to 85 mmHg as an adjusted normal range.

The Earth's atmosphere contains approximately 21% oxygen, which provides ample oxygen for a healthy person to survive. However, several conditions can cause hypoxemia, which may require supplemental oxygen. These conditions fall under the following four categories.

1. *Low levels of atmospheric oxygen.* An example is high altitudes, where the low barometric pressure allows only low oxygen tensions to be available.
2. *Alveolar hypoventilation.* Anything that interferes with the transport of oxygen to the alveoli, thereby decreasing ventilation, may cause hypoxemia. Ventilatory depression due to narcotic overdoses, chronic obstructive pulmonary disease (COPD), neuromuscular disease, chest trauma, or pain are some examples.
3. *Ventilation-to-perfusion (V/Q) mismatching.* Any process that impairs the balance between ventilation reaching the alveolus and perfusion to the surrounding capillary may lead to hypoxemia. For example lung diseases such as emphysema, interstitial pulmonary fibrosis, lung cancer, and pneumonia all create conditions that impair the ventilation process (decreasing V) by either destroying the integrity of the alveolus or impairing diffusion by causing secretion barriers. In addition cardiac diseases that affect the cardiac output, such as heart failure or myocardial infarction, or that interfere with capillary perfusion, such as pulmonary emboli, alter the perfusion (Q) of the capillary and thus may lead to a V/Q mismatch.
4. *Right-to-left shunt.* This occurs when the blood leaving the right heart either bypasses a portion of the pulmonary circulation or flows by nonfunctional alveoli. This blood enters the left heart unoxygenated and therefore lowers the overall PaO_2. Examples of right-to-left shunting include cardiogenic pulmonary edema, acute respiratory distress syndrome (ARDS), and atelectasis, in which the alveolus is totally nonfunctional because of collapse or being completely filled with fluid.

Clinical pearl

Oxygen therapy will help under conditions 1, 2, and 3, but not 4, because in the last case the oxygen never gets to the nonventilated alveolus. Right-to-left shunt requires positive end-expiratory pressure (PEEP) or continuous positive airway pressure (CPAP) in addition to oxygen therapy to reestablish ventilation to these nonfunctional units.

time for review

Why do mountain climbers need supplemental oxygen, and why do airplane cabins need to be pressurized?

12.1c Clinical Manifestations of Hypoxemia

The clinical manifestations of hypoxemia relate to the body's attempts to combat and compensate for the hypoxemic condition. Following is a list of these responses.

- *Tachycardia and systemic hypertension.* The tachycardia is an attempt to speed up oxygen delivery, and hypertension is a result of the increased heart rate. If the heart is weakened by disease, bradycardia and hypotension may result.
- *Tachypnea.* The increased respiratory rate is an attempt to get more oxygen into the blood. The depth will probably also increase, resulting in hyperventilation, as evidenced by a decrease in the pressure of arterial carbon dioxide ($PaCO_2$).
- *Pulmonary hypertension.* Constriction of pulmonary capillaries allows slower blood flow (slows the bus) and therefore more oxygen can be loaded onto the hemoglobin at the lungs.
- *Cerebral and coronary vasodilatation.* This leads to increased blood flow to the vital areas of the heart and brain.
- *Cyanosis, diaphoresis, and pallor.* These may all be present.
- *Restlessness, agitation, and confusion.* Insufficient oxygen to the brain causes these symptoms.
- *Secondary* ***polycythemia***. With chronic hypoxemia, as in COPD or in the case of individuals living at high altitudes, the body stimulates the production of more red blood cells and therefore has higher hemoglobin levels.

Learning Hint

Come back to the bus analogy for the body's response to hypoxemia. The bus will need to speed up (tachycardia) to deliver more blood systemically. However it will slow down (pulmonary vasoconstriction) at the lungs to pick up more oxygen. The roads leading to the heart (coronary artery) and brain (cerebral circulation) will open up (dilate) to enhance delivery to these vital organs. Over time, more buses may be added (secondary polycythemia) if the hypoxemia remains chronic.

12.1d Hypoxia

The presence of hypoxemia does not necessarily mean that you have hypoxia. Hypoxia means low levels of oxygen to the tissue. A patient can have low levels of oxygen in the blood (hypoxemia) but not necessarily have low levels reaching the tissues (hypoxia), because the body may have compensated with tachycardia, pulmonary vasoconstriction, or polycythemia. Conversely a patient can have hypoxia but not hypoxemia. For example a patient may have normal or high PaO_2 (no hypoxemia), yet the hemoglobin may be defective, or the tissues may not be able to utilize the oxygen, leading to hypoxia. Of course hypoxemia and hypoxia can occur at the same time. Let's review some specific types of hypoxia.

Hypoxemic Hypoxia

Sound like a redundant term? Basically, **hypoxemic hypoxia** is caused by anything that interferes with the ability of oxygen to get to the alveoli or diffuse across them. Some examples of causes include atmospheres with insufficient oxygen, such as those that mountain climbers contend with; airway obstructions that do not let oxygen pass; fluid in the alveoli, which acts as a barrier to diffusion; and any situation that leads to hypoventilation, such as muscle weakness/disease, brain injuries, or drug overdoses that suppress the respiratory system. Hypoxemia is always present in these situations, because an adequate oxygen supply never reaches the alveoli.

Anemic Hypoxia

Anemic hypoxia is anything that interferes with the hemoglobin's oxygen-carrying capacity. For example anemic patients or patients with dysfunctional hemoglobin, as in carbon monoxide poisoning or sickle cell anemia, may not be able to carry sufficient oxygen to the tissues. Hypoxemia may or may not be present in these patients, because they may have normal amounts of dissolved oxygen (PaO_2) but be unable to load it properly onto hemoglobin molecules.

Clinical pearl

Carbon monoxide (CO) has 210–250 times oxygen's affinity for hemoglobin. If you are in an atmosphere of carbon monoxide (a burning building or being exposed to car exhaust), your buses will fill up quickly, but they will be filled with carbon monoxide first. Now when the bus comes to the tissue, carbon monoxide is delivered, which the tissues cannot utilize. In addition, because of the high affinity, the kids (CO molecules) don't want to get off the bus and instead continue to occupy a seat an oxygen molecule should have. Patients with CO poisoning look well oxygenated (cherry red) because of the high saturation of hemoglobin with CO.

Stagnant or Circulatory Hypoxia

Stagnant hypoxia is anything that interferes with the circulatory system's ability to transport oxygen. Examples include decreased cardiac output, cardiogenic shock, hypovolemia, and any cardiovascular instability, such as congestive heart failure. In these cases, hypoxemia is almost always present.

Histotoxic Hypoxia

Histotoxic hypoxia is an inability of the tissue to utilize available oxygen, no matter how much is presented. Cyanide poisoning is the classic example. It is rarely accompanied by hypoxemia, but it is nevertheless deadly.

Demand Hypoxia

In hypermetabolic states, the tissue demand for oxygen may exceed the supply. Fever and strenuous exercise are examples of **demand hypoxia** in which hypoxemia will be present.

As you can see, when you assess a patient for hypoxia, you need to look at more than just the PaO_2. You must also look at the oxygen saturation of the hemoglobin (SaO_2), the amount and type of hemoglobin, and the cardiovascular status.

Clinical pearl

Not all patients have a PaO_2 of 80–100 mmHg as their normal range. Premature infants and chronically hypoxemic COPD patients may have lower limits of acceptability.

time for review

Contrast hypoxemia and hypoxia in terms of definition and clinical assessment.

12.1e Goals of Oxygen Therapy

The three major goals of oxygen therapy are to (1) treat hypoxemia, (2) decrease the work of breathing, and (3) decrease myocardial work.

Treating Hypoxemia

The following guidelines are used to assess hypoxemia in adults, children, or infants who are breathing room air at rest. If the patient's ABG shows either a

PaO_2 of less than 60 mmHg or a saturation (SaO_2) of less than 90%, or if pulse oximetry is used and a reading of less than 90% (SpO_2) is obtained, you can document that your patient needs oxygen therapy.

Decreasing the Work of Breathing

A patient who is having a difficult time breathing consumes a lot of oxygen just to survive. The body increases the work of the respiratory muscles by increasing the rate and depth of breathing in order to bring in more oxygen. A clinical assessment of the patient in respiratory distress and in need of oxygen therapy may find an increase in the rate and depth of breathing, accessory muscle use, and cyanosis.

Decreasing Myocardial Work

The heart is the major organ that pumps the blood containing oxygen to the tissues of the body. When there is a decrease in the blood's oxygen levels, the heart attempts to correct this situation by increasing its pumping action and rate. This action also produces an increased need for oxygen for the heart's muscles, because of its increased workload. This can lead to arrhythmias or heart failure. Therefore oxygen therapy should be started in order to assist the heart with this increased work, so that it may safely provide more oxygen to the tissues.

12.1f Oxygen Administration Devices

Before discussing particular devices for oxygen therapy, it is important to talk about the idea of *fractional inspired oxygen* or FIO_2. Our atmosphere consists of approximately 21 parts in 100 oxygen, or 21%; therefore the FIO_2 of room air is 0.21. When supplemental oxygen is delivered to a patient, we increase the FIO_2 in order to provide more oxygen to the body for gas exchange. You can deliver from 22% up to 100% oxygen, depending on the type of device used. Successful oxygen therapy depends on choosing the right type of device and the proper FIO_2. Oxygen therapy that can deliver 100% oxygen at increased atmospheric pressures is called *hyperbaric oxygen therapy* (see Figure 12-2).

FIGURE 12-2 Hyperbaric Chambers

Hyperbaric oxygen is used to treat carbon monoxide poisoning, thermal burns, decompression sickness, air embolism, crush injury, and anaerobic infections. Increasing the barometric pressure greatly increases the amount of oxygen getting to the alveoli, or PaO_2.

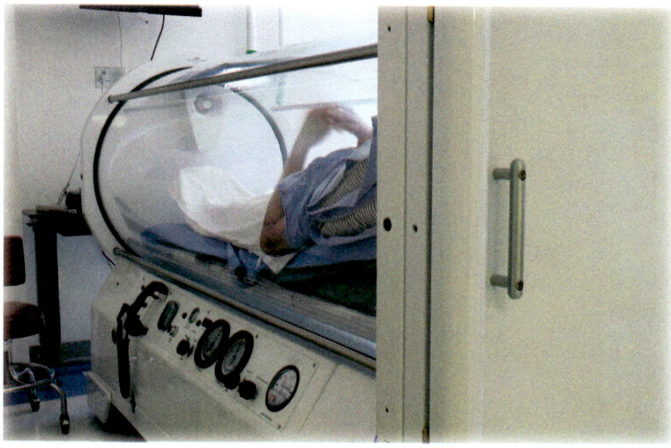

Clinical pearl

Cyanosis is a bluish discoloration of the skin. This bluish color comes from excessive amounts of deoxygenated hemoglobin (a lot of blue buses). Be careful, though; a patient with low hemoglobin levels (anemia) may not show signs of cyanosis because, in essence, the person doesn't have enough hemoglobin to effect a color change in the blood. Nevertheless the patient is probably still suffering from hypoxia and still needs supplemental oxygen.

Clinical pearl

The ultimate goal is to treat the underlying cause of the hypoxia, whether it is hypoxemia that will respond to oxygen therapy, anemia, or cardiovascular instability that may need additional treatments alongside oxygen therapy.

Clinical pearl

Medical oxygen is regulated by the U.S. Food and Drug Administration (FDA) and must be 99% pure. It can be stored as a compressed gas in cylinders or as liquid oxygen that is converted to a gas before being delivered to a patient. Oxygen cylinders and oxygen piping systems are color-coded green in the United States; however, white is the international color for oxygen.

Low-Flow Oxygen Devices

After assessing a patient and determining that oxygen therapy is needed, the next step is to decide what device will provide the amount of oxygen needed for this patient. **Low-flow oxygen systems** provide only a portion of the total amount of gas the patient is breathing. For example, while a portion of what the patient is breathing is coming from the oxygen device, the rest must be added from room air. Common low-flow oxygen devices include the **nasal cannula, simple mask,** and **nonrebreathing mask.**

Clinical pearl

Nasal cannulas should not be run at more than 6 liters per minute, because the high flow over a small surface area will cause excessive drying of the nasal mucosa.

Nasal Cannula One of the most commonly used low-flow oxygen therapy devices is the nasal cannula. The small-bore flexible plastic tubing has two short extensions that insert into the nostrils and direct the oxygen into the nasal cavity. It is well tolerated by most patients and has advantages over a mask for comfort of eating or speaking. The major disadvantage is that, as with all low-flow oxygen devices, as patients increase the rate and/or depth of breathing in a crisis situation, they will pull in more room air but the oxygen delivered will remain fixed, so the FIO_2 will drop because of air dilution. The nasal cannula is frequently used for low FIO_2 ranges in long-term oxygen therapy for COPD patients, to treat mild hypoxemia, and in cardiac intensive care to decrease myocardial work (see Figure 12-3, which shows a nasal cannula).

FIGURE 12-3 Nasal Cannula

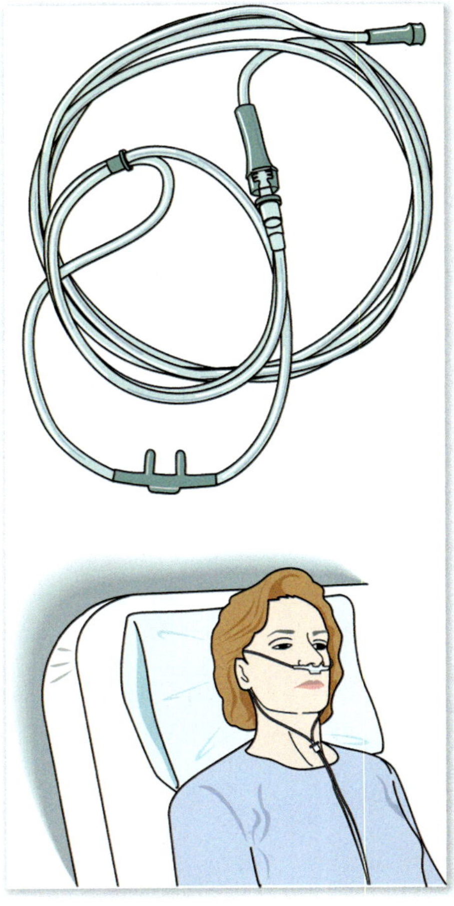

Simple Mask A simple mask is a low-flow oxygen device that fits over the patient's nose and mouth and acts as a reservoir for the next breath. The FIO_2 varies with this device because of a number of factors, including a poor sealing system, variable tidal volumes and breathing rates, and low gas flows. This mask can deliver an FIO_2 between 0.35 and 0.50, depending on the patient's ventilation rate and depth. A simple mask is generally used for emergencies and short-term therapies, which require a moderate FIO_2 (see Figure 12-4).

FIGURE 12-4 Simple Mask

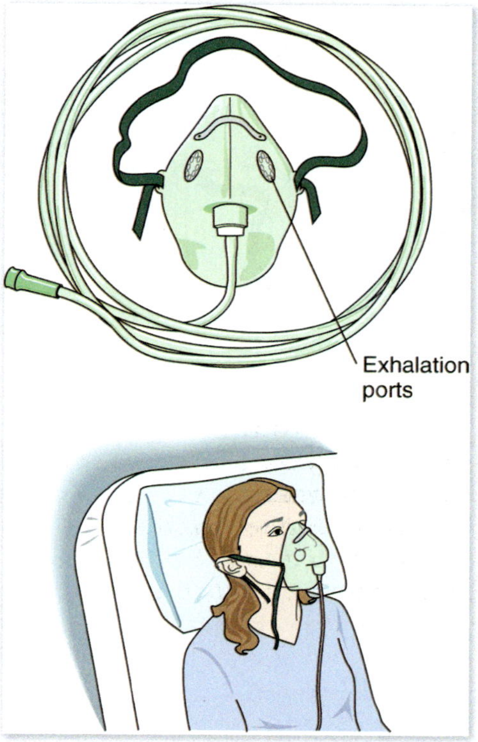

Nonrebreathing Mask A nonrebreathing mask is designed to fit over the patient's nose and mouth as the simple oxygen mask does; however a 500-ml to 1,000-ml plastic bag is added to the mask, which acts as an oxygen reservoir for the next breath. This mask has a series of one-way valves that permit the reservoir bag to fill only with pure oxygen, the exhaled gases being vented outside the mask. This reservoir of 100% oxygen and the exhalation valves on the mask force the patient to take the next breath from the reservoir bag, providing higher FIO_2, in the range of 50% to 70%.

Clinical pearl

The simple mask should be run at a minimum of 5 liters per minute to ensure that the carbon dioxide the patient exhales is washed away and not rebreathed.

Clinical pearl

The oxygen supplied to the patient, whether it comes from an oxygen cylinder or from a bulk system piped into the hospital, is dry and therefore often needs to be humidified so that it is more palatable to the sensitive, moist body tissues.

Clinical pearl

The nonrebreathing mask originally had two one-way valves for exhalation. One of the valves is usually removed in order to prevent suffocation if the flow rate is not adequate or if the patient becomes disconnected from the oxygen source.

CONTROVERSY

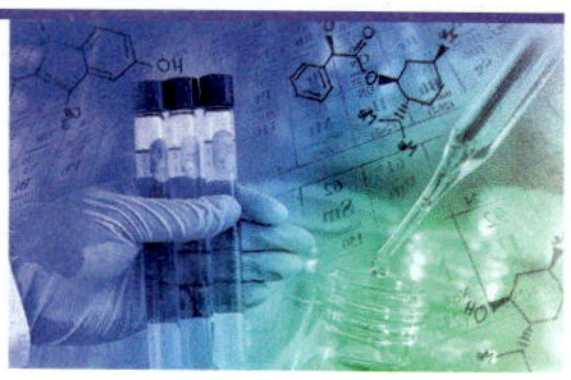

In many textbooks the range for the nonrebreathing mask is given as 70% to 100%, but studies have shown that, owing to removal of one valve for safety and difficulty obtaining a perfect seal, the percentage of oxygen delivered to the patient is lowered.

BVT Lab

Visit www.BVTLab.com to explore the student resources available for this chapter.

It is very important to note that the flow to the reservoir bag must be sufficient that the bag does not deflate more than one-third when the patient inhales. If the flow rate is too low, the patient may suffocate, especially if the mask has a tight seal; if not, the delivered FIO_2 will be decreased if the patient has to breathe around the mask and draw in room air. See Figure 12-5, which illustrates a nonrebreathing mask.

FIGURE 12-5 Nonrebreathing Mask

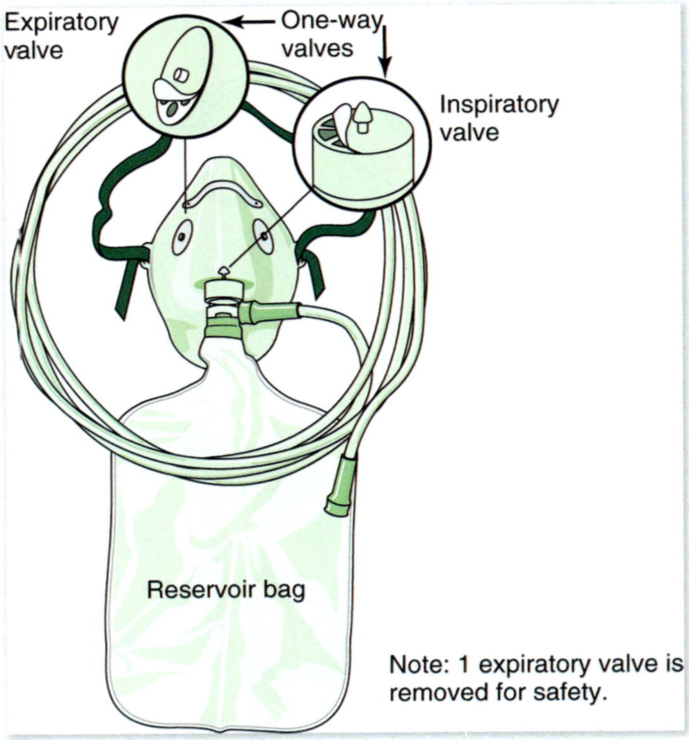

time for review

If a patient on a low-flow device, such as a 2 liters/minute nasal cannula, suddenly experiences respiratory distress and increases his rate and depth of ventilation, what happens to the FIO_2 reaching the lungs?

High-Flow Oxygen Systems

High-flow oxygen systems provide enough gas flow to meet all of the patient's ventilatory demands and thus prevent dilution of the desired FIO_2. **High-flow therapy** (HFT) delivers a precise FIO_2 that does not change with a patient's ventilation rate, breathing pattern, or depth of breathing; so high-flow systems are advantageous when close monitoring of a patient's oxygenation status is needed. **Heated humidified high-flow** (HHHF) **therapy** delivers a high flow of heated and humidified gas through a device such as a nasal cannula. Since a cannula is used, the patient can drink and speak while having a higher FIO_2 delivered, something that previously required special masks or even intubation. Research studies comparing the efficacy of high-flow oxygen with other oxygen delivery systems in acute hypoxemic respiratory failure have been sparse. Several recent studies have found comparable if not superior clinical outcomes with high-flow oxygen therapy when compared to noninvasive ventilation or standard oxygen therapy in adults. Other types of high-flow systems that meet the patient's ventilation demands include the **jet mixing mask** and **large-volume nebulizers.**

Jet Mixing Mask A jet mixing mask (also referred to as an air entrainment mask) is an example of a high-flow device that delivers a total high flow by mixing oxygen with room air. This mask uses the Bernoulli principle to take pure oxygen from a flow meter and mix it with a certain proportion of room air and then deliver oxygen concentrations ranging from 24% to 50% to the patient. Every percentage of oxygen has its own ratio of air to oxygen. The most common proportions are listed in Table 12-2.

Clinical pearl

No humidification is needed for jet mixing masks, because a large amount of room air is pulled in, and air is already humidified by the water molecules in the atmosphere.

TABLE 12-2 Common Oxygen Percentages and Air-to-Oxygen Ratios

Oxygen (%)	Approximate Air : Oxygen Ratio
24	25:1
28	10:1
30	8:1
35	5:1
40	3:1
60	1:1

Large-Volume Nebulizers A large-volume nebulizer is another example of a high-flow system and is typically used for a patient who requires a precise, nonchanging FIO_2 coupled with high moisture levels in aerosol form; for retained secretions; or for a patient whose body's natural humidification system is impaired or bypassed. This device works on the same principle as the jet mixing mask but also provides **bland aerosol therapy** (nonmedicated). The large-volume nebulizer can be connected to a variety of devices, including an aerosol mask, a face tent for patients with facial burns or who cannot tolerate a mask, a T-piece or Briggs adapter for intubated patients, or a tracheostomy mask (collar) for patients with a tracheostomy (see Figure 12-6).

Clinical pearl

Nebulizers produce aerosol particles in sizes that can transmit bacteria into the lungs and thus present an opportunity for health-care-associated infections. Proper maintenance and sterile technique are required with aerosol therapy.

FIGURE 12-6 Bland Aerosol Delivery Devices

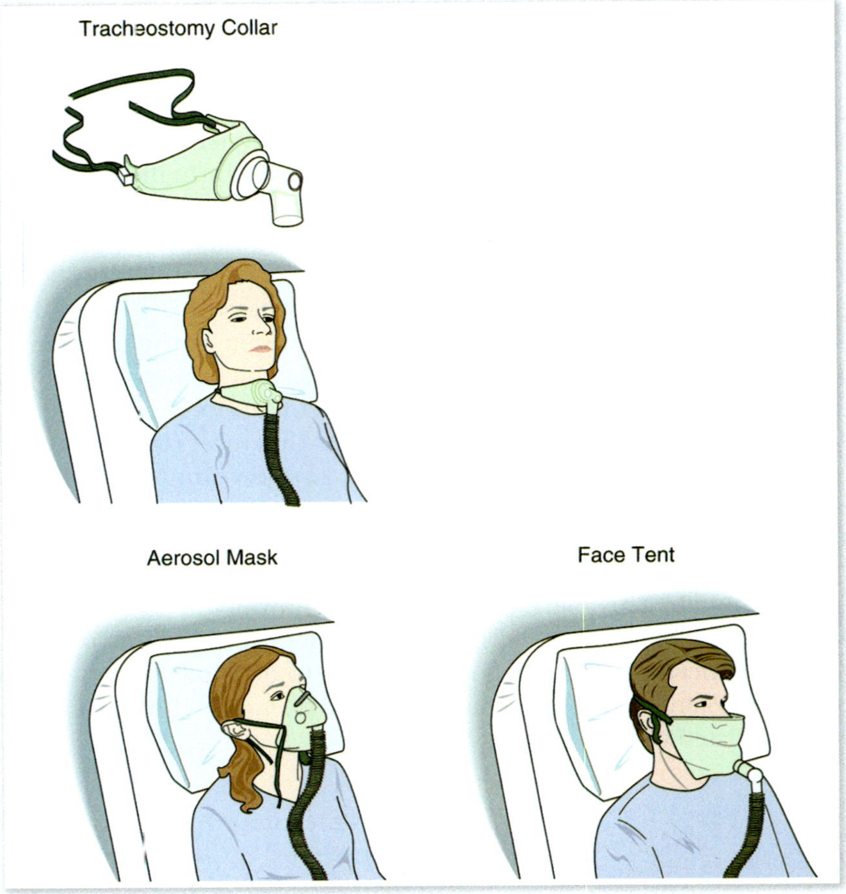

Clinical pearl

Placing patients in certain positions will often help their oxygenation status. For example patients with pulmonary edema and otherwise normal heart function will often be less hypoxemic in Fowler's position (sitting at a 45° angle). Patients with chronic lung disease will also do better sitting up, because it allows better movement of the diaphragm, especially on expiration, when gravity assists it in falling. In addition leaning forward will help patients better utilize their accessory muscles of ventilation.

12.1g Monitoring Oxygen Therapy

Patients on oxygen therapy should be monitored for all of the following:

- *Sensorium*. The patient should think more clearly and become less restless and agitated because more oxygen is being delivered to the brain.
- *Dyspnea*. Shortness of breath should improve, and the patient's accessory muscle use should decrease.
- *Color*. Cyanosis may improve and should be monitored via the skin and nail beds.
- *Vital signs*. Vital signs should return toward normal.
- *PaO_2 value*. The PaO_2 obtained from an ABG should rise toward acceptable limits for that particular patient.
- *Pulse oximetry*. The amount of hemoglobin saturated with oxygen (SaO_2) should show improved values with the proper use of oxygen therapy. A value of 95% to 98% is considered normal, but most physicians will accept a reading of 90% to 92%. See Figure 12-7, which shows a pulse oximeter. Be careful, as patients with dysfunctional hemoglobin can give erroneous readings.

FIGURE 12-7 A Pulse Oximeter

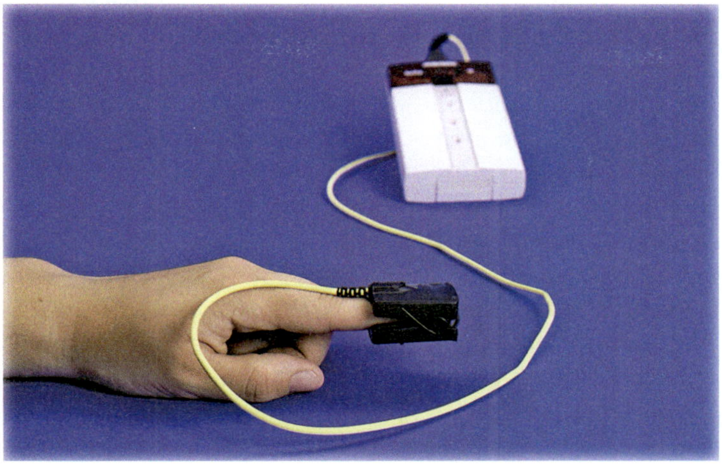

time for review

Name four positive clinical signs that show oxygen therapy is being effective.

12.1h Hazards of Oxygen Therapy

Oxygen is considered a drug, and if proper delivery of this drug is not monitored, some problems could occur that might be harmful. Some of the hazards of oxygen therapy include the following.

- ***Oxygen toxicity*** is a serious condition that may occur if too much oxygen is delivered for too long, and it can potentially lead to death. If a normal person breathes 100% oxygen for longer than 12 to 24 hours, he or she will show early signs of oxygen toxicity, which include a sore throat, dyspnea, cough, and substernal discomfort. If oxygen is continued, then nausea, vomiting, diffuse infiltrates, atelectasis, and eventually ARDS may develop. This is because too much oxygen in this person's system causes the formation of **free radicals** or oxidants, which are charged particles that disrupt tissue formation. However certain mechanically ventilated patients—with severe ARDS, for example—may require 100% oxygen with increased levels of pressure for days just to maintain a reasonable oxygen saturation.
- *Oxygen-induced hypercapnea* may occur in patients who suffer from COPD. These patients may have chronic retention of carbon dioxide ($PaCO_2$), which depresses the respiratory centers in the brain that usually control the stimulus to breathe. When these centers are depressed, the patient's stimulus to breathe is controlled by the **peripheral chemoreceptors**, which respond to arterial $PaCO_2$ and oxygen tension (PaO_2) of less than 60 mmHg. Traditional teaching suggests that this **hypoxic drive** mechanism is solely responsible for the rise

in carbon dioxide when oxygen is administered to patients with chronic hypercapnea. It turns out that two other mechanisms are more important: (1) worsened V/Q mismatch due to reversal of hypoxemic pulmonary vasoconstriction and (2) decreased affinity of hemoglobin for CO_2. A general guideline when applying oxygen therapy to a COPD patient who has *chronic* hypoxemia is to maintain the PaO_2 in the 60 to 70 mmHg range corresponding to an SaO_2 of 88% to 93%, since the patient is more at risk from tissue hypoxia than from hypercapnea.

Clinical pearl

Normal arterial $PaCO_2$ ranges between 35 and 45 mmHg. Higher-than-normal levels of $PaCO_2$ decrease the pH, resulting in an acidotic condition. For example insufficient alveolar ventilation limits the amount of CO_2 exhaled and thus allows levels in the bloodstream to rise, resulting in respiratory acidosis. Conversely alveolar hyperventilation causes the $PaCO_2$ levels to fall below 35 mmHg and produces respiratory alkalosis.

- *Retinopathy of prematurity (ROP),* formerly called *retrolental fibroplasia,* is caused by both prematurity and high PaO_2 levels in premature infants, which causes vasospasm to occur in the retinal area, leading to the formation of fibrous scar tissue behind the lens of the eye (retrolental fibroplasia), causing vision impairment or blindness.
- **Absorptive atelectasis** can occur when high concentrations of oxygen wash out the inert nitrogen in the lungs. With subsequent absorption of oxygen into the circulatory system, the lower pressures in the airways become subatmospheric and lead to atelectasis.
- Environmental hazards can occur because oxygen promotes combustion, causing a fire to burn hotter and faster. This is why oxygen is used in welding to increase the temperature. Therefore, if a facility is not a smoke-free environment, a "No Smoking—Oxygen in Use" sign must be posted, and the danger of fire must also be emphasized in the home care setting. Because of the extensive use of oxygen in the hospital, all health-care personnel should know where all oxygen shut-off valves and fire extinguishers are located as well as how to use them.

Clinical pearl

If the patient has carbon monoxide (CO) poisoning, you can accept higher-than-normal PaO_2 and SaO_2 levels. CO has 210 to 250 times more affinity for hemoglobin than oxygen, and this means the hemoglobin will first want to load up all the seats on the bus with CO so oxygen can't get on board—even if there is a large amount waiting outside the bus (i.e., high PaO_2).

Although these hazards may be present, oxygen therapy should not be withheld from patients in critical need. For example patients may require 100% oxygen to survive a cardiopulmonary arrest or carbon monoxide poisoning, and the resulting possible hazards are less ominous than the resulting death if high levels of oxygen are withheld.

In summary the oxygen amount in the blood tension (PaO_2) and the length of exposure determine if a toxic response is likely. Generally speaking an FIO_2 of less than 50% should not result in a meaningful amount of toxic response in adults. The best advice when administering oxygen therapy is to follow this general rule: Administer oxygen at the lowest possible FIO_2 to get the desired PaO_2 or SaO_2.

Patient & Family Education

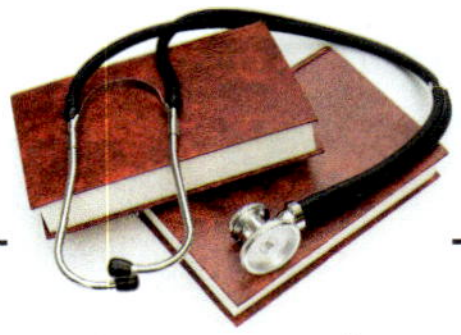

Oxygen should never be used while smoking. Fires causing severe burns or death have been reported in patients attempting to smoke while on oxygen. Of course family members should also be instructed not to smoke near oxygen-dependent patients.

12.2 HELIUM THERAPY

Helium (He) is an odorless and tasteless gas that is very light and low in density. This is why helium balloons float so well and why inhaled helium allows the vocal cords to vibrate much more easily, giving a high-pitched, cartoonish sound to the voice. Helium is also physiologically inert and poorly soluble in water and therefore does not react within the body.

Clinical pearl

Helium is an excellent heat conductor and can be used during laser airway surgery to absorb the heat from the laser beam, thereby lessening the surrounding tissue damage in the airway. Breathing helium/oxygen diving mixtures minimizes the risk of oxygen toxicity and decompression sickness (the bends). Helium is also used in certain pulmonary function tests.

12.2a Indications for Helium Therapy

Helium does not support life, and the practice of inhaling helium to cause vocal distortion is dangerous. Helium must be mixed with oxygen to form a **heliox** mixture. This mixture has been demonstrated to be effective in treating patients with upper-airway obstructions. The airway obstruction enhances the rough turbulent flow already present in the larger airways. The low-density helium/oxygen mixture favors a smoother, more laminar flow through the airways, thus reducing the airway resistance and work of breathing and allowing more flow beyond the obstruction. Helium/oxygen mixtures are less useful in lower-airway obstruction, where flow is laminar and independent of gas density. Heliox may also be beneficial for asthma with impending respiratory failure, postoperative stridor, and severe COPD exacerbations. It is important to keep in mind that the clinical evidence with helium/oxygen mixtures is very limited since most of the clinical trials were conducted with fewer than 30 subjects.

12.2b Administration of Helium/Oxygen

The helium/oxygen mixture is compressed in cylinders color-coded brown (helium) and green (oxygen), with a percentage mixture of either 80% He and 20% O_2 or 70% He and 30% O_2. Helium/oxygen is administered via a well-fitting nonrebreathing mask or through patient artificial airways.

12.2c Hazard of Helium/Oxygen Therapy

Although it's not a true hazard, the patient should still be told that his or her voice will change temporarily to a higher pitch and will return to normal shortly after the therapy. It has been suggested that breathing helium/oxygen mixtures may affect the cough mechanism, because an effective cough requires turbulent flow in the larger airways to generate the explosive pressure. However this will be only a temporary diminishment of cough effectiveness; it will return within minutes after the treatment, when the helium is cleared from the airways.

time for review

What is the main indication for heliox therapy?

12.3 NITRIC OXIDE THERAPY

Certain conditions and disease states can lead to increased pulmonary hypertension. This increase in pulmonary vascular resistance not only puts a strain on the heart but can also cause damage and leakage of the pulmonary capillaries, which will greatly impair gas exchange capabilities. All blood vessels have a single cell layer that lines their inner lumen; this is referred to as the endothelial layer or endothelium. The capillary vessels contain only a single endothelium layer and are void of the smooth muscle and collagen layers that the veins and arteries contain. In the early 1980s it was discovered that the endothelium produces a chemical substance that is a very potent vasodilator and can reduce pulmonary vascular resistance. This chemical was originally termed endothelium-derived relaxing factor (EDRF) but was later shown to be equivalent to nitric oxide (NO).

Clinical pearl

Nitric oxide is not exclusively a vascular smooth muscle relaxant; it also relaxes bronchial smooth muscle, so it is a bronchodilator and may have potential future use.

12.3a Physiology of Nitric Oxide

Nitric oxide binds to the enzyme guanyl cyclase and increases levels and stability of cGMP, which causes vasodilation within blood vessels. However, nitric oxide is rapidly metabolized on contact with blood and reacts with hemoglobin to form methemoglobin. In essence, contact with blood destroys nitric oxide's vasodilation effects. Although this may seem like a disadvantage, it is actually advantageous in treating pulmonary hypertension. **Inhaled nitric oxide** (INO) diffuses across the alveoli and *first* comes in contact with the endothelium layer of the capillaries and pulmonary arterioles, producing vasodilation and decreasing pulmonary vascular resistance. Further diffusion of nitric oxide now causes it to enter the bloodstream and neutralizes its effect so that it does not cause systemic vasodilation. Therefore, INO is a *selective* pulmonary vasodilator.

Learning Hint

Do not confuse nitric oxide (NO)—the potent inhaled vasodilator—with nitrous oxide (N_2O), the anesthetic gas commonly referred to as laughing gas.

INO can travel only to well-ventilated alveoli, so it will improve the ventilation/perfusion ratio and thus oxygenation by redistributing capillary blood to well-ventilated lung units, causing enhanced gas exchange. In addition the decreased pulmonary vascular resistance reduces the stress on the right heart, which is pumping into the pulmonary vascular bed. Table 12-3 summarizes the beneficial effects of INO.

TABLE 12-3 Beneficial Effects of INO

Lowers pulmonary hypertension
Reduces pulmonary vascular resistance with no change in systemic vascular resistance
Enhances right-heart function
Improves arterial oxygenation by enhancing ventilation/perfusion ratio

12.3b INO Administration and Dosage

Nitric oxide combined with oxygen is rapidly oxidized into toxic substances; therefore it is combined with inert nitrogen in compressed-gas cylinders. It is generally provided through the inspiratory line of the ventilator, and continuous monitoring for NO and nitrogen dioxide (NO_2) levels should be performed. Many studies have demonstrated that inhaled nitric oxide seems to be relatively effective and safe at doses between 20 and 80 parts per million (ppm), although a specific dosage has not been approved by the FDA.

12.3c Therapeutic Indications for Inhalation of Nitric Oxide

INO has been shown to be effective in treating patients with increased pulmonary vascular resistance secondary to severe pulmonary hypertension. Inhalation of nitric oxide has proven beneficial for the following conditions:

- Acute respiratory distress syndrome (ARDS)
- Infant respiratory distress syndrome (IRDS)
- Persistent pulmonary hypertension of the neonate (PPHN)
- Other conditions that cause pulmonary hypertension

12.3d Monitoring Nitric Oxide Therapy

Although studies have suggested that short-term, low-dose inhalation of nitric oxide is a relatively safe procedure, continuous monitoring of the NO should be maintained to ensure that it remains within the prescribed dose. In addition the toxic metabolites of nitric oxide, when combined with oxygen (NO_2, NO_3), along with methemoglobin levels, should be monitored. Premature infants may be more prone to higher methemoglobin levels than adults during nitric oxide therapy.

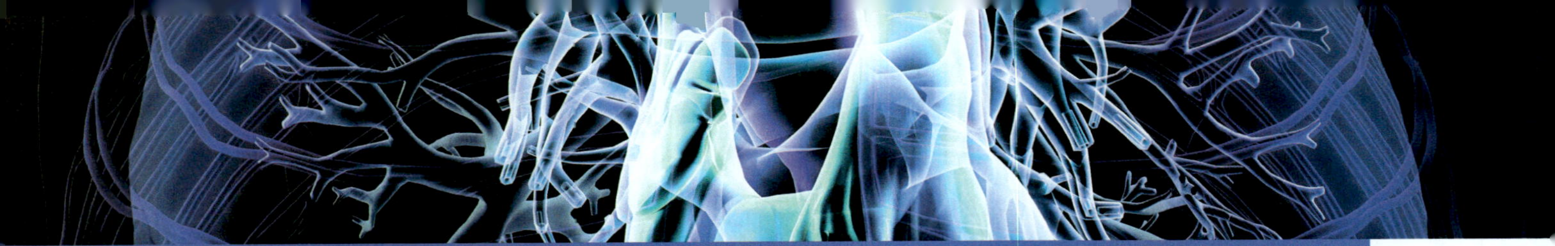

Summary

Medical gases are indicated for a variety of clinical conditions. Oxygen therapy is one of the most frequently prescribed drugs in medicine and is delivered via a host of devices. The major goals of oxygen therapy include treating hypoxemia, decreasing the work of breathing, and decreasing myocardial work.

In addition to oxygen therapy, other medical gases are used, including helium and nitric oxide therapy. Low-density helium is mixed with oxygen primarily to treat airway obstruction. Inhaled nitric oxide is used to lower pulmonary hypertension, which also serves to enhance right-heart function.

REVIEW QUESTIONS

1. Hypoxemia is
   (a) low levels of tissue oxygen
   (b) low levels of arterial oxygen
   (c) low levels of hemoglobin
   (d) low levels of red blood cells

2. Which of the following are clinical manifestations of hypoxemia?
   I. tachycardia
   II. cerebral vasodilation
   III. tachypnea
   IV. pulmonary hypotension

   (a) all
   (b) I and III
   (c) I, II, and III
   (d) II and IV

3. Which of the following medical gases need(s) to be mixed with oxygen before delivering to a patient?
   (a) nitric oxide
   (b) argon
   (c) helium
   (d) (a) and (c)

4. Inhaled nitric oxide (INO) will
   (a) increase pulmonary hypertension
   (b) increase systemic vascular resistance
   (c) decrease pulmonary hypertension
   (d) decrease arterial oxygenation

5. Classify the following PaO_2s:
   100 mmHg ____
   55 mmHg ____
   39 mmHg ____
   45 mmHg ____
   125 mmHg ____
6. Classify the type of hypoxia:
   Low hemoglobin levels ____
   CNS drug overdose ____
   Severe hypotension ____
   Fever ____
7. List and explain the three major goals of oxygen therapy.
8. Explain how a patient can have hypoxemia but not hypoxia.
9. Contrast low-flow and high-flow oxygen delivery devices.
10. Give three positive clinical responses expected with effective oxygen therapy.
11. List the indication for heliox therapy and what properties of helium make it useful for this purpose.

CASE STUDY 1

A 68-year-old woman

A 68-year-old woman with heart failure has a PaO_2 of 41 mmHg. Pharmacologic treatment of the heart failure is begun. She has tachycardia and tachypnea and is showing signs of acrocyanosis. What oxygen therapy recommendations would you make at this time?

How would you monitor the treatment's effectiveness?

What would be your response to an order that read, "Simple oxygen mask at 2 liters per minute"?

PART 3

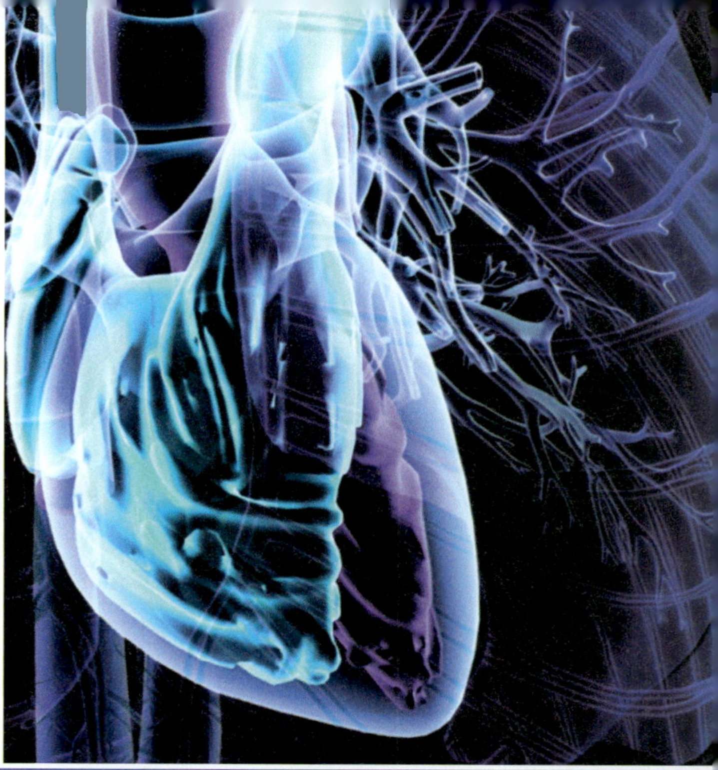

Putting It All Together

Chapter 13

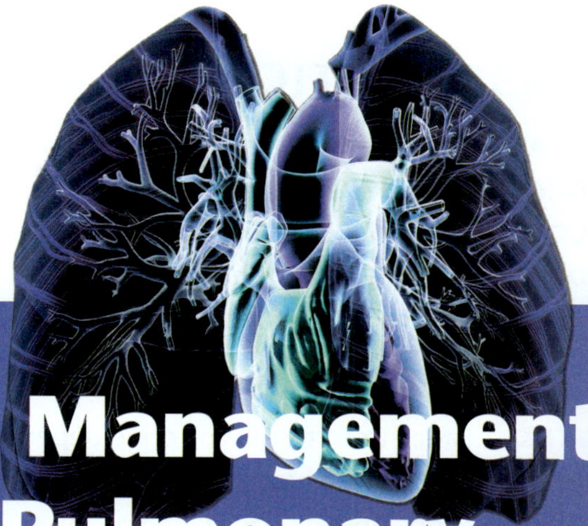

Pharmacologic Management of Obstructive Pulmonary Disease: Asthma, Chronic Bronchitis, and Emphysema

OBJECTIVES

Upon completion of this chapter you will be able to

- Explain the pathophysiology of asthma and chronic obstructive pulmonary disease (COPD).
- Contrast asthma and COPD.
- Distinguish among the various forms of COPD.
- Recognize the importance of treatment guidelines in the management of asthma and COPD.
- Develop a pharmacologic regimen for asthma, chronic bronchitis, or emphysema.
- Develop a monitoring and educational plan for asthma, chronic bronchitis, or emphysema.

KEY TERMS

asthma
asthma COPD overlap syndrome
chronic bronchitis
chronic obstructive pulmonary disease
dyspnea
emphysema
long-term control
quick-relief medication

ABBREVIATIONS

α_1-AT alpha$_1$-antitrypsin
ACOS asthma COPD overlap syndrome
COPD chronic obstructive pulmonary disease
DPI dry-powder inhaler
FEV$_1$/FVC forced expiratory volume in 1 second divided by the total forced vital capacity; known as FEV$_1$/FVC ratio
FTND Fagerstrom test for nicotine dependence
GERD gastroesophageal reflux disease
GINA Global Initiative for Asthma
GOLD Global Initiative for Chronic Obstructive Lung Disease
ICS inhaled corticosteroid
IgE immunoglobulin E
LABA long-acting β_2-agonist
LAMA long-acting muscarinic antagonist
MDI metered-dose inhaler
mMRC Modified Medical Research Council
NAEPP EPR-3 National Asthma Education and Prevention Program, Third Expert Panel Report
NHLBI National Heart, Lung, and Blood Institute
NRT nicotine replacement therapy
$PaCO_2$ arterial partial pressure of carbon dioxide
PaO_2 arterial partial pressure of oxygen
PDE-4 phosphodiesterase-4
PEFR peak expiratory flow rate
RSV respiratory syncytial virus
SABA short-acting β_2-agonist
SAMA short-acting muscarinic antagonist

Obstructive pulmonary disease is a global term used to describe abnormal pulmonary conditions associated with cough, sputum production, dyspnea, airflow obstruction, and impaired gas exchange. It is the fourth leading cause of death in the United States. Specific **chronic obstructive pulmonary disease** (COPD) conditions such as **emphysema** and **chronic bronchitis** are delineated on the basis of clinical, anatomic, or physiologic criteria and can coexist, making diagnosis very difficult. COPD is not fully reversible and is progressive, whereas asthma is an obstructive disease with reversibility and therefore is not considered COPD. See Table 13-1, which gives definitions for the various obstructive pulmonary disease states.

These overlapping disease states can sometimes lead to a state of confusion in diagnosis because of their many common features and the fact that patients may have more than one disease state. In fact the latest Global Initiative for Chronic Obstructive Lung Disease (GOLD-2015) has identified an **asthma COPD overlap syndrome** (ACOS) that has combined features of both asthma and COPD in some patients. In addition drug therapies for each condition overlap; this can also be confusing in terms of developing a therapeutic plan for an individual patient. Therefore it is very important to start this discussion with an understanding of how these disease entities are defined and how they can be differentiated. Patients with asthma, chronic bronchitis, or emphysema all share features of airway obstruction, and their treatment modalities will have similar goals. **Asthma** is distinguished by having reversible airway narrowing and airway hyperreactivity; it is most commonly characterized as an inflammatory process. Patients with emphysema or chronic bronchitis, on the other hand, *may* have airway hyperreactivity. Inflammation plays some role in the development of COPD, but it has a different underlying cause and responds differently to medications than the inflammation of asthma.

TABLE 13-1 Definitions of Obstructive Pulmonary Disease States

Disease	Description
Chronic Asthma	A chronic inflammatory disorder of the airways in which many cells and cellular elements play a role, in particular mast cells, eosinophils, T lymphocytes, neutrophils, and epithelial cells. In susceptible individuals, this inflammation causes recurrent episodes of wheezing, breathlessness, chest tightness, and cough, particularly at night and in the early morning. These episodes are usually associated with widespread but variable airflow obstruction that is often reversible either spontaneously or with treatment. The inflammation also causes an associated increase in the existing bronchial hyperresponsiveness to a variety of stimuli.
Chronic Bronchitis	Usually defined in clinical terms as the presence of productive cough during 3 months of the year for 2 consecutive years, provided that other causes of chronic sputum production such as tuberculosis and bronchiectasis are excluded. Airway hyperreactivity may be present, but airflow limitation is not fully reversible.
Emphysema	A pathologic diagnosis marked by destruction of alveolar walls, with resultant loss of elastic recoil in the lung. Dyspnea on exertion is the predominant clinical feature, and airway hyperreactivity may also be present.

Emphysema is characterized anatomically as the permanent, abnormal enlargement of distal airway spaces and destruction of the alveolar wall. Chronic bronchitis is associated with a productive cough, enlargement of mucous glands, and hypertrophy of the airway smooth muscle. Although asthma, emphysema, and chronic bronchitis can all be termed "chronic obstructive pulmonary disease," asthma is distinguished from the other two by the presence of inflammation with the participation of complex cellular and chemical mediators, as described in Chapter 7. Asthma is generally characterized by reversibility of bronchospasm, and COPD by its *limited* reversibility. For the purposes of our discussion, we will generally refer to chronic bronchitis and emphysema as COPD and discuss asthma as a separate disease entity.

13.1 ASTHMA

13.1a Background

Asthma is a chronic inflammatory illness of the airways that affects nearly 25.7 million people in the United States, including 7 million children. Asthma is the most common chronic disease in children and younger adults, with about 80% of cases developing before the age of 45. In addition to direct dollar costs of patient care, asthma results in 14.7 million missed school days and 11.8 million days of missed work per year. Furthermore there are approximately 5,000 deaths due to asthma annually, the majority of which are preventable. These factors, plus its ongoing rise in incidence, make the understanding of asthma treatment and prevention a high priority. Because of the magnitude of this problem, interest in asthma management increased dramatically in the late 1980s. This interest led to the development of programs to increase asthma awareness and treatment guidelines to improve patient management. Two major sources of guidelines are the National Heart, Lung, and Blood Institute (NHLBI) branch of the National Institutes of Health (NIH) and the World Health Organization (WHO). Guidelines from the NHLBI were developed as part of the National Asthma Education and Prevention Program (NAEPP) and

Learning Hint

A key point to keep in mind is that asthma is a disease of inflammation and reversibility.

will be referred to frequently throughout the asthma section of this chapter. Guidelines from Global Initiative for Asthma (GINA) were prepared through a collaboration between the NHLBI and the WHO.

13.1b Differential Diagnosis

Wheezing is the most prominent clinical feature of asthma, especially in the early morning and after exposure to cold air or exercise. As already mentioned, COPD patients (bronchitis and emphysema) can present with many of the same symptoms, as can patients with chronic cough, hyperventilation syndromes, heart failure, pulmonary embolism, gastroesophageal reflux disease, allergies, Sjögren syndrome, and others. Asthma medication is effective for some of these diseases, but not all. Therefore it is important to have the correct diagnosis for effective pharmacotherapy. If you are uncertain that your patient has been evaluated fully for these other diseases, or if your patient's response to appropriate asthma medication is not optimal, refer him or her back to his or her physician for further evaluation and workup.

Clinical pearl

An increase in forced expiratory volume in 1 second (FEV_1) of ≥12% or ≥200 ml after a bronchodilator (demonstrating that obstruction is reversible), diurnal variation in peak expiratory flow rate (PEFR) ≥20%, and a positive methacholine test are the primary diagnostic criteria for asthma.

Table 13-2 lists the differential diagnostic markers for COPD and asthma. No one marker is conclusive, so the entire clinical picture must be assessed for correct diagnosis and treatment. Because asthma is an inflammatory disorder, patients should be assessed for markers of inflammation such as episodic attacks related to irritant or allergen exposure, variable peak expiratory flow rate (PEFR), eosinophilia, and improvement on corticosteroids.

TABLE 13-2 Diagnostic Markers to Differentiate COPD and Asthma

Diagnostic Markers	COPD	Asthma
Age	Patient age typically over 40	Asthma typically presents at an early age
Smoking history	Smokers and ex-smokers	No direct correlation between smoking and asthma
Dyspnea	Shortness of breath, especially on exertion	Episodic attacks, especially on exposure to allergen/irritant/exercise
Cough	Productive cough, typically in the morning	Cough, typically in the evening
Triggers (allergens, exercise, temperature, humidity, etc.)	None usually identified for attacks	Exposure leads to attacks; allergic rhinitis and/or eczema may be present
Spirometry	FEV_1/FVC ratio ≤70%	FEV_1/FVC ratio low during attacks only
Daily variation in peak expiratory flow rate (PEFR)	Little	Morning dip and day-to-day variability
Effect of corticosteroid trial	Inconclusive (<20% of patients are successful)	Improvement
Eosinophilia	No	Maybe
Chest X-ray	Hyperinflation	Hyperinflation during attacks

time for review

Explain this clinical statement: "All that wheezes is not asthma."

13.1c Asthma Symptoms

The most common symptoms of asthma include episodic wheezing, shortness of breath, cough, and chest tightness. These symptoms are often worse at nighttime or in the early morning, because of diurnal variations in muscle tone of the airways. The degree of wheezing is used as a major criterion for judging the severity of an asthmatic episode, although in severe attacks, wheezing may diminish or be absent due to decreased airflow. Cough, although it is a common asthmatic symptom, is also the third most common presenting symptom in the ambulatory care setting. When a patient presents with cough, a thorough history, identification of triggers, and pulmonary function testing will make the diagnosis of asthma more clear.

The patient's history can be very helpful, as many asthmatic patients have a family history of allergies such as asthma, eczema, or hay fever. Usually the patient or the patient's parents can identify exposures or circumstances that trigger the patient's symptoms. Asthma is a chronic disease, even though certain disease triggers may wax and wane, leading to episodic attacks. Therefore patients and their caregivers need to understand the chronic nature of asthma and the underlying inflammatory process. It is important that patients be able to identify and control their exposure to environmental allergens or other types of triggers. Persons with asthma develop bronchospasm upon exposure to specific sensitizing substances usually described as "triggers." Common triggers include allergens, inhalants, viruses, cold air, and exercise. Although it may seem strange to have this discussion on preventive measures in a pharmacology text, the authors believe that *preventing the use of medications* is in fact an important pharmacologic intervention and mindset. See Table 13-3, which lists triggers for asthmatic attacks.

Allergies

Seasonal, indoor, and outdoor allergen exposure can lead to asthma symptoms. One of the most common allergens is the domestic dust mite, which is found throughout our households and businesses. It is difficult to limit exposure to this allergen, but the World Health Organization recommends frequent washing of bed linens and blankets in hot water, encasing pillows and mattresses in airtight covers, and removing carpets, especially in bedrooms. The use of vinyl, leather, or plain wooden furniture is encouraged over fabric-upholstered furniture. Allergies to animals should be identified and, if found, animals should be removed from the home or at least from the sleeping area. Cockroach allergen is another very common triggering substance for asthma. Houses and work areas should be cleaned thoroughly and often. An appropriate pesticide should be used regularly, but not while the patient is nearby. Many patients also experience triggers from outdoor pollens and both outdoor and indoor molds. To avoid exposure to the outdoor triggers, patients may need to remain inside, with windows and

BVT Lab

Flashcards are available for this chapter at www.BVTLab.com.

TABLE 13-3 Triggers for Asthmatic Attacks

Allergens
Animal dander (pets with fur or feathers)
Pollen (grass, trees, weeds)
House dust mites (in mattresses, pillows, upholstered furniture, carpets)
Mold
Cockroaches
Inhaled irritants
Tobacco smoke
Wood smoke
Sulfur dioxide
Air pollution
Strong odors or sprays (perfumes, paint fumes, pesticides, hair sprays, cleaning agents)
Occupational inhalants
Viral respiratory infections (rhinovirus, influenza, parainfluenza, corona virus, respiratory syncytial virus [RSV])
Cold air
Exercise
Strong emotions
Menses
Drugs
Aspirin
NSAIDs
β-Adrenergic blockers (oral or ophthalmic)
Preservatives (sulfites and benzalkonium chloride)
Methacholine (used to provoke bronchoconstriction during diagnostic testing)
Histamine (alternative agent to provoke bronchoconstriction during testing)
Other factors that can aggravate asthma
Allergic rhinitis
Rhinosinusitis
Gastroesophageal reflux disease (GERD)

doors closed, when pollen and mold counts are highest. To avoid exposure to indoor molds, dampness in the home should be reduced, and damp areas should be cleaned and disinfected regularly. Air conditioning will help to reduce both types of exposure. Patients may also want to consider specific immunotherapy ("allergy shots") if exposure cannot be controlled.

Exercise

Most asthmatic patients experience a decrease in airflow with exercise, commonly referred to as "exercise-induced asthma." In fact some patients only have asthma attacks when they exercise. It is not necessary for patients with exercise-induced asthma to avoid exercise. Rather symptoms can be prevented through the use of a short- or long-acting bronchodilator inhaled immediately before exercising.

Gastroesophageal Reflux

Gastroesophageal reflux disease (GERD) has long been recognized in association with wheezing and asthma symptoms. The reflux of acidic stomach contents into the esophagus is thought to initiate a reflex bronchoconstriction. This condition can also be controlled with medication.

Infections

Viral infections of the upper respiratory tract are a common cause of asthma attacks in both adults and children. This may occur because of damage to the respiratory epithelium and inflammation that increase airway hyperreactivity. It isn't very easy to avoid respiratory viral infections, but asthmatics should be aware of good hand-washing techniques and other ways to reduce viral transmission. If patients develop an upper respiratory tract infection or a sinus infection, they should closely monitor their peak flow rates and begin appropriate bronchodilator and/or anti-inflammatory therapy as soon as indicated. Recommendations vary, but the Centers for Disease Control and Prevention (CDC) recommends that children and adults with asthma be vaccinated for influenza yearly.

Irritants

Inhalation of irritants can trigger bronchospasm. Irritants are likely to stimulate receptors along the respiratory tract and include things like perfumes, detergents, smoke, strong smells, dust, and air pollution. The general mechanisms are not known, but it is presumed that these irritants cause epithelial damage and inflammation in the airway mucosa. If patients identify any of these substances as triggers, they should try to minimize their exposure to them, or when exposure is unavoidable, they should begin treatment with appropriate bronchodilator therapy. Tobacco smoke is a particularly common irritant and should be avoided. Neither patients nor family members should smoke. If there are family members who do smoke, they should restrict smoking to areas outside the house.

Clinical pearl

Emotion and stress can also be precipitating factors for asthma in some patients.

time for review

What type of assessment would you perform for indoor air pollution in a home or office?

13.1d Asthma Treatment Goals

Several broad goal categories for the management of asthma have been established along with ways to determine if the goals are met. According to the NAEPP Third Expert Panel Report (EPR-3), the goals are

1. Reduce impairment
   a. Prevent troublesome and chronic symptoms
   b. Infrequent use of a short-acting β-agonist (SABA) ($\leq$2 days/week)

   c. Maintain near-normal pulmonary function
   d. Maintain normal activity levels
   e. Meet patients' and families' expectations of satisfaction with asthma care
2. Reduce risk
   a. Prevent exacerbations and the need for emergency department visits and/or hospitalizations
   b. Prevent progressive loss of lung function; for children, prevent reduced growth
   c. Provide optimal pharmacotherapy with minimal or no adverse effects

Achieving control of asthma requires selecting appropriate medications, stopping asthma attacks, identifying and avoiding triggers that make asthma worse, educating patients to manage their condition, and monitoring and modifying asthma care for effective long-term control. Drug therapy must be selected carefully, monitored closely, and optimized for the individual patient. This requires extensive patient education and close cooperation among all health-care providers.

13.1e Classification of Asthma Severity

Patients with asthma are usually classified into one of four levels of severity, which is used as the basis for determining pharmacologic interventions. The NAEPP EPR-3 broadly classifies asthma as either intermittent (symptoms no more than two times per week) or persistent (symptoms occurring more frequently). Persistent asthma is further subdivided into mild, moderate, or severe, based on frequency of symptoms, episodes of nocturnal asthma, and PEFR. See Table 13-4 for the levels of asthma severity.

TABLE 13-4 Levels of Asthma Severity

Level	Frequency of Symptoms	Nocturnal Asthma Attacks	PEF/FEV_1
Intermittent	≤2 times/week PEF normal between attacks	≤2 times/month	≥80% of best PEF/FEV_1 variability <20%
Mild persistent	3–6 days/week Attacks may affect activity	3–4 times/month	≥80% of best PEF/FEV_1 variability <20%–30%
Moderate persistent	Daily Attacks affect activity	>1 time/week	>60 but <80% of best PEF/FEV_1 variability >30%
Severe persistent	Continual Limits physical activity	Frequent	≤60% of best PEF/FEV_1 variability >30%

Source: Modified from GINA and NAEPP EPR-3

Patients with *intermittent* asthma can generally control their asthma with medications on an as-needed basis but need to understand how to avoid allergic triggers for their disease. Patients with *mild persistent* asthma have symptoms more often than twice a week but not as often as daily. Patients in both of these asthma categories (intermittent/mild persistent) have normal pulmonary function between episodes. Patients with *moderate persistent* asthma have daily symptoms, with exacerbations (flare-ups) of the disease affecting daily activity. In addition nighttime asthma symptoms are more frequent. In moderate asthma, pulmonary function does not always return to normal on its own.

Patients in all categories of persistent asthma should be on anti-inflammatory medication to prevent their symptoms from occurring. Asthma is considered *severe* if symptoms are continuous, with frequent exacerbations and more nighttime symptoms. In severe asthma, the patient's pulmonary activity is persistently abnormal, and the patient needs fairly regular use of inhaled bronchodilators. Patients in this category may have life-threatening episodes of bronchoconstriction and usually require therapy with oral corticosteroids at doses of up to 60 to 80 mg/day of prednisone. Additional therapy needs may include a mast cell stabilizer such as cromolyn, a leukotriene-modifying agent, or a methylxanthine derivative. In patients who have positive allergy skin tests or serum IgE levels within a certain range, and who are inadequately controlled on inhaled long-acting β-agonists (LABAs) and high-dose inhaled glucocorticoids, the addition of omalizumab may be considered.

13.1f Asthma Medications

The NAEPP EPR-3 groups asthma medications into two general categories: (1) agents for **long-term control**, used to prevent symptoms and achieve and maintain control of persistent asthma; and (2) **quick-relief medications**, used to provide rapid relief in treating asthma symptoms and exacerbations. Quick-relief medications include short-acting β_2-agonists (SABAs) and short-acting inhaled anticholinergics, also known as short-acting muscarinic antagonists (SAMAs). The β_2-agonists are preferred for most patients, while an inhaled anticholinergic can be added to a β_2-agonist for increased effect during an acute attack. See Table 13-5, which lists quick-relief asthma medications.

Because asthma is primarily an inflammatory disease, the most effective agents for long-term control are those with anti-inflammatory properties, particularly corticosteroids. For long-term use, inhaled corticosteroids (ICS) are preferred over oral corticosteroids because of their lower risk for side effects. There are other agents with anti-inflammatory effects, such as mast cell stabilizers—which inhibit mediator release (cromolyn and nedocromil)—and the leukotriene modifiers (zileuton, zafirlukast, and montelukast), but these agents are less effective than inhaled corticosteroids. Long-acting β_2-agonists can also be used as long-term preventive medications and are especially useful when added to an inhaled corticosteroid. Finally methylxanthines are classified as long-term-control medications, but they are rarely used because of their side effects and lesser effectiveness. Long-term-control agents help prevent acute exacerbations with regular use and are also thought to be helpful in minimizing the need for oral corticosteroid therapy. See Table 13-6, which compares long-term asthma control medications.

Clinical pearl

Remember that inhaled corticosteroids should always be administered with a handheld spacer. Use of spacers reduces the risk of oropharyngeal candidiasis (i.e., thrush), which often develops when the aerosol particles are deposited in the mouth. Also remember to rinse your mouth.

TABLE 13-5 Quick-Relief Asthma Medications

Medication	Generic Name	Mechanism of Action	Side Effects (risk for serious adverse effects)	Long-Term Effect	Quick-Relief Effect
Short-acting β_2-agonists (SABAs)	albuterol	Bronchodilator	Inhaled β_2-agonists have fewer, and less significant, side effects than tablets or syrups.	+/–	+ + +
	metaproterenol pirbuterol terbutaline levalbuterol		Tablet or syrup β_2-agonists may cause cardiovascular stimulation, skeletal muscle tremor, headache, and irritability.	+/–	+ +
Anticholinergics (SAMAs)	ipratropium bromide	Bronchodilator	Minimal mouth dryness or bad taste in mouth.	0	+ +
Short-acting theophylline	aminophylline	Bronchodilator	Side effects include nausea and vomiting. At higher serum concentrations, side effects can also include: seizures, tachycardia, and arrhythmias. Monitoring of theophylline blood levels is required.	+/–	+
epinephrine/ adrenaline injection		Bronchodilator	Similar, but more significant effects than β_2-agonists. Generally not used in adults for asthma.	Not recommended for long-term treatment.	In general, not recommended for treating asthma attacks if β_2-agonists are an available treatment.

13.1g Asthma Management

In recent years much attention has been directed toward asthma management. As mentioned previously, treatment guidelines are available to aid in managing these patients. Both the NAEPP EPR-3 and GINA guidelines include recommendations for the pharmacologic treatment of asthma. It is important to note that both of these sets of guidelines are based on scientific evidence to the greatest extent possible and are updated regularly. The NAEPP EPR-3 guidelines came out in 1997, with a partial update in 2002 and 2007. GINA guidelines were published in 2002 and have been updated annually. Readers are strongly encouraged to visit the NHLBI and GINA websites for access to the complete guidelines. These guidelines provide recommendations for managing all levels of asthma in children and adults as well as for the treatment of acute attacks. Information is also available for the management of asthma during pregnancy. In addition in 2003, the NAEPP developed a related guide especially for respiratory therapists (also available on the NHLBI website). Treatment recommendations in both sets of guidelines are very similar.

Table 13-6 Long-Term Asthma Control Medications

Medication/Route Administered	Generic Name	Mechanism of Action	Side Effects (risk for serious adverse effects)
Inhaled corticosteroids (ICS)	beclomethasone budesonide ciclesonide flunisolide fluticasone triamcinolone mometasone	Anti-inflammatory agent	Inhaled corticosteroids have few known adverse effects. Use of spacers and mouth washing after inhalation help prevent oral candidiasis. Doses above 1 mg/day may be associated with skin thinning, easy bruising, and adrenal suppression.
Corticosteroids available as tablets, syrups, or parenteral formulations	prednisolone prednisone methylprednisolone hydrocortisone dexamethasone cortisone		Tablet or syrup corticosteroids used long term may lead to diabetes, osteoporosis, hypertension, cataracts, growth suppression in children, hypothalamic–pituitary–adrenal axis suppression, obesity, skin thinning, or muscle weakness.
Mast cell stabilizers for inhalation	cromolyn sodium	Anti-inflammatory agent (inhibits mediator release)	Minimal side effects. Cough may occur with inhalation.
	nedocromil	Anti-inflammatory agent (inhibits mediator release)	Minimal side effects. Cough may occur upon inhalation
Long-acting β_2-agonists (LABAs)	Inhaled salmeterol Inhaled formoterol Inhaled arformoterol Inhaled indacterol Inhaled olodaterol	Bronchodilator	Inhaled β_2-agonists have fewer, and less significant, side effects than tablets.
β_2-agonists available as sustained-release tablets	terbutaline albuterol		Tablet β_2-agonists may cause cardiovascular stimulation, anxiety, skeletal muscle tremor, headache, or hypokalemia.
Sustained-release methylxanthines	theophylline aminophylline	Bronchodilator with uncertain anti-inflammatory effect	Nausea and vomiting are most common. Serious effects occurring at higher serum concentrations include seizures, tachycardia, and arrhythmias. Theophylline blood level monitoring is required.
Leukotriene modifiers, tablets	montelukast zafirlukast zileuton	Block effects of leukotrienes that contribute to bronchospasm and inflammation	Minimal side effects with montelukast and zafirlukast. Drug interactions and possible liver toxicity with zileuton
Monoclonal antibody, for subcutaneous injection	omalizumab	Blocks IgE from activating mast cells in patients with severe allergic asthma	Injection site reactions are common, usually occurring within an hour of injection.

BVT Lab

Visit www.BVTLab.com to explore the student resources available for this chapter.

It is recommended that a stepwise approach be used in the pharmacologic management of asthma. A key to the treatment algorithm is to remember which agents are for long-term preventive care and which are quick-relief medications. Quick-relief medications are used to treat acute symptoms and exacerbations in patients with intermittent and persistent asthma. All patients should have a quick-relief medication. Long-term medications are to prevent asthma attacks, and all patients with persistent asthma should be taking one of these medications daily. Inhaled corticosteroids are the preferred agents for long-term management. They are the most effective agents we have, and they are generally well tolerated. They can be given in low, medium, or high doses based on the severity of asthma. In the past there have been concerns about using inhaled corticosteroids in children. However the most recent information shows them to be safe, and they are now recommended.

For *moderate persistent* asthma, a long-acting β_2-agonist should be added. (Note that long-acting β_2-bronchodilators such as salmeterol are recommended only as long-term medications and not for quick relief, because their onset of action is too slow.) In 2010, the FDA proposed specific labeling changes for LABAs due to the possibility of an increased risk of asthma-related deaths. These include a warning that contraindicated the use of LABAs in asthma without the use of a corticosteroid; advocated stopping the use of LABAs, if possible, once asthma is controlled; recommended against starting a LABA in patients whose asthma is adequately controlled on low- to medium-dose corticosteroids; and recommended the use of fixed-dose combination products to ensure LABAs are used together with corticosteroids. Products such as Symbicort® and Advair® contain both a long-acting β_2-agonist and an inhaled corticosteroid. Higher levels of therapy should be initiated to achieve control in persistent asthma, and once control is achieved, therapy should be stepped down to the lowest level needed to control symptoms.

Remember that quick-relief medications can also be used to prevent symptoms. For example a patient with exercise- or cold-induced asthma should use a quick-relief medication 15 to 30 minutes before a triggering event. Patients should track and report their use of inhaled β_2-agonists, as this may indicate the need for additional long-term medications or may signal an acute exacerbation. See Figure 13-1 for a summary of treatment recommendations for chronic asthma. Keep in mind that patient education, in addition to pharmacologic therapy, is a crucial component of management.

FIGURE 13-1 Stepwise Approach to Asthma Management Based on Level of Asthma Severity (for adults and children >5 years of age)

Source: Modified from NAEPP 2007 update and GINA.

Quick-relief medications

- All patients, regardless of severity, should have a short-acting inhaled β_2-agonist for as needed use.
- Intensity of treatment depends on severity of exacerbation.
- Use of short-acting inhaled β_2-agonist on a daily basis or increasing use indicates the need for additional long-term control therapy.

Level of Asthma Severity	Preferred Daily Medication for Symptom Control	Other Treatment Options (may be used in any order of preference)	Education
Step 1: Mild intermittent asthma	No daily medication needed		• Teach basic facts about asthma • Teach inhaler spacer or holding chamber technique • Discuss roles of medications • Develop self-management plan • Develop action plan for when and how to take rescue actions, especially for patients with a history of severe exacerbations • Discuss appropriate environmental control measures to avoid exposures to known allergens and irritants
Step 2: Mild persistent asthma	Low-dose inhaled corticosteroids	Mast cell stabilizer, leukotriene modifier, *or* sustained-release theophylline	*Step 1* actions plus: • Teach self-monitoring • Refer to group education if available • Review and update self-management plan
Step 3: Moderate persistent asthma	Low-dose inhaled corticosteroids *and* long-acting inhaled β_2-agonist	Medium-dose inhaled corticosteroids *or* low-dose inhaled corticosteroids *and* leukotriene modifier *or* sustained-release theophylline	*Step 1* actions plus: • Teach self-monitoring • Refer to group education if available • Review and update self-management plan
Step 4: Severe persistent asthma	Medium-dose inhaled corticosteroids *and* long-acting inhaled β_2-agonist	Medium-dose inhaled corticosteroids *and* sustained-release theophylline *or* leukotriene modifier	*Step 1* and *2* actions plus: • Individualized education and counseling
Step 5: Severe persistent asthma (uncontrolled by Step 4)	High-dose inhaled corticosteroids *and* long-acting inhaled β_2-agonist	Add anti-IgE for patients who have allergies	
Step 6: Severe persistent asthma (uncontrolled by Step 5)	High-dose inhaled corticosteroids *and* long-acting inhaled β_2-agonist *and* oral corticosteroids	Add anti-IgE for patients who have allergies	

1. *Review treatment every 3 to 6 months. If control is sustained for at least 3 months, a gradual stepwise reduction in treatment may be possible.*
2. *If control is not achieved, consider a step up, but first review the patient's medication technique, compliance, and environmental control (avoidance of triggers).*

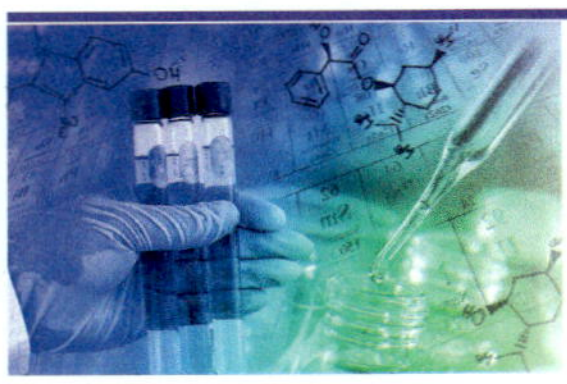

CONTROVERSY

Sustained-release theophylline has also been used in patients with asthma for many years, but its utility has been questioned more recently, because the agent has many side effects and a narrow therapeutic range.

time for review

In lay terms, how would you explain to a patient when to use quick-relief versus when to use long-term-control medication?

13.1h Management of Acute Asthma Exacerbations

It is essential that patients be able to recognize when their asthma is getting worse and know what to do. The NAEPP EPR-3 guidelines recommend that all patients have a written action plan, to enhance awareness and monitoring of asthma. We have included a sample monitoring plan in Figure 13-2; it utilizes personal peak flow meter measurements and symptom recognition to assist the patient.

FIGURE 13-2 Sample Action Plan for Management of Asthma

Addressograph here	Asthma Action Plan for ______ Physician: ______ Date: ______ Provider name and phone number: ______ ______	
Green Zone (Optimal) Peak flow = ______	**Yellow Zone (Caution)** Peak flow = ______	**Red Zone (Alert)** Peak flow = ______
No symptoms Able to do daily activities with little difficulty	Coughing Sleep disturbed by symptoms Short of breath/wheezing Difficulty doing normal daily activities	Symptoms are worse even while resting Very short of breath Trouble walking or talking Unable to do normal daily activities
Peak flow reading (80–100% of personal best)	Peak flow reading: (50– 80% of personal best)	Peak flow reading: (<50% of personal best)
☐ Review trigger control	☐ Rest	☐ Call your physician
☐ Take quick-relief medications ______ ______ as needed	☐ Increase dosage of: ______ ______	☐ Add or increase your oral steroid: ______
☐ Before exercise or exposure to other triggers, take: ______ ☐ Annual flu vaccination	☐ Continue other **green** zone medications ☐ Add: ______ ______	☐ Continue other **green** and **yellow** zone medications ☐ Special notes: ______ ______

What happens when your patient becomes too sick to follow her or his action plan and needs hospitalization? The NAEPP EPR-3–recommended algorithm for emergent asthma exacerbations is shown in Figure 13-3. Patients with mild or moderate exacerbations (pulmonary function >50% of predicted) can be treated with a metered-dose inhaler (MDI) or nebulized short-acting β_2-agonists administered three times during the first hour at home or in the emergency department. Patients with more severe exacerbations (pulmonary function <50% predicted) should be treated with nebulized medications in an emergency department, as they are probably not able to breathe deeply enough and may be too agitated over the event to benefit from the MDI. Supplemental oxygen is indicated if the patient is hypoxemic.

FIGURE 13-3 Management of Acute Asthma Exacerbations

Source: Modified from the NAEPP EPR-3.

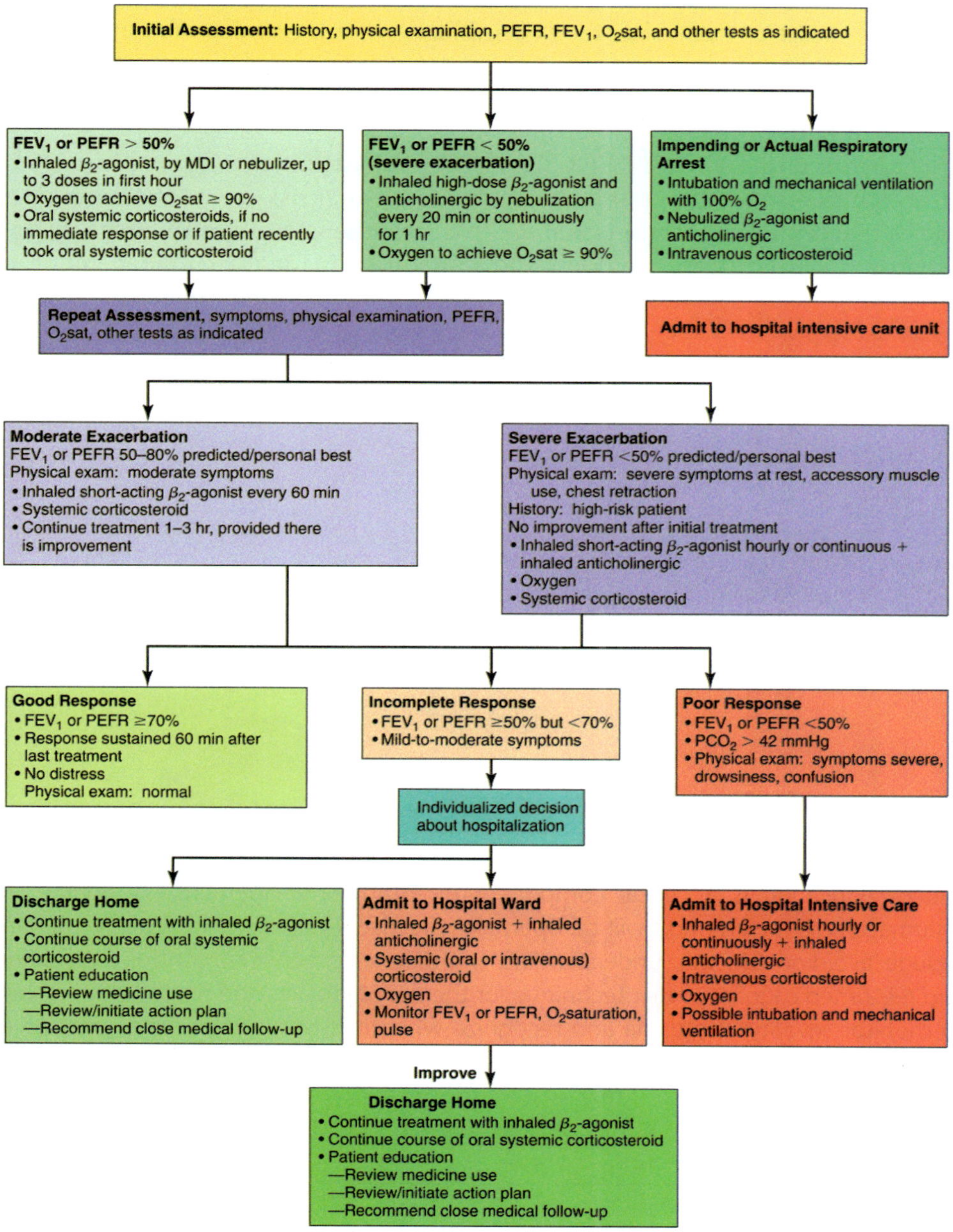

Clinical pearl

Magnesium is a weak bronchodilator, and there are case reports of magnesium preventing respiratory failure in patients presenting with severe asthma exacerbations.

If symptoms persist beyond the initial treatment, systemic corticosteroids are indicated, and short-acting anticholinergic agents may be used if the prescriber considers the symptoms to be severe. Inhaled corticosteroids act much too slowly to be used in these situations and should be considered only as long-term preventive agents. All patients whose symptoms are severe enough to require treatment in the emergency department should receive a course of oral corticosteroids.

If patients are not recovered after the initial emergency department therapy, they may require admission to the hospital. These patients should continue to receive treatment with frequent inhaled β_2-agonists plus inhaled anticholinergics and systemic corticosteroids. Antibiotics are not generally indicated, as the cause of exacerbation is more frequently viral.

If symptoms persist and the patient requires therapy in an intensive care unit (ICU), he or she should also continue to receive β_2-agonist therapy via the inhaled or subcutaneous route. It is generally believed that the inhaled route is equal in effectiveness to systemic administration and preferred whenever possible. Patients may also receive inhaled or intravenous magnesium and aggressive therapy with oxygen. In general patients may be discharged from the hospital when their pulmonary function returns to 70% of their predicted normal or better.

According to the NAEPP EPR-3, 80%–90% of asthma deaths are preventable. Although the factors that put an individual patient at risk are still being debated, one well-accepted risk factor is inability to assess the severity of an attack by both patients and health-care providers and subsequent inadequate management.

time for review

A patient in acute respiratory distress with a respiratory rate of 34 should receive what type of inhaled medication? What would be the best delivery device, an MDI or a spontaneous nebulized treatment?

Patient & Family Education

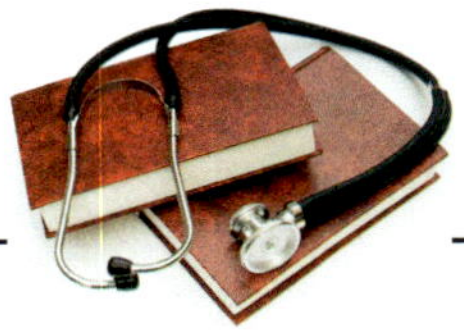

Patient education is a critical component of asthma management. Without it, no pharmacologic intervention will be optimally effective. Important concepts for patients include avoiding triggers, understanding the difference between control medications and relief medications, proper technique for the use of inhalers and related devices, how to monitor severity of asthma and recognize when it is becoming worse, what to do should this happen, and when to seek help. It is important for all health-care personnel to assess patient knowledge and reinforce these concepts at each encounter. Moderate to severe persistent asthma or history of exacerbations should have a written plan of action, with daily peak flow monitoring.

13.2 COPD

Official estimates from 2011 are that 11.8 million persons in the United States have COPD, but this is likely an underestimate, because patients typically don't present for diagnosis until they have moderate to severe disease. Based on data from population surveys, it is estimated that 24 million persons in the United States may have some degree of COPD. Regardless COPD is a major cause of disability in adults and is estimated to have direct economic costs of $18 billion annually and indirect economic costs (lost earnings, etc.) of over $14 billion in the United States.

13.2a Background

Although the death rates for COPD have declined for men (57 per 100,000 in 1999 versus 47.6 per 100,000 in 2010), there has been no significant change in death rates for women (35.3 per 100,000 in 1999 versus 36.4 per 100,000 in 2010). This is believed to be the result of the increased number of women smoking starting in 1940. Because we have seen a decrease in smoking frequency these past 30 years, it is believed that the COPD death rate will also decrease in the coming decades.

Clinical pearl

Men have a higher incidence of COPD than women do, and Caucasians have a higher incidence than blacks.

13.2b Etiology

The primary etiology for COPD is exposure to tobacco smoke. Smokers have higher death rates from both chronic bronchitis and emphysema. Smokers also have more lung function abnormalities, show more respiratory symptoms, and experience all forms of COPD at a much higher rate than nonsmokers. Age of starting, total pack-years, and current smoking status are predictive of COPD mortality. Passive smoking (the exposure of nonsmokers to cigarette smoke) also seems to increase the risk of COPD-related disease. Children of parents who smoke have a higher prevalence of respiratory symptoms than children of nonsmokers. Exposure to smoke at an early age may impair the attainment of maximal lung function in adult life. Air pollution, occupational exposure, asthma, and nonspecific airway hyperresponsiveness may all play a role in the development of COPD.

Emphysema

In the past, it was customary to divide persons with COPD into two categories: those with emphysema (the "pink puffer") and those with chronic bronchitis (the "blue bloater"). However most persons with COPD have features of both of these diseases. We are going to keep the distinctions (even though the GOLD definition has eliminated them), partially to help you categorize when to use certain therapies; so we'll begin with the description and treatment of emphysema.

Clinical pearl

Most persons with α_1-AT deficiency are Caucasians of northern European descent.

About 2 million persons in the United States are estimated to have emphysema. Of these, 60,000 to 100,000 have a genetic deficiency of α_1-antitrypsin (α_1-AT) as their underlying etiology. α_1-AT is a glycoprotein found in extracellular and intracellular fluid. It is essential in protecting the lung against naturally occurring proteases that have the ability to break down the elastin and macromolecules in lung tissue. Patients with this deficiency tend to develop emphysema at a younger age (in their 40s or 50s) than do patients with emphysema from other causes. Smoking further accelerates the process, by stimulating the release of neutrophil elastase. The syndrome of α_1-AT deficiency is perceived by most clinicians as being rare, but the reality is that most patients with α_1-AT deficiency go undiagnosed and are treated simply as people with emphysema. Manifestations of severe α_1-AT deficiency involve the lungs, the liver, and the skin, and the major clinical feature is emphysema. The disorder is detected by a decrease in the level of α_1-AT to below a so-called protective value of 80 mg/dl. This is in comparison to normal serum levels of 150 to 350 mg/dl.

Clinical Presentation

The primary clinical features distinguishing emphysema from asthma and bronchitis are **dyspnea** (labored or difficult breathing) on exertion and nonproductive cough. Emphysemic patients tend to have the "pink puffer" appearance, breathing with all of their accessory muscles. They exhale through "pursed" lips to maintain airway pressure and prevent airway collapse, but maintain a pink skin color. The work of breathing for severely emphysemic patients is much like running a marathon. They must continually work to maintain airway pressure in their abnormally large airspaces and must maintain a rapid respiratory rate. Weight loss is typical with severe emphysema. Think how much weight you'd lose if you ran a marathon each day!

Chronic Bronchitis

Chronic bronchitis is more common than emphysema, with a prevalence of over 9 million persons in the United States. Cigarette smoking is the major causative factor in up to 90% of cases. Patients with chronic bronchitis have an increase in size and number of the mucus-secreting glands, narrowing and inflammation of the small airways, obstruction of airways caused by narrowing and mucus hypersecretion, and bacterial colonization of the airways. Acute episodes are usually brought on by a respiratory tract infection. The usual clinical presentation of chronic bronchitis begins with morning cough productive of sputum. The patient may report a decline in exercise tolerance, although he or she may not have appreciated this decline until questioned. Wheezes may be present, and an increase in the anterior–posterior diameter of the chest (the classic "barrel chest") may be present in both emphysema and chronic bronchitis. The patient who has predominantly chronic bronchitis symptoms may undergo repeated episodes of respiratory failure and frequently develop right-sided heart failure.

Respiratory infections trigger acute exacerbations in the COPD patient, especially in elderly patients with chronic bronchitis. Patients present with hypersecretion of mucus and then, owing to their decreased removal of bronchial secretions by ciliary activity, are far more likely to develop pneumonia and significant lung damage from the infection.

Clinical Presentation

Wheezing and prolonged forced expiratory time strongly suggest airflow obstruction. If this is accompanied by decreased breath sounds, it is likely that the patient has at least moderately severe disease. Most patients with COPD are short of breath, especially with any exertion, and usually have a productive morning cough. It is unlikely that the patient will be able to identify triggers that make his or her disease worsen. Patients with classic features of chronic bronchitis are sometimes referred to as "blue bloaters." They may have cyanosis and suffer from morning headaches, which can suggest nighttime hypercapnea (CO_2 retention). These patients tend to be overweight, although patients with advanced disease may experience weight loss, which can also be a prominent symptom associated with bronchogenic carcinoma. Many COPD patients have a somewhat characteristic physical appearance, with a hyperinflated barrel chest, wheezing on forced expiration, subcutaneous fat wasting on their extremities and lower torso, and adoption of positions that relieve their dyspnea. Their accessory respiratory muscles of the neck and shoulder girdle may be in full use, and they may exhale through pursed lips to maintain alveolar inflation.

In patients with COPD, spirometry will be diagnostic if the FEV_1/FVC ratio drops below 70%, thus confirming airflow limitations. Unlike with the reversibility found in asthma, this value should be a fairly consistent finding and will not improve between acute attacks. The sputum of most patients with chronic bronchitis is typically colonized with bacteria, making it difficult to interpret a Gram stain.

Table 13-7 describes some of the ways that chronic bronchitis differs from emphysema in clinical presentation. Much of the therapy of these diseases is aimed at symptom control, so delineating which disease the patient has is not really necessary. However because the two terms are in common usage, you may want to review Table 13-7 so that you will have a good understanding of the patients' presentation when they are described as having emphysema or chronic bronchitis. Of the two clinical diagnoses, emphysema is the more disabling.

Learning Hint

Chronic progressive breathlessness occurs often in COPD, whereas asthmatic patients usually have a more episodic occurrence of these symptoms. Although inflammation plays some role in COPD, it is different from the inflammation in asthma and is less likely to respond to corticosteroids. Asthma occurs in all age groups, but COPD is usually a disease of older patients.

Clinical pearl

Smoking history is the most important initial screening the clinician can perform, as it may help to clinically distinguish COPD from asthma. The impact of smoking can be quantified by calculating a pack-year history. A pack-year history is calculated by multiplying the number of packs smoked per day by the number of years smoked.

TABLE 13-7 Clinical Features of the Two Major Types of COPD

Feature	Emphysema	Chronic Bronchitis
Sputum	Minimal	Copious
Dyspnea	Relatively early	Relatively late
Cor pulmonale	Rare	Common
Weight	Marked weight loss, cachectic appearance	Obesity common
Smoking history	Common	Common
Chest X-ray findings	Hyperinflation	Increased markings
Hematocrit	Normal	May be increased
Blood gases	Normal or slightly low PaO_2 Normal pH or mild respiratory acidosis Normal or slightly high $PaCO_2$	Low PaO_2 Respiratory acidosis Elevated $PaCO_2$
Respiratory failure	Rare until end stage	Repeated episodes
Pulmonary function tests	Decreased FEV_1	Decreased FEV_1
	Decreased FVC	Decreased FVC
	Greatly increased residual volume	Increased residual volume

13.2c Prevention: The Key to Treatment of COPD

Smoking Cessation

The only method known to prevent or slow the progression of COPD is to stop smoking. All patients who smoke need to be regularly encouraged to stop. Cigarette smoking kills nearly 440,000 Americans each year and debilitates nearly one-half of all long-term smokers. In addition to its effects on the lungs, it contributes substantially to both cardiovascular and cerebrovascular disease. Tobacco dependence is a powerful addiction and one that is extremely difficult to break. Some patients can be successful on their own, but most require behavioral counseling and encouragement in addition to pharmacologic therapy. Tobacco relapse rates are high, and most successful quitters have made at least five attempts to stop before achieving that goal. Therefore all health-care providers must continually offer help and support to patients who are willing to try to stop smoking. A number of clinical practice guidelines are available to aid health professionals in helping persons to stop smoking. One popular approach centers on the "5 As": ask, advise, assess, assist, and arrange. See Table 13-8 for a description of these five steps.

TABLE 13-8 The "5 As" of Smoking Cessation

Ask	Screen all patients for tobacco use.
Advise	Strongly advise all smokers to quit.
Assess	Assess the patient's readiness to quit.
Assist	Assist patients in quitting. Help patients to identify a plan for quitting, determine pharmacotherapy, recommend counseling options, support group options.
Arrange	Monitor patients' progress with quitting and arrange for patient follow-up.

Many therapies are available to help smokers to quit. Health-care providers should help patients identify what therapies will best suit them. They should be given written instructions on the use of the option selected. The dose and duration of therapy should be individualized. Patients should be contacted frequently and/or return to the office for encouragement and motivation and to monitor their use of the therapies chosen. The patient should be encouraged to enter a formal smoking-cessation program, and the health-care provider should be aware of what programs are available in the community and how the patient can enter one. Finally the health-care provider needs to congratulate the patient on success.

Smoking Cessation Therapies Pharmacologic therapy is an extremely important adjunct to behavioral interventions for smoking cessation. When choosing the appropriate therapy, the clinician needs to consider what the patient wants, whether he or she has had any adverse reactions to any of the therapies, whether the side effects are tolerable, whether the medication is effective, and how addicted the patient is to nicotine.

It is important to somehow quantify the patient's addiction to nicotine. The Fagerstrom test for nicotine dependence (FTND; see Figure 13-4) is a good tool to help you do this. A score of 6 or higher on the FTND indicates a high level of nicotine dependence. Patients in this category will have difficulty overcoming the initial withdrawal symptoms of nicotine and will benefit the most from pharmacotherapy to aid cessation. Even a person with a lower score may benefit from nicotine replacement therapy or bupropion (Zyban®) to aid in cessation since the success rate from unaided quit attempts is only about 3% to 6% a year later. The patient's preference will also have a great deal to do with which drug therapy (if any) is chosen. The best pharmacotherapy will not be successful until the patient has truly decided to quit. Pharmacotherapy alone is rarely a means to successful cessation in the nicotine-addicted patient. Patients should be encouraged to seek educational and behavioral modification therapy for smoking cessation and to use pharmacotherapy as an aid to these programs since the combination of counseling and pharmacotherapy produces greater quit rates.

Nicotine replacement therapy (NRT) works for many patients, because it can be adjusted to substitute partially for the nicotine the patient inhales through smoking cigarettes. In general you will adjust the NRT to deliver less nicotine than is received through smoking, but enough will be given to decrease the intensity of nicotine withdrawal symptoms. Even though nicotine is still being ingested, the carcinogens that would be delivered through smoking are not. Additionally NRT produces more consistent blood levels of nicotine than smoking a cigarette, therefore decreasing the craving that occurs when the smoker's blood levels of nicotine drop between cigarettes. Currently there are four methods of NRT: the patch, nicotine gum/lozenge, nicotine nasal spray, and the nicotine oral inhaler. Table 13-9 gives some details about these dosage forms. Experts recommend using the patch as the primary form of NRT with the use of additional short-acting products to control cravings.

Clinical pearl

Patients who use nicotine replacement therapy need to be cautioned about proper disposal of the "used" dosage forms. The patches, gum, and sprays all contain enough residual nicotine to be toxic to children and pets. It is also important that patients have completely stopped smoking before starting NRT.

FIGURE 13-4 The Fagerstrom Test for Nicotine Dependence

Questions and Possible Answers	Score
How soon after you wake up do you smoke your first cigarette?	
≤ 5 minutes	3
6 – 30 minutes	2
31 – 60 minutes	1
≥ 60 minutes	0
Do you find it difficult to refrain from smoking in places where it is forbidden (e.g., in church, at work, in the library, in a cinema)?	
Yes	1
No	0
What cigarette would you hate most to give up?	
The first in the morning	1
Any other	0
How many cigarettes per day do you smoke?	
≤ 10	0
11 – 20	1
21 – 30	2
≥ 31	3
Do you smoke more frequently during the first hours after waking than the rest of the day?	
Yes	1
No	0
Do you smoke if you are so ill that you are in bed most of the day?	
Yes	1
No	0

TABLE 13-9 Nicotine Replacement Therapies, Bupropion, and Varenicline

Dosage Form	Dosing	Adverse Effects	Rx or OTC?	Cautions
Nicotrol® Patch (for patients who smoke >10 cigarettes a day)	15 mg/day for 6 wks	Skin irritation, insomnia	OTC	Avoid if pregnant and have heart disease
Nicoderm CQ® (21, 14, 7 mg/24 hr)	<10 cigarettes/day: 14 mg/24 hr for 16–24 hr/day × 6 wks, then one 7 mg/24 hr for 16–24 hr/day × 2 wks	Skin irritation, insomnia	OTC	Avoid if pregnant and have heart disease
	>10 cigarettes/day: 21 mg/24 hr for 6–24 hr/day × 6 wks, then 14 mg/24 hr for 16–24 hr/day × 2 wks, then one 7 mg/24 hr for 16–24 hr/day × 2 wks			
Nicorette® gum Original and flavored (2 and 4 mg)	2 mg (4 mg for highly dependent patients who request it, or for those who failed the 2 mg), chewed and held between the cheek and gum intermittently over 30 min every 1–2 hrs for 6 wks, then every 2–4 hrs for 3 wks, then every 4–8 hrs for 3 wks; do not exceed 30 pieces/day.	Mouth irritation, sore jaw, dyspepsia, nausea, hiccups	OTC	Avoid in denture wearers, pregnancy, heart disease
Commit® lozenge (2 mg and 4 mg)	2 mg for patients who smoke their first cigarette more than 30 min after waking up, use 4 mg if first cigarettes within 30 min of waking up. Dose schedule same as for gum. Not to exceed 20 lozenges/day.	Mouth irritation, dyspepsia, nausea, hiccups	OTC	Avoid in pregnancy, heart disease
Nicotrol NS® nasal spray 10 mg/ml	One or two 1-mg doses (each dose is two 0.5-mg sprays, one in each nostril) per hour initially, increased as needed. Do not exceed 5 doses/hr or 40 doses/day. Full dose for up to 8 wks, then taper dose over 4–6 wks.	Rhinitis, sore throat, sneezing, coughing	Rx	Avoid in rhinitis, common cold symptoms, pregnancy, heart disease
Nicotrol® oral inhaler (10-mg nicotine cartridges, 4 mg delivered)	Cartridge must be inserted into mouthpiece and activated. Initial use is 6–16 cartridges/day. Patient controls depth and frequency of inhalation.	Dyspepsia, coughing, mouth irritation, burning	Rx	Avoid in COPD, asthma, pregnancy, heart disease
Zyban® (bupropion)	Start at least 1 week before quitting cigarettes; begin with 150 mg/day x 3 days. If needed, increase to 150 mg twice daily; use for 7–12 wks.	Headache, insomnia, dry mouth	Rx	Several possible drug interactions—avoid in seizure disorders, bulimia, anorexia, CNS disorders, or alcoholism
Chantix® (varenicline)	0.5 mg daily for 3 days, then 0.5 mg b.i.d. for 4 days, then 1 mg b.i.d.	Nausea, abnormal dreams, insomnia	Rx	Suicidal behaviors, aggressive thoughts

Bupropion (Zyban®) is an FDA-approved non-NRT treatment for nicotine addiction. This agent is also used for the treatment of depression, under the brand name Wellbutrin®. We do not know how this medication treats nicotine addiction, but it is speculated that the drug's brain adrenergic and dopaminergic activity plays some role in easing nicotine withdrawal. Bupropion has several drug interactions and some significant side effects, so patients must be carefully screened before beginning this therapy. Some patients may benefit from combining NRT and bupropion.

Varenicline (Chantix®) became available a few years ago. This medication is a partial agonist of the nicotinic acetylcholine receptor, and its efficacy may be related to two mechanisms. First it binds to and stimulates the receptor thereby reducing the craving for nicotine; second, since it binds to the receptor with high affinity, it may block inhaled nicotine from working. The most common adverse effect of varenicline is nausea. This may be easily treated by cutting back on the dosage. Serious neuropsychiatric symptoms including mood disturbances, psychosis, and hostility have been rarely reported.

Two other medications that might be considered for smoking cessation are clonidine (an antihypertensive agent) and nortriptyline (an antidepressant). These agents are rarely recommended, however. They are less effective than standard therapies for smoking cessation, and they have quite a few more side effects.

Life Span Considerations

Even though the prevalence of smoking in teens has gradually declined in the United States since the late 1990s, in 2011, 23% of twelfth-grade students reported smoking in the last 30 days. It is important to treat adolescent smoking aggressively since 90% of adult smokers reported smoking their first cigarette before their 18th birthday and most adolescent smokers report that they want to quit smoking.

It is important to counsel adult smokers willing to quit that if they are successful in quitting, they will reduce their chances of dying from smoking-related diseases even if they already have COPD and cardiac disease.

Vaccinations

Annual influenza vaccination is essential for all COPD patients. Influenza vaccination has been shown to decrease serious illness and mortality in COPD patients by about 50%. Chemoprophylaxis with oseltamivir should be considered in nonimmunized patients in the case of an outbreak, when there is an inadequate amount of time for immunization to become effective, or in patients for whom the vaccine is contraindicated. Contraindications include patients who have had a serious reaction in the past or who have a serious allergic reaction (e.g., anaphylaxis) to eggs.

Although there is less evidence for its effectiveness, pneumococcal vaccine is also recommended for COPD patients. There are now two vaccines approved for use in the United States. Pneumococcal polysaccharide vaccine (Pneumovax® 23) incorporates the antigens of 23 strains of bacteria that are responsible for 90% of the pneumococcal pneumonia that occurs in the United States. Pneumococcal conjugate vaccine (Prevnar 13®) contains capsular polysaccharides from 13 common strains. The indications and vaccination schedules for both vaccines are dependent upon pneumococcal disease risk factors and age. The pneumococcal polysaccharide vaccine may be administered IM or SC, while the conjugate vaccine is given IM only. Vaccination schedules are constantly updated as new information becomes available. Health-care professionals should consult the United States advisory Committee on Immunization Practices for current recommendations. Side effects of both vaccines are generally mild and consist of minor redness and pain at the injection site.

13.2d COPD Treatment Goals

As with asthma, there has been an increased focus on improving the diagnosis and management of patients with COPD worldwide. As a result there are now practice guidelines available to aid the clinician. The GOLD Guidelines, prepared by the Global Initiative for Chronic Obstructive Lung Disease, are one such resource. Their objectives are to increase awareness of COPD in both health professionals and the general public.

According to these guidelines, there are four components to patient management: assessing and monitoring the disease, reducing risk factors, managing stable disease, and managing exacerbations. Goals of therapy are to prevent disease progression, relieve symptoms, improve exercise tolerance, improve overall health status, prevent and treat exacerbations and other complications, and reduce mortality. While the following discussion represents a synopsis of the 2015 report, you can visit www.goldcopd.org for the latest information.

time for review

What are some key COPD prevention methods?

13.2e Assessment of COPD

It is important to determine the severity of COPD, its impact on a patient's health status, and the risk of future events. This assessment helps to guide therapy. The following items should be included in the assessment:

- *Assess the current level of patient's symptoms.* There are several validated assessment tools that can be used to provide an objective measure of symptoms. These include the COPD Assessment Test (CAT; http://catestonline.org), Clinical COPD Questionnaire (CCQ; http://www.ccq.nl), and the mMRC Breathlessness Scale.
- *Assess the degree of airflow limitation with spirometry.* See Table 13-10 for classification of COPD severity as suggested by the GOLD guidelines.
- *Assess the risk of exacerbations.* Patients who have experienced two or more exacerbations within the last year, who have a $FEV_1 < 50\%$ predicted, and/or who have had one or more hospitalizations for COPD exacerbation should be considered high risk
- *Assess other chronic health problems (comorbidities).* Lung cancer, bronchiectasis, diabetes, cardiovascular disease, anxiety and depression, respiratory infections, and osteoporosis have all been found to influence the chance of death in patients with COPD and should be looked for and treated when found.

TABLE 13-10 Classification of COPD Severity in Terms of Airflow Limitations: GOLD Classification

Stage	Severity	Diagnostic Features
GOLD I	Mild COPD	• FEV_1/FVC <70%
		• FEV_1 ≥80% predicted
		• With or without chronic symptoms
		• Patient may or may not be aware of decreased lung function
GOLD II	Moderate COPD	• FEV_1/FVC <70%
		• FEV_1 ≥50% but <80% predicted
		• With or without chronic symptoms, although shortness of breath on exertion is common
		• Stage at which patients will begin seeking medical attention for symptoms
GOLD III	Severe COPD	• FEV_1/FVC <70%
		• FEV_1 ≥30% but <50% predicted
		• With or without chronic symptoms, although at this stage, patient may have repeated exacerbations
GOLD IV	Very severe COPD	• FEV_1/FVC <70%
		• FEV_1 <30% predicted
		• Quality of life is severely affected; symptoms of heart failure may be present; exacerbations may be life-threatening

Note: FEV_1 is measured postbronchodilator.

Source: Modified from the GOLD Global Strategy for the Diagnosis, Management, and Prevention of Chronic Obstructive Pulmonary Disease 2015 Update.

After being assessed patients can be graded, according to GOLD standards, in four categories, as shown in Table 13-11.

TABLE 13-11 Patient Grading in COPD

Patient Grade	Patient Characteristics
A	Low risk, fewer symptoms
B	Low risk, more symptoms
C	High risk, fewer symptoms
D	High risk, more symptoms

COPD severity increases as a patient moves through the alphabet. Adapted from GOLD 2015.

13.2f Drugs Used to Treat COPD

The following medications are therapeutic options in the treatment of COPD:

- Short- and long-acting β-agonists (SABAs and LABAs)
- Short- and long-acting muscarinic antagonists (SAMAs and LAMAs)
- Combinations of SABA and SAMA in one inhaler
- Combinations of LABA and LAMA in one inhaler
- Inhaled corticosteroids (ICS)
- Combinations of LABA and ICS

- Methylxanthines
- Systemic corticosteroids
- Phosphodiesterase-4 inhibitors

β_2-Agonists and Anticholinergics

Pharmacologic options for COPD are very similar to those for asthma, but certain differences need to be emphasized. The β_2-agonists will produce less bronchodilation in COPD than in asthma. Also COPD patients tend to be older than asthmatic patients and will probably be less tolerant of the sympathomimetic effects (tremor, nervousness, palpitations, etc.) of the β_2-agonists. On the other hand patients with COPD respond better to anticholinergic agents than do patients with asthma. (It is believed that cholinergic nerve fibers in the airways play a larger role in COPD than in asthma.)

Current thinking is that β_2-agonists and anticholinergic agents are equally effective as bronchodilators in COPD, although a given patient may respond better to one or another. However the side-effect profile of anticholinergics may be less troublesome for the older COPD population. Anticholinergic drugs have a slower onset and longer duration than β_2-agonists and are better for use on a regular basis, not "as needed." The use of a combination product containing both albuterol and ipratropium (e.g., Combivent®) in the same MDI may help the patient by simplifying therapy. Long-acting are more effective than short-acting bronchodilators for symptom relief and they reduce exacerbations and hospitalizations more, as well. Combinations of bronchodilators from different classes may improve therapy and reduce side effects instead of increasing the dose of a single agent.

Theophylline

Theophylline, at one time, was probably the most common agent used in this patient population. However its potent toxicities and the availability of newer agents have caused it to fall from favor. The agent is still of value for the management of both asthma and COPD in patients who are not capable of using an MDI effectively or who are inadequately controlled with their inhaled medications. A peak theophylline level between 5 and 15 mcg/ml is considered to be a therapeutic level. As the theophylline level increases, toxicities such as tachycardia and nausea can progress to seizures and coma. Theophylline and other xanthine derivatives help to improve respiratory muscle function, stimulate the respiratory center, and enhance activities of daily living in patients who are severely limited by their COPD and who also have cardiac disease. Careful dosing is required, and blood levels of the drug must be monitored regularly, especially when any other medication is started or the patient has coexisting diseases.

Anti-Inflammatory Drugs

In sharp contrast to the therapy of asthma, anti-inflammatory drugs are of far less benefit in COPD patients. Although inflammation plays a role in the development of COPD, it is not allergic in nature and responds to therapy differently than in asthma. Medications such as cromolyn, nedocromil, and leukotriene inhibitors have no established use unless the patient has coexisting asthma. Inhaled corticosteroids improve symptoms, lung function, and quality of life, and decrease exacerbations in patients with an $FEV_1 < 60\%$ predicted. Unfortunately the benefits come at a cost of an increased chance of developing pneumonia. Inhaled corticosteroids are not used alone in COPD, but when combined with long-acting β_2-agonists they result in improved lung function and health status, and a decrease in exacerbations in patients with moderate to severe COPD. When this combination is added to a long-acting, inhaled anticholinergic agent, additional benefits may be seen.

Oral corticosteroids are recommended only for short-term use in patients with moderate to severe exacerbations. Because the COPD patient population is typically older than the asthma population, it is important to remember the side effects of oral corticosteroid use. Complications such as skin damage, cataracts, diabetes, osteoporosis, gastric ulceration, muscle wasting, and secondary infection are more likely to occur in the COPD population. Therefore it is important that oral corticosteroid use be minimized; only short "burst" therapy should be used, if possible.

Phosphodiesterase-4 Inhibitors

Roflumilast (Daliresp®) is a phosphodiesterase-4 inhibitor that leads to an intracellular accumulation of cyclic AMP. This results in an anti-inflammatory effect. The dose is 500 mg orally once daily. It has been studied in patients with severe and very severe COPD (GOLD III and IV). It has been shown to decrease the number of exacerbations requiring corticosteroid treatment. Side effects include headache, dizziness, weight loss, and diarrhea. Table 13-12 summarizes the pharmacologic bronchodilator and anti-inflammatory options used in COPD.

Mucokinetic Agents

Mucokinetic agents (organic iodide, guaifenesin, acetylcysteine, etc.) have had little objective information published supporting their value in the treatment of COPD. Their use is far more accepted in Europe, where they are favored for their antioxidant effects in addition to their action of decreasing the viscosity of the mucus.

Antibiotics

Infection is a common cause of exacerbation in patients with COPD. Therefore antibiotics are recommended for patients who are showing signs of exacerbation and are having an increase in sputum purulence thought to be due to an infection. The organisms most frequently responsible for infection are *Streptococcus pneumonia*, *Haemophilus influenzae*, and *Moraxella catarrhalis*. Because most patients with COPD have chronic colonization of their sputum with these bacteria, it is sometimes difficult to know whether the patient is acutely infected and, if so, which organism is responsible. Other bacteria besides the ones above may be responsible for acute infection in patients with more serious illness or who have been hospitalized or recently treated with antibiotics. For milder exacerbations, older, less costly antibiotics should be used, such as amoxicillin, tetracycline, doxycycline, or trimethoprim–sulfamethoxazole. Decisions should be made on the basis of local bacterial resistance patterns, stage of COPD, and severity of the exacerbation. In the past prophylactic antibiotics were prescribed for some patients to prevent exacerbations; however, in an attempt to prevent the development of resistant organisms, this practice is now discouraged.

TABLE 13-12 Pharmacologic Bronchodilator and Anti-Inflammatory Options for COPD

Pharmacologic Category	Generic, Trade Name	Route of Administration
SABA	albuterol, Proventil® HFA	Inhalation
	levalbuterol, Xopenex®	Inhalation
	metaproterenol	Oral
	pirbuterol	Inhalation
	terbutaline	Oral, SubQ
LABA	arformoterol, Brovana®	Inhalation
	indacaterol, Arcapta®	Inhalation
	formoterol, Foradil®	Inhalation
	olodaterol, Striverdi®	Inhalation
	salmeterol, Serevent®	Inhalation
SAMA	ipratropium, Atrovent®	Inhalation
LAMA	aclidinium, Tudorza®	Inhalation
	tiotropium, Spiriva®	Inhalation
	umeclidinium, Incruse®	Inhalation
ICS	beclomethasone, Qvar®	Inhalation
	budesonide, Pulmicort®	Inhalation
	ciclesonide, Alvesco®	Inhalation
	flunisolide, Aerospan®	Inhalation
	fluticasone, Flovent®	Inhalation
	mometasone, Asmanex®	Inhalation
ICS & LABA	budesonide & formoterol, Symbicort®	Inhalation
	fluticasone & salmeterol, Advair®	Inhalation
	fluticasone & vilanterol, Breo® Ellipta®	Inhalation
	mometasone & formoterol, Dulera®	Inhalation
LABA & LAMA	umeclidinium & vilanterol, Anoro® Ellipta®	Inhalation
Methylxanthines	theophylline, Theo-24®	Oral, IV
Systemic corticosteroids	methylprednisolone, Solu-Medrol™	IV, oral
	prednisone, Rayos®	Oral
Phosphodiesterase-4 enzyme inhibitor	roflumilast, Daliresp®	Oral

α_1-Antitrypsin

Augmentation therapy with α_1-AT is accomplished by administering α_1-proteinase inhibitor (Prolastin®-C, Aralast®, Zemaira®). This therapy is appropriate for nonsmoking, younger patients with severe α_1-AT deficiency and associated emphysema. These products must be given by intravenous infusion on a weekly basis and are very costly. Therapy is generally well tolerated and is considered safe.

Oxygen

Oxygen therapy is often needed to maintain normal PaO_2 levels and to decrease the work of breathing associated with COPD. In addition COPD causes associated cardiac stress, which oxygen therapy also helps to treat. For patients with chronic hypoxia, continuous oxygen therapy (> 15 hours per day) has been shown to decrease mortality by half when compared to nocturnal oxygen therapy.

13.2g Step-by-Step Approach

Therapy of the patient with COPD is multifaceted. *The importance of smoking cessation cannot be overemphasized.* It is the single intervention that will slow the rate of decline in pulmonary function and improve the patient's quality of life. Additionally therapy goals should include prevention of acute exacerbations, improvement of chronic obstruction, reduction in the rate of disease progression, and improvement in both the physical and the psychological states of the patient.

Smoking cessation and annual influenza vaccinations remain cornerstones of COPD therapy. Recently updated pneumococcal vaccination guidelines should be applied to all patients with COPD. For symptom control, bronchodilators form the cornerstone of therapy for patients with COPD. For patients with intermittent symptoms, a short-acting bronchodilator (either a β_2-agonist or an anticholinergic) may be prescribed as needed (GOLD Class A). The β_2-agonists may offer an advantage in this instance, because they have a more rapid onset of action.

For patients with more persistent symptoms, scheduled use of either a short-acting or long-acting bronchodilator is indicated (GOLD Class B). Short- and long-acting options are available for both the β_2-agonist and anticholinergic bronchodilators. For patients who do not receive adequate symptom relief, it is more effective to use a combination of bronchodilators with different mechanisms than a single agent alone. Even though patients might not demonstrate a significant improvement in their pulmonary function tests with bronchodilators, they may still experience an improvement in exercise tolerance, dyspnea, or other quality-of-life measures. Thus these agents should be continued if the patient notes improvement. Theophylline can be considered if inhaled bronchodilators are inadequate, although inhaled bronchodilators are always preferred as first-line therapy. For the inhaled route, MDI and DPI are preferred over nebulizers. Mucokinetic agents are generally not recommended.

Patients with more advanced disease (GOLD class C or D, $FEV_1 < 60\%$ predicted) can benefit from the addition of inhaled corticosteroids. Even though patients may not show an improvement in FEV_1, they may experience a decrease in the number of exacerbations as well as subjective improvement. Chronic use of oral corticosteroids is not recommended. See Table 13-13 for a recommended GOLD approach to managing stable COPD according to the assessment of patient grade.

TABLE 13-13 Therapeutic Options for Stable COPD According to GOLD Classification

Patient Grade	Recommended First Choice	Alternative Choice	Other Options
A	SAMA or SABA prn	LAMA or LABA with SABA and/or SAMA	theophylline
B	LAMA or LABA	LAMA and LABA	SABA and/or SAMA
C	ICS and LABA	LAMA and LABA	SABA and/or SAMA
	LAMA	LAMA and PDE-4 inhibitor	theophylline
		LABA and PDE-4 inhibitor	
D	ICS and LABA and/or LAMA	ICS and LABA and LAMA	SABA and/or SAMA
		ICS and LABA and PDE-4 inhibitor	N-acetylcysteine
		LAMA and LABA	
		LAMA and PDE-4 inhibitor	theophylline

Note: SABAs should always be available as a rescue inhaler for patients no matter what their grade for acute exacerbations.
Source: Modified from GOLD guidelines 2015 update.

Learning Hint

Because the mainstay of asthma and COPD treatment is inhaled medications, a key part of the success of therapy is that patients understand the proper technique for using an MDI well enough that they can demonstrate it to you. It is best to recommend the use of a spacer with MDI products as the most predictable way of delivering a consistent dose.

Exacerbations are common as the underlying stage of COPD becomes more severe. The most common causes of an acute exacerbation are bronchitis, pneumonia, and air pollution. In some cases these exacerbations can precipitate acute respiratory failure and may be fatal. Treatment is based on the severity of the exacerbation and whether the patient needs to be hospitalized. Factors influencing the decision to hospitalize include initial response to increased bronchodilator therapy, presence of worsening hypoxemia or respiratory acidosis, presence of comorbid disease states, severity of symptoms, stage of COPD before the exacerbation, and degree of home support.

The first step in managing an acute exacerbation is to increase the patient's bronchodilator therapy. This may mean increasing doses or frequency of inhaled agents, combining a β_2-agonist with an anticholinergic, and/or switching to nebulizer therapy. Antibiotics may also be added if the patient is showing signs of an increase in sputum purulence and either an increase in dyspnea or an increase in sputum volume. Oral or intravenous corticosteroids are usually considered at the same time. Corticosteroids are most likely to benefit patients whose baseline FEV_1 is ≤50%. In these cases corticosteroids have been shown to shorten the patient's recovery time. Oxygen therapy is a key component of therapy for hospitalized patients, and in some cases, ventilatory support is needed.

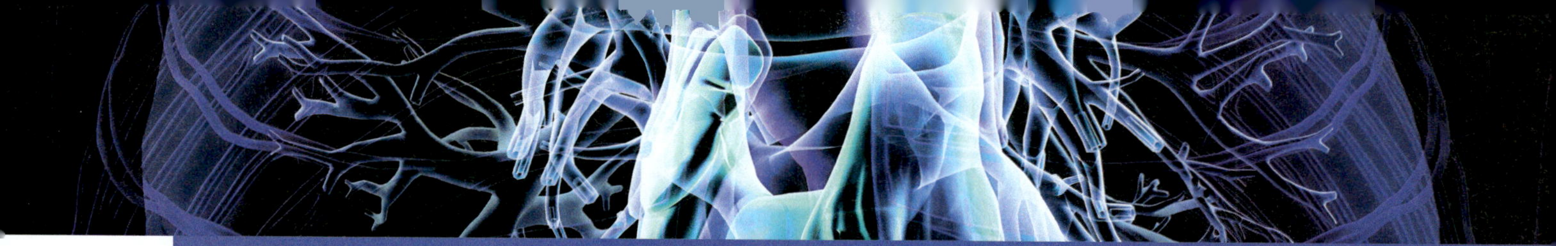

Summary

Asthma and COPD include a spectrum of diseases characterized by cough, sputum production, dyspnea, airflow limitation, bronchospasm, airway hyperreactivity, and impaired gas exchange. Pharmacologic management of these symptoms and diseases begins with an awareness of risk factors and identification of at-risk patients. Once a disease is recognized, patients and families need education about the disease and how to control it. Smoking cessation is key to stopping progression of this entire range of diseases. Appropriate drug therapy should be selected according to the patient's symptomatology and application of the accepted standards of care for the disease. Exacerbations and infections should be minimized, bronchodilation should be maximized, and anti-inflammatory drugs should be used when appropriate. In partnership with the patient, health-care providers can help to improve the patients' quality of life and maximize their pulmonary function.

REVIEW QUESTIONS

1. Match the level of asthma with its definition:

mild intermittent	continuous symptoms with frequent exacerbations
moderate persistent	daily symptoms with flare-ups affecting daily activity
severe persistent	self-limited, brief symptoms up to twice a week

2. Check the category that describes the medication:

albuterol	____ quick relief
	____ long term
cromolyn	____ quick relief
	____ long term
prednisone	____ quick relief
	____ long term

3. Smoking is the most important initial screening that can clinically distinguish COPD from asthma.
   true ____
   false ____

4. The following are generally of less benefit to COPD patients than asthma patients:
   (a) oral steroids
   (b) inhaled steroids
   (c) cromolyn
   (d) all of the above
   (e) none of the above

5. Chronic bronchitis is characterized clinically by
   (a) decreased FEV_1
   (b) common smoking history
   (c) minimal sputum
   (d) (a) and (b)
   (e) all of the above
6. Explain the differences among emphysema, asthma, and chronic bronchitis.
7. Describe some goals for an asthma patient, as recommended by the NAEPP EPR-3.
8. Discuss the role of an asthma action plan and what it may include.
9. Contrast the roles of MDIs versus spontaneous aerosol treatment of β_2-agonist delivery in emergency asthma exacerbations.

CASE STUDY 1

A 25-year-old man

A 25-year-old man with a history of asthma and GERD presents to the emergency room with a chief complaint that when he woke up, he couldn't breathe. He reports breathing fine before he went to bed. On the way to the hospital, he was given albuterol nebs and oxygen via nasal cannula.

Atrovent 2 puffs q.i.d.
Albuterol 2 puffs b.i.d prn.
VS: 110/48, RR 28, P 132
Skin: no cyanosis
Chest: decreased breath sounds, bilateral wheezes

1. What other pharmacotherapy choices are available to treat this acute asthma attack?
2. What are short-term and long-term goals for this patient's pharmacotherapy?
3. What would you recommend for this patient on discharge?

Chapter 14

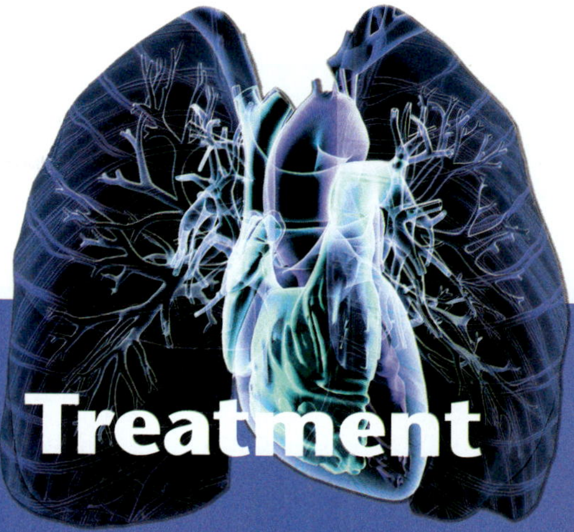

Pharmacologic Treatment of Respiratory Infectious Disease

OBJECTIVES

Upon completion of this chapter you will be able to

- Discuss pathogens associated with and diagnosis of:
  - Community-acquired pneumonia
  - Hospital-acquired pneumonia
  - Ventilator-associated pneumonia
  - Health-care-associated pneumonia
  - Otitis media
  - Sinusitis
  - Pharyngitis
  - Croup
  - Epiglottitis
  - Tuberculosis
  - PJP pneumonia
  - Bronchitis
  - Bronchiolitis
  - Avian influenza
- Describe goals of pharmacotherapy and monitoring parameters for:
  - Community-acquired pneumonia
  - Hospital-acquired pneumonia
  - Ventilator-associated pneumonia
  - Health-care-associated pneumonia

OBJECTIVES (CONTINUED)

- Describe goals of pharmacotherapy and monitoring parameters for:
  - Otitis media
  - Sinusitis
  - Pharyngitis
  - Croup
  - Epiglottitis
  - Tuberculosis
  - PJP pneumonia
  - Bronchitis
  - Bronchiolitis
  - Avian influenza
- Ask and find the answers to questions necessary to develop a therapeutic plan for an individual with a respiratory infectious disease.
- Discuss controversies in pharmacologic treatment of respiratory infectious disease.
- Discuss chemical terrorism as it relates to the role of antibiotics.

KEY TERMS

antibiogram
bronchiolitis
bronchitis
community-acquired pneumonia
cross-allergenicity
croup
culture
empiric therapy
epiglottitis
otitis media
pharyngitis
pneumonia
sinusitis
tuberculosis

ABBREVIATIONS

CAP community-acquired pneumonia
CMV cytomegalovirus
DOT directly observed treatment
GAS Group A β-hemolytic *Streptococcus*
HAP hospital-acquired pneumonia
HCAP health-care-associated pneumonia
HCW health-care worker
Hib *Haemophilus influenza* type B
IDSA Infectious Diseases Society of America
PJP *Pneumocystis jiroveci* pneumonia
PPD purified protein derivative
TB tuberculosis
TMP–SMX trimethoprim–sulfamethoxazole
VAP ventilator-associated pneumonia

Respiratory tract infections are among the most common infectious diseases seen in health care today. Any area of the respiratory tract can become infected, and because it is a continuous system, disease can easily spread to other areas of the respiratory tract. Respiratory infections are generally differentiated on the basis of anatomy. Acute otitis media, sinusitis, and pharyngitis are the primary infectious processes of the upper airways, whereas bronchitis and pneumonia occur in the lower respiratory tract.

In treating these infections, several questions need to be answered. First and foremost we need to consider whether an antibiotic is really necessary. Viral infections do not respond to antibiotics, and the use of antibiotics in viral syndromes negatively influences bacterial resistance patterns and puts the patient at unnecessary risk for adverse effects that can be caused by antimicrobials. Second, if antimicrobial therapy is necessary, we need to consider what the likely infecting organisms are, how serious the infection is, and what the antibiotic susceptibility/resistance patterns in the locality are. We can try to get cultures, but these are not always conclusive. Finally we need to consider the patient. Does the patient require a procedure to control the source of the infection (e.g., an empyema would require a chest tube to drain the pus from the pleural space)? Will the antibiotic reach the site of infection? What drug(s), dose(s), administration route(s), and schedule(s) are best suited to the patient? What symptomatic treatment is necessary, and when is prophylactic antibiotic therapy appropriate? This chapter offers insights into these questions and the treatment of respiratory infectious diseases.

This chapter presents what seems like a host of organisms that cause respiratory infections, along with a corresponding host of antimicrobial agents to treat them. The total may seem overwhelming, but reference tables simplify the material whenever possible. You received a basic foundation for learning about anti-infective agents in Chapter 8, and this chapter builds on that knowledge by integrating major respiratory infectious diseases with overall effective therapy. Keep in mind that most treatment depends ultimately on identifying the causative microorganism and then selecting an antimicrobial that is effective against that particular microorganism.

14.1 DEVELOPING A THERAPEUTIC PLAN FOR RESPIRATORY INFECTIOUS DISEASES

14.1a Empiric Treatment

To deliver effective therapy, you must develop a specific therapeutic plan. There are many steps to developing the therapeutic plan. You may be actively involved in several of these and not so involved in others. Here's a review of some of the things to consider for any respiratory infectious disease.

Much of the treatment of respiratory tract infections is **empiric therapy**, meaning that antibiotic therapy is begun without identifying the pathogenic organism or without a positive **culture** from a specimen. However we do have knowledge of specific pathogens that are common in respiratory infections. In addition we can list empirically some antibiotics that have usually been effective against these suspected pathogens. We can then develop a table that lists the site of infection and suggested "best-guess" antibiotics. See Table 14-1, which lists and matches the commonly suspected respiratory pathogens for the disease states covered in this chapter with their best-guess effective antibiotics. Of course, if treatment of respiratory infectious disease were this easy, we could end this chapter right here; therefore it is important to note that, although Table 14-1 does establish the background for this chapter, there is more to the story.

TABLE 14-1 Respiratory Infectious Diseases, Suspected Pathogens, and Initial Antimicrobial Recommendations

Disease	Suspected Pathogen(s)	Initial Antimicrobial
Childhood otitis	*Streptococcus pneumoniae, Haemophilus influenzae, Moraxella catarrhalis*	amoxicillin, azithromycin, or trimethoprim–sulfamethoxazole cefuroxime or amoxicillin clavulanate
Sinusitis	*Streptococcus pneumoniae*	amoxicillin or trimethoprim–sulfamethoxazole, azithromycin, telithromycin
Pharyngitis	Group A *Streptococcus*	penicillin
Epiglottitis	*Haemophilus influenzae*	cefuroxime or cefotaxime or ceftriaxone
Croup*	Parainfluenza viruses, respiratory syncytial virus (RSV), coronavirus, *Mycoplasma pneumoniae*	Nebulized epinephrine and glucocorticoids, azithromycin for *Mycoplasma pneumoniae*
Acute bronchitis	Viruses (most common cause), *Mycoplasma pneumoniae, Chlamydophila pneumoniae, Bordetella pertussis*	azithromycin, clarithromycin
Acute exacerbaitions of chronic bronchitis	Viral, *Haemophilus influenzae, Moraxella catarrhalis, Streptococcus pneumoniae*	azithromyin, trimethoprim-sulfamethoxazole, doxycycline, fluoroquinolones, cefpodoxime
Bronchiolitis	RSV	ribavirin for severe cases
Community-acquired pneumonia	*Streptococcus pneumoniae, Haemophilus influenzae*	See Table 14-7
Pneumonia (ventilator-associated, hospital-acquired, health-care-associated)	Gram-negative aerobic rods, *Staphylococcus aureus*	See Table 14-7

*Croup (laryngotracheitis) is usually caused by viruses. Bacterial infection may occur as a consequence of the croup. The most commonly found bacteria include *Staphylococcus aureus, Strepotococcus pneumoniae,* and *Streptococcus pyogenes* (Group A streptococcus).

14.1b Local Resistance Patterns (the Antibiogram)

Once identification of the suspected common respiratory infection's pathogens and initial choice of antibiotics have been determined, the next step is to customize that information for the particular health-care setting and practice site. Some facilities may have different resistant strains, and the first- or second-choice drug may not be effective. Many factors must be considered in choosing empiric therapy, but a key element is understanding how effective antibiotics are against the likely infecting organisms in your local community or practice setting. Most health-care systems regularly provide something called an **antibiogram**. The antibiogram is a compilation of the culture results received by the local laboratory and is usually updated yearly. It gives the types of organisms and numbers of isolates, along with a comparison of the antibiotics that are both effective and noneffective in that particular institution. You can use this to make a "best guess" of which antibiotic to use for the suspected causative infecting organism.

BVT Lab

Flashcards are available for this chapter at www.BVTLab.com.

14.1c Individualizing Therapy

With the infectious process and likely pathogen identified, you are one step closer to empiric treatment. An antibiogram from your practice setting can help narrow the antimicrobial choices. However a few more steps are still necessary. You will need several more pieces of information before you'll know what, if any, antibiotic to use. Here are some further questions you should ask:

1. Is an antibiotic really necessary?
2. Does the patient have any allergies?
3. Are there any age restrictions for the antibiotic you wish to use?
4. How might the dosage form affect your choice of antibiotic?
5. Will the antibiotic reach the site of infection?

Clinical pearl

It is important to carefully determine how many isolates or samples from the infection site were tested, from what sources the isolates were obtained, and in what physical areas in the health-care system the infected patients were located. Intensive care units (ICUs) may have very different microbial flora and antibiotic sensitivities than more general medical/surgical areas. Also specialty facilities, such as a pediatrics hospital, will not present the same picture as an adult inpatient facility.

Is an Antibiotic Really Necessary?

Many patients present with respiratory symptoms and request treatment with antibiotics. A major question all clinicians must address is whether the patient really needs antibiotics to treat the condition. Many of the conditions discussed in this chapter are viral in origin and will not respond to antibiotics. Patients who have previously recovered well after receiving an antibiotic will request antibiotics for their next illness; in fact their main reason for seeing a health-care provider may be to get an antibiotic.

Overuse of antibiotics has contributed to the rise in antibiotic resistance in the United States and throughout the world. Fortunately this rise in resistance has been met with advances in antibiotic development. However we have reached a point where new antibiotic discovery has slowed, and the antibiotics we have aren't always effective against the infectious agent, resulting in a "perfect storm" situation. It is also possible to cause a patient harm by overusing antibiotics. Some of our newer antibiotics have the potential for more significant side effects and morbidity.

Clinical pearl

It's important for both the patient and the health-care worker to understand that not all patients who have previously recovered after receiving an antibiotic did so solely because of the antibiotic. Infections sometime resolve regardless of what we do or do not do.

Does the Patient Have Any Allergies?

Penicillin allergy is fairly common, and allergies to other antibiotics are becoming more common. We must also be aware of the incidence of **cross-allergenicity**. Cephalosporins and some other β-lactam antibiotics may cause an allergic reaction in patients who are allergic to penicillins, so they should be avoided if possible in penicillin-allergic patients, especially if the reaction was severe. You need to be certain of the description of the patient's allergic reaction, as that will give you an idea of the risk to the patient. The patient needs to be questioned about the time, course, and symptoms of the allergic reaction, and this information should be carefully documented in the patient's medical record. Patients who have a history of rash to penicillin are less likely to react to the other β-lactam antibiotics and often can be safely given even penicillin. Patients who have anaphylactic reactions, or even hives, with one medication are more likely to experience cross-allergenicity (a similar severe reaction) with chemically related compounds.

Clinical pearl

There are always exceptions. Quinolone antibiotics, for example, are usually equally effective when given orally or intravenously.

Are There Any Age Restrictions for the Antibiotic You Wish to Use?

Children cannot be given all of the same antibiotics that adults can. Tetracyclines cause tooth staining and affect bone growth in developing children younger than age 8; thus they are contraindicated. Quinolones may cause bone joint disease (arthropathy) with erosions of cartilage in weight-bearing joints, so they are not recommended for children under 18 years old. The increasing development of bacterial resistance has caused some experts to recommend this class of antibiotics in children with certain diseases such as cystic fibrosis.

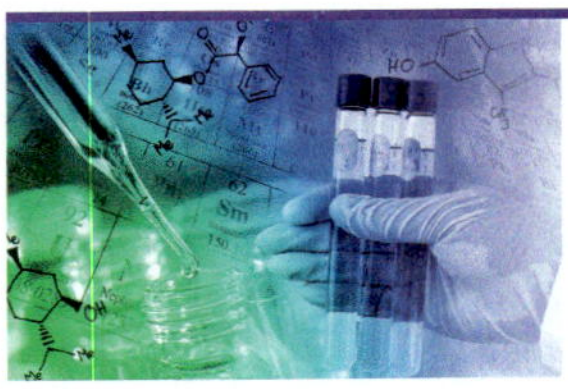

CONTROVERSY

The effects on bone joints in children relate to cartilage and are based on animal data from beagle dogs. In certain situations the benefit from using a quinolone in a child may outweigh the risk of cartilage damage.

How Might the Dosage Form Affect Your Choice of Antibiotic?

If the patient is clinically ill and requires hospitalization, you may wish to choose an intravenous dosage form. This is especially necessary if the patient is nauseated or otherwise unable to take a medication orally. In general, with the exception of quinolone and antibiotics that have oral and IV equipotent serum levels, intravenous forms give higher, faster blood levels of the antibiotic and may work more quickly.

time for review

If a patient is acutely ill and in urgent need of an antibiotic, why is it still important to check the chart for medication allergies before administering an antibiotic?

If the patient is a child, you might want a chewable or suspension form of the antibiotic if an oral dosage form is to be used. You may also want to see how these forms are flavored, as the taste of many antibiotics is very unpleasant.

Clinical pearl

Daptomycin is an example of an antibiotic that should not be used for the treatment of pneumonia because distribution to the lung is poor and the drug is inactivated by pulmonary surfactant.

Will the Antibiotic Reach the Site of Infection?

Depending on the pharmacokinetic characteristics of the antibiotic, it might not reach the site of infection at an adequate concentration to eradicate the infecting organisms. This is especially problematic when treating pneumonia. Many antibiotics do not penetrate the pulmonary or pleural tissue very well, especially when the infectious process is affecting blood flow to the area. This doesn't necessarily preclude using the antibiotic, but it may mean that a higher-than-normal dose will be required. This may be important with sinus or otitis inner ear infections as well.

Now that you know the questions to ask and the basics for developing a therapeutic plan, it's time to get more specific about different respiratory infectious diseases pertinent to the pulmonary system, starting from the top anatomically and progressing to the lower respiratory tract.

14.2 UPPER-AIRWAY INFECTIOUS DISEASES

14.2a Otitis Media

Although one may not consider ear infections pertinent to a discussion of respiratory infectious diseases, the ears' communication with the nasal passageways make them a common site for the spread of respiratory infections. **Otitis media** (see Figure 14-1), or inflammation of the middle ear, is one of the most common causes of morbidity in infants and children, even with all of the antibiotic choices available. It is estimated that more than 60% of children will have at least one episode of acute otitis media by their first birthday, and about 75% will have had an episode by age 3.

FIGURE 14-1 **Otoscopic View of Otitis Media**

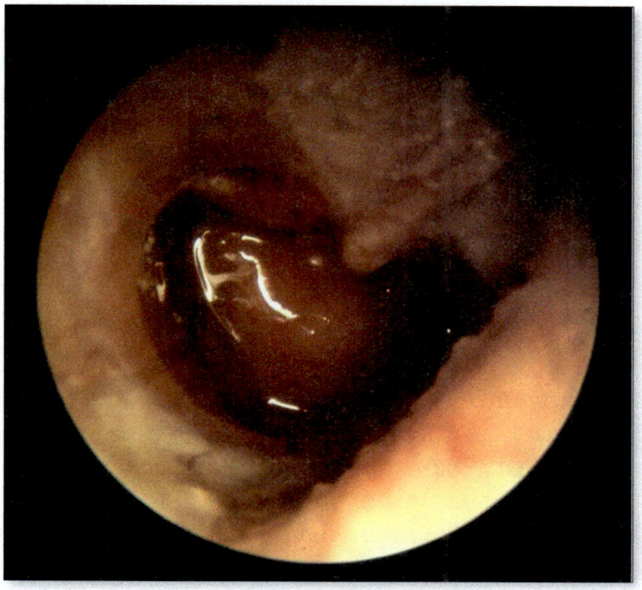

Source: Welleschik (Own work) Wikimedia Commons

Acute otitis media is most common in infancy and early childhood, peaking in incidence between the ages of 6 and 18 months. It is more common in males and in certain ethnic groups, including Native Americans and Alaskan and Canadian Eskimos. An estimated $3 billion to $4 billion are spent annually on the medical and surgical treatment of otitis media in the United States. Table 14-2 lists the factors that increase the risk of acute otitis media in children.

Diagnosis and Treatment

The clinical course of otitis media may include nonspecific symptoms, particularly in young children. Typical symptoms include irritability, ear tugging, lethargy, anorexia, fever, and/or vomiting. These usually occur in a child who has had cold symptoms of runny nose, nasal congestion, or cough.

TABLE 14-2 Factors That Increase the Risk of Otitis Media in Children

Male gender
Sibling in the home
Early age at onset of acute otitis media
Bottle feeding
Group daycare
Exposure to tobacco smoke
Nationality—Native American and Alaskan and Canadian Eskimo
Use of pacifier

The accurate diagnosis of acute otitis media is very important. The physician examines the child, looking for bulging of the tympanic membrane and/or other signs of acute inflammation and middle ear effusion. An accurate diagnosis is extremely important so antibiotics may be prescribed for children who need them and avoided when not necessary. Ibuprofen or acetaminophen may be used in all children to reduce the pain and fever. When the diagnosis is made it is reasonable to treat children under 2 years of age with appropriate antibiotics. For children over 2, the decision to treat with antibiotics can be individualized.

The use of the conjugate polysaccharide *Haemophilus influenzae* type B vaccine has been very effective at decreasing the incidence of this organism as a pathogen for otitis media and gives us proof that prevention is important in this disease. Measures should be taken to avoid exposure to allergens, irritants, and other sick individuals.

Microbial Causes

Table 14-3 lists the typical causes and their prevalence. Protection of the middle ear from microbial or viral invasion depends on the length of the eustachian tube, the pressure difference between the middle ear and the nasopharynx, and the angle of the eustachian tube opening. Infants are most likely to get otitis media, because their eustachian tubes are shorter and wider and are at a flatter angle relative to the nasopharynx than in older children or adults. Acute otitis media generally occurs when an infant develops a viral respiratory tract infection, which results in edema and congestion of the entire respiratory tract. Middle ear secretions cannot be drained into the nasopharynx because of inflammatory obstruction of the eustachian tube. These accumulated secretions become an excellent environment for the growth of bacteria.

time for review

What are some risk factors for development of otitis media?

TABLE 14-3 Microbial Causes of Acute Otitis Media

Pathogen	Percent of Cases
Streptococcus pneumoniae	~40%
Haemophilus influenzae	~20%
Moraxella catarrhalis	~20%
Streptococcus pyogenes	~3%
Staphylococcus aureus	~2%
Viral	~40%
No bacteria found	~20%

Pharmacologic Treatment

The first decision in the management of acute otitis media is whether to treat the patient with antibiotics. Children and adults with acute otitis media should receive therapy for associated symptoms; as mentioned previously, ibuprofen or acetaminophen may be used for relief of pain and fever, but these medications have not been shown to help hasten recovery from acute otitis media, nor do they help resolve effusions. Effusions are important, because they can result in hearing loss, which may also impair speech. Effusions are also relevant because the presence of fluid in the ear decreases antibiotic penetration.

Analgesics and antipyretics, such as acetaminophen or nonsteroidal anti-inflammatory agents (ibuprofen, naproxen, etc.), or aspirin, are helpful in relieving the fever and ear pain that are often present with otitis media. Aspirin is not used in children because of its association with Reye's syndrome. A significant percentage of children recover from their acute episode of otitis media with symptomatic treatment only. Clinically, there is no way to know which patients need antibiotics and which will recover on their own; therefore, as mentioned previously, the decision can be based on age and how sick the individual appears.

Most cases of acute otitis media are treated empirically, and the causative organisms are not typically isolated. Therefore, as with many common infections, it is very important to know the likely pathogens and the local resistance patterns. If treatment fails, it is likely that the infection was caused by a virus, or else the bacterium is either resistant to the drug therapy or is one that does not typically cause otitis media. The development of resistance is rapidly becoming an all-too-common problem, and all health-care providers must carefully evaluate the antibiotics to be used. An additional challenge is to use an antibiotic that will achieve a "killing" level in the fluid in the middle ear.

The three most common bacterial pathogens in acute otitis media are *Streptococcus pneumoniae, Haemophilus influenzae,* and *Moraxella catarrhalis.* Resistant strains of these bacteria have emerged and complicated the therapy choices for otitis as well as for other respiratory tract infections. There is no one preferred antimicrobial for all children or adults with acute otitis media. Amoxicillin is usually used as a first-line agent in young children. Amoxicillin achieves the highest concentrations in the middle ear effusions and should be the first choice in young children with no penicillin allergy or recurrent infection. Older children are more likely to harbor resistant organisms, owing to their prior treatment with antibiotics. First-line therapies in children over 3 years of age and adults include high-dose amoxicillin, cefuroxime axetil (Ceftin®),

Clinical pearl

Do you know someone who has had "tubes" put in his or her ears? A frequent nonpharmacologic treatment for recurrent otitis media is myringotomy and insertion of tympanostomy tubes. This procedure reduces the recurrence of otitis media by approximately 50%. The insertion of tympanostomy tubes interrupts the cycle of recurrent infections and helps prevent hearing loss.

amoxicillin–clavulanate (Augmentin®), cefpodoxime proxetil (Vantin®), and cefdinir (Omnicef®). These agents have good coverage against resistant pneumococcal infections. Patients who have received a course of antibiotics within the previous 3 months are classified as high-risk for resistance. Higher doses may be recommended in these cases.

Table 14-4 details the dosage and regimens that should be used with each of these antibiotics.

TABLE 14-4 First- and Second-Line Antibiotic Therapy for Acute Otitis Media

Antibiotic	Trade Name	Dosage Forms[a]	Dosage (for children)	Duration (days)
amoxicillin	Many	c, ch, s	40 mg/kg/day in 3 divided doses, 80–90 mg/kg/day for drug-resistant *Streptococcus pneumoniae*	10
trimethoprim sulfamethoxazole	Bactrim®, Septra®	t, s	10 mg/kg/day (trimethoprim) in 2 divided doses	10
amoxicillin clavulanate	Augmentin®	t, ch, s	80–90 mg/kg/day (amoxicillin) in 3 divided doses	10
azithromycin	Zithromax®	c, s	10 mg/kg on day 1, 5 mg/kg on days 2–5	5
cefpodoxime proxetil	Vantin®	t, s	10 mg/kg/day in 1 or 2 divided doses	10
cefprozil	Cefzil®	t, s	30 mg/kg/day in 2 divided doses	10
ceftriaxone	Rocephin®	i	50 mg/kg IM × 1 dose	1
cefuroxime	Ceftin®	t, s	30 mg/kg/day in 2 divided doses	10
clarithromycin	Biaxin®	t, s	15 mg/kg/day in 2 divided doses	10

[a]t, tablet; c, capsule; i, injectable; s, suspension; ch, chewable.

14.2b Sinusitis

Clinical pearl

The classification of acute versus chronic, while it may seem minor, is an important distinction that in itself can affect antibiotic choice in treating sinusitis and several other infections. The definitions of acute versus chronic are not consistent for all infections.

Acute **sinusitis**, an inflammation of the mucosal lining of the paranasal sinuses, affects both children and adults. It is estimated to affect 31 to 35 million Americans per year and can exacerbate asthma attacks and trigger other pulmonary disease. Children experience an average of six to eight viral infections of the upper respiratory tract each year; adults experience two to three. Of these upper respiratory tract infections, approximately 0.5% will be complicated by acute sinusitis. Bacterial sinusitis can be either acute or chronic. Chronic sinusitis is defined as lasting more than 3 months. It is not known if this is due to more virulent pathogens or an immune function decrease in the patient.

Sinusitis occurs when the mucociliary transport mechanism of the ciliary pseudocolumnar epithelium is impaired and pathogens are allowed to remain in the sinus cavities. Mucopurulent rhinorrhea (discharge from the nasal passages consisting of mucus and pus), postnasal drip, facial pain, maxillary toothache, cough, fever, nausea, and congestion preceded by an upper respiratory infection are typical complaints of patients with acute sinusitis. The persistence of nasal discharge and a cough for more than 10 days following an upper respiratory infection are indicative of sinusitis. Previously clear, thin nasal discharge may become mucoid or purulent, with an increase in both viscosity and quantity.

A poor response of these symptoms to decongestant medication gives clues that sinusitis may be the culprit. Headaches caused by sinusitis respond poorly to analgesics, and the pain usually corresponds directly to the sinuses affected. Adults typically experience the feeling of fullness or dull ache associated with an infection in the frontal sinuses.

Nasal allergies contribute to the edema and swelling of the nasal mucosa, but little evidence is available that actually links allergy to acute sinusitis. Barotrauma from deep-sea diving and airplane travel are also recognized precipitating factors for sinusitis. Chemical irritants such as chlorine may impair secretion clearance and thus foster development of sinusitis.

Clinical pearl

Children under the age of 5 most likely will not have frontal sinusitis symptoms, as their frontal sinuses have not fully developed. (This is also why they have those cute round faces.)

Diagnosis and Treatment

A computerized tomography (CT) scan is considered the "gold standard" for evaluating sinusitis but is a very expensive diagnostic tool. Sinus aspiration is the only definitive way of determining the presence of infection. Sinus X-rays can help the physician detect mucosal thickening, air–fluid levels, or sinus opacification. However a normal sinus X-ray does not rule out sinusitis, and sinus films have high false-positive and false-negative rates. Transillumination of the frontal and maxillary sinuses is a simple and inexpensive test that is done in a darkened room with a high-intensity light source. The presence of an opacified sinus can be detected in this fashion and is diagnostic of acute sinusitis in a patient with previously normal sinuses. The diagnosis is most often made clinically based on the history and physical exam.

Microbial Causes

Most cases of acute sinusitis are due to viruses. As noted in Table 14-5, the most common bacterial causes of sinusitis in both children and adults are *Streptococcus pneumoniae* and *Haemophilus influenza*. Empiric antibiotic coverage is generally focused on these organisms.

TABLE 14-5 Etiology of Acute Sinusitis

Type	Species	Adults
Bacteria	*Streptococcus pneumoniae, Haemophilus influenzae*	70%
	Moraxella catarrhalis	30%

time for review

Are *Streptococcus pneumoniae* and *Staphylococcus aureus* gram-positive or gram-negative organisms?

Pharmacologic Treatment

Clinical pearl

Rebound congestion occurs when topical decongestants are used for more than 3 days in a row. Use beyond the recommended time frame makes the congestion worse, not better. The fancy medical term for this is *rhinitis medicamentosa.*

The treatment of sinusitis is most effective when the cause is clearly identified, yet sinus aspiration isn't often done. It is controversial whether antimicrobial treatment should be used for sinuses, because viruses are the most frequent culprit. Therapies for chronic sinusitis are focused on control of symptoms, whereas antibiotics are required for acute bacterial sinusitis. The medications used for symptomatic relief have not been proven to reduce the duration of the illness, but at least they can make the patient feel better until the infection resolves. Intranasal cromolyn, antihistamines, intranasal corticosteroids, and topical decongestants are all used to treat or prevent symptoms. Intranasal cromolyn can help to protect the sinus mucosa from an allergic response that would contribute to the sinusitis. Oral first-generation antihistamines can also help prevent an allergic response but should be used cautiously, as they can make the nasal secretions more viscous, interfering with the clearance of purulent mucous secretions. Intranasal corticosteroids are very effective for allergic rhinitis and may help control chronic sinusitis symptoms. The topical decongestants (phenylephrine and oxymetazoline) may facilitate nasal drainage but should only be used for less than 72 hours, because they induce tolerance and rebound congestion. Irrigation of the nasal cavity with a saline solution is also effective for providing symptomatic relief, especially when the nasal mucosa are dry.

A 2012 guideline from the Infectious Diseases Society of America (IDSA) recommends withholding antimicrobials and observing patients with mild symptoms for up to 3 days. If symptoms worsen, antimicrobials should be initiated promptly. Empiric therapy should be directed at the common organisms *Streptococcus pneumoniae* and *Haemophilus influenzae.* Many antibiotics are effective against sinusitis, but we must always consider bacterial resistance and choose therapies that are effective without inducing resistance. Amoxicillin and, in a penicillin-allergic patient, trimethoprim–sulfamethoxazole have long been and are still considered first-line therapies for acute sinusitis when treatment with antimicrobials is recommended. Amoxicillin will be ineffective against β-lactamase–producing microorganism and/or *Streptococcus pneumoniae* that is highly resistant to penicillin. *Streptococcus pneumoniae* has also developed significant resistance to macrolides and may require treatment with an oral second- or third-generation cephalosporin such as cefuroxime axetil or cefpodoxime, respectively.

If the patient does not respond in 72 hours to amoxicillin or trimethoprim–sulfamethoxazole, antibiotic therapy should be changed to an agent that is less likely to have developed bacterial resistance. Usually this means changing to high-dose amoxicillin, amoxicillin clavulanate, a second- or third-generation cephalosporin (cefuroxime axetil, cefixime, cefaclor), or an antistreptococcal quinolone (levofloxacin is generally the preferred quinolone, as ciprofloxacin and ofloxacin have poor *S. pneumoniae* activity). Macrolides (azithromycin, telithromycin, and clarithromycin) are also effective against the common pathogens and are rapidly becoming the drugs of choice. Health-care professionals should use local resistance patterns (e.g., antibiogram discussed previously) to understand resistance trends within the community. Table 14-6 describes the antibiotics generally used for acute sinusitis. Duration of therapy recommendations are for 10 to 14 days or at least a week after signs and symptoms are controlled.

Clinical pearl

The current 2012 IDSA guideline recommends that antimicrobial regimens for sinusitis should be continued for 5 to 7 days.

TABLE 14-6 Antimicrobial Regimens for Adult Acute Sinusitis

Antimicrobial Agent	Brand Name	Oral Dose in Adults
amoxicillin	Various	500 mg q 8 hrs
amoxicillin clavulanate	Augmentin®	500 mg q 8 hrs or 875 mg q 12 hrs
azithromycin	Zithromax®	500 mg/day, then 250 mg/day × 4 days
cefuroxime	Ceftin®	250–500 mg q 12 hrs
cefaclor	Ceclor®	250–500 mg q 8 hrs
cefixime	Suprax®	200–400 mg q 12 hrs
clarithromycin	Biaxin®	250–500 mg q 12 hrs
levofloxacin	Levaquin®	500 mg q 24 hrs
trimethoprim–sulfamethoxazole	Bactrim® DS, Septra® DS*	trimethoprim 160 mg, sulfamethoxazole 800 mg (per tablet) q 12 hrs

*Each Bactrim® DS or Septra® DS tablet contains 160 mg of trimethoprim and 800 mg of sulfamethoxazole.

14.2c Pharyngitis

Pharyngitis (sore throat) is an inflammation of the pharynx and surrounding lymphoid tissue that may be caused by bacteria or viruses (see Figure 14-2). The evaluation, diagnosis, and treatment of patients with pharyngitis is a common problem in primary care. The occurrence of a sore throat is associated with more than 10% of physician office visits, while less than 20% of those patients who experience a sore throat actually seek care.

Clinical pearl

Acetaminophen is the preferred agent for sore throat pain because of some association of nonsteroidal anti-inflammatory drugs with toxic shock syndrome.

Microbial Causes

Viruses cause most pharyngitis; they are generally the same ones that cause the common cold (rhinovirus, coronavirus, adenovirus, and parainfluenza virus). Other viral causes include herpes simplex virus, influenza virus, coxsackievirus, Epstein-Barr virus, and cytomegalovirus (CMV). However some pharyngitis (10% to 30%) is the result of bacterial infection, most commonly with Group A β-hemolytic streptococci such as *Streptococcus pyogenes*. Acute bacterial pharyngitis can also be caused by Group C and G streptococci, *Arcanobacterium haemolyticum*, and, possibly, *Mycoplasma pneumoniae* or *Chlamydophila pneumoniae*.

FIGURE 14-2 Severe Pharyngitis

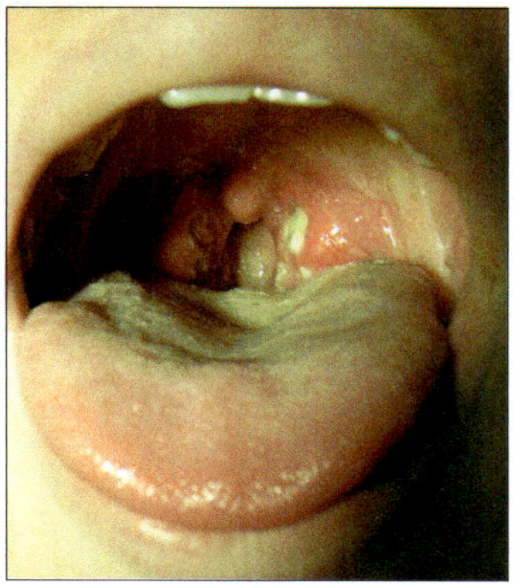

Source: By James Heilman, MD (Own work) Wikimedia Commons.

BVT Lab

Visit www.BVTLab.com to explore the student resources available for this chapter.

Diagnosis and Treatment

Most often pharyngitis is self-limiting, lasting from 2 to 7 days. The major symptom is sore throat, with or without associated dysphagia (difficulty swallowing). Fever is typically present. Examination usually reveals erythema and possible exudate (white patches), and mucosal congestion is present. The presence of an exudate with fever usually suggests a bacterial infection, but a culture or rapid antigen detection test ("quick strep test") should be obtained to confirm the causative organism. The rapid antigen detection test allows the diagnosis of Group A β-hemolytic *Streptococcus* (GAS) infection within 5 minutes. This test is very specific for Group A β-hemolytic *Streptococcus,* and patients with a positive test can be treated immediately without waiting for culture results. Unfortunately a negative test does not rule out the possibility of a GAS infection, and a throat culture may be necessary. Bacterial eradication occurs in 48 to 72 hours of treatment, which is important in decreasing transmission.

time for review

How long should children be kept home when they have strep throat, and why?

Complications of untreated pharyngitis include spread of the infection to the tonsils, retropharyngeal abscess, cervical lymphadenitis, otitis media, sinusitis, and mastoiditis. Another complication is acute rheumatic fever (common before the second half of the twentieth century and the advent of antibiotics). The most serious of the sequelae of acute rheumatic fever is heart valve damage.

Pharmacologic Treatment

Penicillin has long been the antibiotic of choice for pharyngitis. Even with the development of antimicrobial resistance, Group A *Streptococcus* remains susceptible to penicillin, and penicillin remains the drug of choice for this infection. Children younger than 12 years of age should receive 50 mg/kg/day, divided into three doses, of penicillin V for 10 days; or an injection of benzathine penicillin, 50,000 U/kg IM, as a single dose. For adolescents and adults, penicillin V, 500 mg twice daily for 10 days, should be given. In the penicillin-allergic patient, azithromycin 500 mg orally on day 1, followed by 250 mg daily on days 2 through 5 (12 mg/kg/day in kids under 27 kg) or clindamycin are acceptable alternatives. See Figure 14-3 for a sample protocol for treating pharyngitis.

FIGURE 14-3 Protocol for Treating Pharyngitis

Question the patient:

- Absence of cough?
- Exudate present?
- History of fever >38°C or >100°F?
- Swollen, tender anterior cervical nodes?

Number of Criteria Met	Likelihood of Group A β-Hemolytic *Streptococcus*	Suggested Action
0 1	2% – 3% 3% – 7%	No culture indicated and no antibiotics required
2 3	8% – 16% 19% – 34%	Culture, treat if culture is positive
4	41% – 61%	Culture, treat with antibiotics if clinically indicated regardless of culture results[a]

[a]If patient has a high fever, is clinically unwell, and presents early in disease course.

time for review

Why might it be appropriate for you, the health-care worker, to encourage a patient with a history of respiratory disease and a sore throat to see a physician?

14.3 OTHER UPPER-AIRWAY INFECTIONS

14.3a Epiglottitis

Epiglottitis is an airway emergency whereby *Haemophilus influenzae* type B causes acute airway obstruction. It is most prevalent in children ages 2 to 6 and requires rapid recognition and treatment. Since the introduction of the universal *Haemophilus influenza* type B (Hib) vaccine, the incidence is decreasing.

Learning Hint

Respiratory distress, drooling, dysphagia, and dysphonia are the four Ds that are signs of the dangerous disease, epiglottitis.

Diagnosis and Treatment

Onset is fast, and fever and sore throat are usually the first symptoms. Epiglottitis is nonseasonal, and recurrence is rare. Respiratory distress, drooling, inspiratory stridor, loss of voice, and intercostal retractions are common manifestations.

Microbial Causes

Airway maintenance is the mainstay of treatment, with antibiotic therapy empirically selected against *H. influenzae* type B, although other pathogens, such as penicillin-resistant *Pneumococcus*, β-hemolytic *Streptococci*, and *Staphylococcus aureus* (including MRSA), can still cause the disease.

Pharmacologic Treatment

The preferred treatments are cefotaxime (150–225 mg/kg/day) or ceftriaxone (80–100 mg/kg/day) + clindamycin or vancomycin (added in severely ill patients for staphylococcal coverage).

14.3b Croup

Learning Hint

Clinical presentation of croup is that of a barking cough and inspiratory stridor.

Croup is different from epiglottitis but also results from infections of the laryngeal area. It, too, can cause airway obstruction and is characterized by noisy breathing, especially on inspiration. The medical term for croup is laryngotracheitis (now you know why it's easier to just call it croup).

Microbial Causes

Croup is usually caused by viruses, while bacterial infection may occur after a previous viral infection. Bacterial causes include *Staphylococcus aureus,* Group A β-hemolytic *Streptococci,* and *Pneumococci,* while milder cases may be caused by *Mycoplasma*. Parainfluenza types I and II cause viral croup.

Diagnosis and Treatment

Croup progresses slowly, usually at night. Fever is uncommon. It is most common in late spring and late fall. Children younger than 3 years old most commonly get croup. It is characterized by stridor and no drooling. Treatment consists of air humidification and oxygen.

Pharmacologic Treatment

Pharmacologic therapy starts with nebulized racemic epinephrine and corticosteroids to decrease swelling and inflammation. If a subsequent bacterial infection develops, empiric antibiotic treatment for the bacteria may be necessary after appropriate cultures are obtained with a regimen that would be similar to the one recommended above for epiglottitis.

Now that we have discussed upper respiratory tract infections, we will move down to lower respiratory tract infections, including bronchitis, bronchiolitis, pneumonia, and tuberculosis.

LIFE SPAN CONSIDERATIONS

Bordetella pertussis is a highly contagious infection that is often not considered as a cause of upper respiratory tract infections. It should be considered as a potential cause of a prolonged upper respiratory infection and cough that fails to resolve after 2 weeks. This is true even if the childhood DTP vaccination was given. Erythromycin is still the antibiotic of choice and is given for at least 14 days.

14.4 LOWER RESPIRATORY TRACT INFECTIONS

14.4a Acute Bronchitis and Bronchiolitis

Acute **bronchitis** and **bronchiolitis** are inflammatory conditions of the large and small airways of the tracheobronchial tree. They are usually associated with a respiratory infection. The inflammatory/infectious process in these two conditions does not extend to the alveoli. The treatment of chronic bronchitis was covered in Chapter 13, as it is primarily an inflammatory process. Acute bronchitis occurs in all ages and is seen most commonly in the winter months, following a pattern very similar to that of other acute respiratory tract infections. Damp, cold climates, the presence of respiratory pollutants in the air, or cigarette smoke can precipitate acute attacks. Bronchiolitis is the term for this disease in infants.

Diagnosis and Treatment

Acute bronchitis is usually a self-limiting illness and rarely leads to further complications. In general, infection in the trachea and bronchi leads to increased bronchial secretions and may affect bronchial mucociliary function. The secretions may become thick and tenacious, further affecting mucociliary activity. Acute bronchitis generally begins in the upper airways, and patients present with nonspecific complaints including headache, malaise, and sore throat.

Clinical Pearl

Cough is the hallmark symptom that distinguishes bronchitis from other upper-airway infections, such as pharyngitis.

The cough may develop slowly or rapidly and the symptoms persist despite resolution of the preceding nasal symptoms or sore throat. The cough usually progresses, becoming productive, with mucopurulent sputum. Fever is not usually present. The chest exam may reveal rhonchi and coarse crackles bilaterally, and the chest X-ray is usually normal. This respiratory condition is almost always caused by a virus, so cultures are not useful.

Most infants have symptoms suggestive of an upper respiratory tract infection for 2 to 7 days before the onset of bronchiolitis. These infants are usually irritable and restless, with a mild fever. Again the most common clinical sign is cough. As the infection progresses, the infant may experience vomiting, diarrhea, noisy upper-airway breathing, and an increased respiratory rate. Infants who require hospitalization have noisy, labored breathing, with tachypnea and tachycardia. Many of these infants have a mild conjunctivitis, and 5% to 10% may also have otitis media. Because of their increased work of breathing and coughing, combined with fever, the infants are frequently dehydrated. Diagnosis is made according to clinical symptoms and history. There are several other diseases in infants (asthma, foreign body obstruction, gastroesophageal reflux, etc.) that can present with similar clinical symptoms.

In adults acute bronchitis is almost always self-limiting, and the goals of therapy should be to provide comfort to the patient. Guidelines from the Centers for Disease Control and Prevention state that the only indication for antibiotics is acute bronchitis due to pertussis. Unfortunately antibiotic prescriptions for this condition are common. In the well infant, bronchiolitis is also usually a self-limiting disease, and all that is necessary is to wait for the underlying viral infection to resolve. Hospitalization is necessary for a child suffering from respiratory failure or dehydration.

Microbial Causes

Viruses are the most common infectious agents that cause bronchitis. The common cold viruses, influenza virus, adenovirus, respiratory syncytial virus (RSV), and coronavirus are most often involved. In infants and children, the same pathogens are usually involved. Even though it has been suggested that the same bacterial pathogens that cause pneumonia such as *Streptococcus pneumoniae, Moraxella catarrhalis, Haemophilus influenzae,* and *Staphylococcus aureus* can cause bronchitis, there is no convincing evidence that this is the case.

Bronchiolitis is an acute viral infection of the lower respiratory tract of infants. The peak attack age for children is between the ages of 2 and 10 months. Incidence spikes in the winter months and persists through the spring. Bronchiolitis is one of the major reasons that infants under the age of 6 months require hospitalization. RSV is the most common cause of bronchiolitis, accounting for over 50% of cases. Certain times of the year can bring almost epidemic incidence of RSV, with over 80% of bronchiolitis cases during those times caused by the virus. Parainfluenza virus types 1, 2, and 3 cause most of the rest of the cases of bronchiolitis. Bacteria only rarely cause this disease.

Pharmacologic Treatment

Clinical pearl

Patients should be cautioned not to use any of the over-the-counter combinations that might dry secretions (mostly those containing antihistamines), as they could aggravate the condition and prolong the recovery time.

Acute Bronchitis The most common medications used are for symptomatic therapy. Analgesics, antipyretics, or acetaminophen are helpful in reducing the malaise, lethargy, and fever in adults. Patients with acute bronchitis frequently self-medicate with over-the-counter cough and cold remedies, although there is no evidence that any of these various combination therapies are effective.

Persistent cough may require nighttime suppression with dextromethorphan. More severe cough may require intermittent treatment with codeine- or hydrocodone-containing cough mixtures. One should avoid suppressing a productive cough except when it is persistent enough to disrupt sleep.

Bronchiolitis Aerosolized β-adrenergic therapy has been used to treat bronchiolitis. It is probably best used in the child who has shown some symptoms of bronchospasm, and the response should be monitored before and after therapy. Inhaled or systemic corticosteroids have not been shown to be conclusively beneficial. Because bacteria rarely cause bronchiolitis, antibiotics should not be used routinely. Ribavirin may offer benefit to a small number of bronchiolitis cases. This agent is effective against respiratory syncytial virus (RSV). Use of the aerosolized drug requires special nebulizer equipment (small-particle aerosol generator) and specifically trained personnel for administration via an oxygen hood or mist tent. Special care must be taken to avoid drug particle deposition and clogging of respiratory tubing and valves in mechanical ventilators.

Controversy

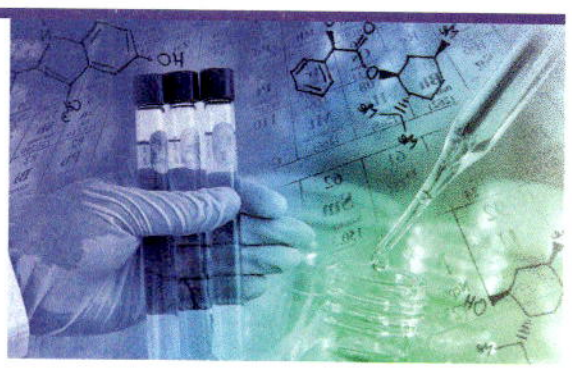

Use of antibiotics for acute bronchitis is not recommended. Unfortunately antibiotic prescriptions for this condition are common. The clinician should stay vigilant for a bacterial infection such as pneumonia that may develop later. It is important to remember that the cough from acute bronchitis lasts from 1 to 3 weeks. Acute bronchitis from *Bordetella pertussis* would respond to antibiotics but is only responsible for about 1% of U.S. cases.

Most experts recommend reserving ribavirin for severely ill and/or immunocompromised children, especially those with serious underlying disorders such as bronchopulmonary dysplasia, congenital heart disease, prematurity, or immunodeficiency disorders.

14.4b Pneumonia

Pneumonia is the sixth-leading cause of death in the United States as well as one of the most common causes of hospitalization. It is defined as an inflammation of the lung tissue and may be caused by bacteria, viruses, or even noninfectious agents such as drugs or chemicals. The principal site of infection is in the alveoli and surrounding interstitial tissue.

Individuals with pneumonia classically present with high white blood cell counts, high fevers, crackles, rhonchi, bronchial breath sounds, and dullness to percussion over the involved areas of the lung. Patients with pneumonia may have pleural effusions, and their chest X-rays usually reveal infiltrates or signs of consolidation. Patients with pneumonia are far more likely to experience complications such as hypoxia, cardiopulmonary failure, local abscesses or empyemas, and possible spread of infection to other organs by way of the bloodstream. There are several well-defined categories of pneumonia that help to define appropriate therapy, and we will review this disease according to these subclassifications.

Community-Acquired Pneumonia

Community-acquired pneumonia (CAP) is an infection of the lung tissue that, in its purest definition, is contracted outside the institutional setting (institutional meaning nursing homes, hospitals, or any other place that might encourage the transmission of bacteria between compromised individuals). This definition by setting has evolved to be more a description of the likely pathogens than a delineation of where the disease was contracted. *Streptococcus pneumoniae, Haemophilus influenzae, Mycoplasma pneumoniae, Chlamydophila pneumoniae,* a variety of respiratory viruses, and *Legionella* spp account for the majority of cases of CAP, with *S. pneumoniae* responsible for a majority of the cases of acute CAP. Gram-negative bacteria and *Staphylococcus aureus* are uncommon causes of CAP but are more likely in patients who have taken antibiotics or have underlying respiratory diseases.

The most significant problem in the treatment of CAP is the growing resistance of *Streptococcus pneumoniae* to antimicrobials. This increasing resistance, combined with the much wider variety of organisms causing the disease, has made diagnosis and treatment a much greater therapeutic challenge.

Atypical Pneumonia The term *atypical pneumonia* has been in use in the medical literature for over a century to refer to a subset of CAP organisms (e.g., *Legionella* spp, *Chlamydophila pneumoniae, Mycoplasma pneumoniae*). Since there is no way to distinguish "typical vs. atypical" CAP pathogens clinically, this term should no longer be used.

Over the years many other organisms, including viruses and fungi, have been found to cause pneumonia. All of these causes other than *S. pneumoniae, M. catarrhalis,* and *H. influenzae* were lumped into the classification of atypical pneumonia. Before the outbreak and identification of a new organism, *Legionella pneumophila,* at the 1976 Philadelphia convention of the American Legion, and the increasingly common incidence of *Chlamydophila pneumoniae* and *Mycoplasma* infections, atypical pneumonia was generally mild and self-limiting, with very low mortality. These new atypical pneumonias were much more deadly and made the "atypical" classification very imprecise. Physicians had to rethink the diagnosis and treatment of community-acquired pneumonia to allow for the presence of these atypical organisms.

Mycoplasma pneumoniae infections tend to follow epidemic patterns, with outbreaks every 4 to 8 years making it hard to define its true incidence. *Legionella* tends to infect older and more immunocompromised patients. It also has a more seasonal occurrence, tending to break out in the spring, when air conditioning is started. *Chlamydia* tends to infect young people such as college students and military recruits.

When you analyze the signs, symptoms, and chest X-rays of patients infected with these three atypical pathogens, very little difference can be seen between atypical and typical pneumonia. *Mycoplasma* may be more slow and insidious and *Legionella* more rapidly progressive, but that is not standard for all. The only real difference between the atypical organisms (*Chlamydia, Legionella,* and *Mycoplasma)* and the typical pneumonia organisms (*S. pneumoniae, M. catarrhalis,* and *H. influenzae*) is that the atypical organisms cannot be cultured with standard microbiologic media or techniques, and they do not respond to treatment with penicillins or other antibiotics classically used for typical pneumonia.

Whereas "typical" pneumonia tends to affect patients with some other chronic illness and who are older than 50 years of age, atypical pneumonia tends to affect young adults with no underlying illness. Typical pneumonia tends to have a rapid onset and high fever, whereas atypical pneumonia may be more insidious in onset. However, it has become very difficult to distinguish atypical infections from typical infections clinically as the atypical organisms have become more virulent and *S. pneumoniae* has become more resistant to therapy. Current recommendations from the American Thoracic Society and Infectious Diseases Society of America for the treatment of CAP recommend that empiric therapy should cover both the "typical" and "atypical" causative organisms.

Therapy Recommendations for CAP and Atypical Pneumonias In the past, antibiotic therapy for CAP was fairly simple. It was quite likely that *S. pneumoniae* was the causative organism, and the pneumococcus responded very well to treatment with penicillin. However as early as 1967, resistant pneumococcus began to show up. We are now faced with 20% to 40% of *S. pneumoniae* strains showing resistance to penicillin. *S. pneumoniae* still accounts for the majority of CAP cases, but other organisms are creeping up in incidence. Because eradication of the offending organism is one of our major treatment goals in pneumonia, appropriate empiric antibiotic therapy is a major challenge. Therapy should minimize any associated morbidity and not cause any drug-induced side effects or organ dysfunction.

The first priority in the treatment of pneumonia is to evaluate the patient's respiratory function and to determine if the patient requires hospitalization or can be treated as an outpatient. Patients may require intravenous fluids, oxygen, bronchodilators, chest physiotherapy with postural drainage, or even mechanical ventilation. The second priority in hospitalized patients is to obtain cultures of the sputum and to use other diagnostic procedures to determine the microbiologic cause of the acute disease. Assessing the patient's clinical setting can help the choice of empiric therapy once you understand what pathogens are likely in specific patient populations. Table 14-7 can help you consider these circumstances.

TABLE 14-7 Empiric Antibiotic Choices for Adult Pneumonias

Clinical Setting	Likely Pathogen	Therapy
Elderly patient, from nursing home or other care facility (health-care-associated pneumonia)	*Streptococcus pneumoniae, Moraxella catarrhalis, Haemophilus influenzae, Klebsiella pneumoniae, Staphylococcus aureus, Pseudomonas aeruginosa*	piperacillin-tazobactam, third- or fourth-generation cephalosporin, imipenem-cilastatin, or meropenem
History of chronic obstructive pulmonary disease (COPD)	*Streptococcus pneumoniae*	azithromycin, doxycycline or clarithromycin plus either cefpodoxime or cefuroxime, respiratory fluoroquinolone (levofloxacin or moxifloxacin)
Alcoholic	*Streptococcus pneumoniae, Klebsiella pneumoniae, Staphylococcus aureus, Haemophilus influenzae,* possibly anaerobes from the oral cavity	ampicillin-sulbactam, piperacillin-tazobactam plus aminoglycoside, imipenem-cilastatin or meropenem, fluoroquinolone, vancomycin (if MRSA suspected)
Previously healthy, ambulatory patient (CAP)	*Streptococcus pneumoniae, Mycoplasma pneumoniae*	clarithromycin, azithromycin, or doxycycline
Aspiration pneumonia	Anaerobes from the oral cavity, *Staphylococcus aureus,* gram-negative enteric organisms	penicillin, clindamycin, ampicillin-sulbactam
Ventilator-associated (VAP) or hospital-acquired (HAP) pneumonia	Gram-negative bacilli such as *Klebsiella pneumoniae, Enterobacter* spp, *Pseudomonas aeruginosa, Staphylococcus aureus*	piperacillin-tazobactam, imipenem-cilastatin or meropenem, or expanded-spectrum cephalosporins such as ceftazidime or cefepime plus an aminoglycoside, fluoroquinolone

The empiric antibiotic choices for the treatment of community-acquired pneumonia are no longer very simple. In the past all patients with the clinical picture of pneumonia were started on penicillin, because *S. pneumoniae* was the most likely and the most aggressive of the likely organisms causing the infection. As *S. pneumoniae* continues to become more resistant to penicillin and the offending agent is often not identified, empiric therapy is guided by local resistance patterns in addition to considering the patient's clinical setting, prior exposure to antibiotics, clinical condition, chest X-ray, and underlying state of health.

Guidelines for the treatment of CAP continue to be revised, and the clinician must be careful to review current literature for the most up-to-date recommendations. The American Thoracic Society and the Infectious Diseases Society of America published a joint guideline in 2007. They recommend macrolides (erythromycin, clarithromycin, or azithromycin) or doxycycline (or tetracycline) for children aged 8 years or older, or an oral β-lactam with good antipneumococcal activity (cefuroxime axetil, amoxicillin, amoxicillin clavulanate) as the first-line therapies for CAP. An oral fluoroquinolone with improved activity against *S. pneumoniae* (levofloxacin, moxifloxacin, gatifloxacin) may be used for the treatment of adults for whom one of these regimens has already failed, or who are allergic to the alternative agents, or who have a documented infection with a highly drug-resistant pneumococcus. The fluoroquinolones should not be used in children. For children younger than 5 years, in whom atypical pathogens are uncommon and for whom doxycycline and fluoroquinolones should be avoided, β-lactams are the best choice.

Health-Care-Associated (HCAP), Ventilator-Associated (VAP), or Hospital-Acquired (HAP) Pneumonia

The common thread for these types of pneumonias is exposure to or frequent contact with various health-care settings. Pneumonia is the second most common hospital-acquired infection in the United States and is associated with substantial morbidity and mortality. Most patients who have so-called VAP, HAP, or HCAP are persons who have severe underlying disease, are immunosuppressed, are comatose, or are otherwise incapacitated and have cardiopulmonary disease. In addition some health-care-associated pneumonia patients are persons who have had thoracic or abdominal surgery. Although patients receiving mechanical ventilation do not represent a major proportion of patients who have pneumonia, they are at highest risk for acquiring a VAP.

Pneumonias caused by *Legionella* spp, *Aspergillus* spp, and influenza virus are often caused by inhalation of contaminated aerosols. RSV infection usually occurs after viral inoculation of the conjunctivae or nasal mucosa by contaminated hands. Traditional preventive measures for VAP, HCAP, or HAP include taking precautions to decrease aspiration by the patient, preventing cross-contamination or colonization via hands of personnel, appropriate disinfection or sterilization of respiratory therapy devices, use of available vaccines to protect against particular infections, and education of hospital staff and patients. Figure 14-4 describes the pathogenesis of pneumonia acquired from health-care settings.

Clinical pearl

Because intubation and mechanical ventilation alter first-line patient respiratory defenses, they greatly increase the risk for health-care-associated bacterial pneumonia. There are VAP protocols for mechanically ventilated patients to try to lessen or prevent pneumonia occurrence; these include increasing the head of the bed, peptic ulcer disease and deep venous thrombosis (DVT) prophylaxis, daily oral care with chlorohexadine, closed system suctioning, and changing the ventilator circuit when needed.

FIGURE 14-4 Pathogenesis of Health-Care-Associated Bacterial Pneumonia

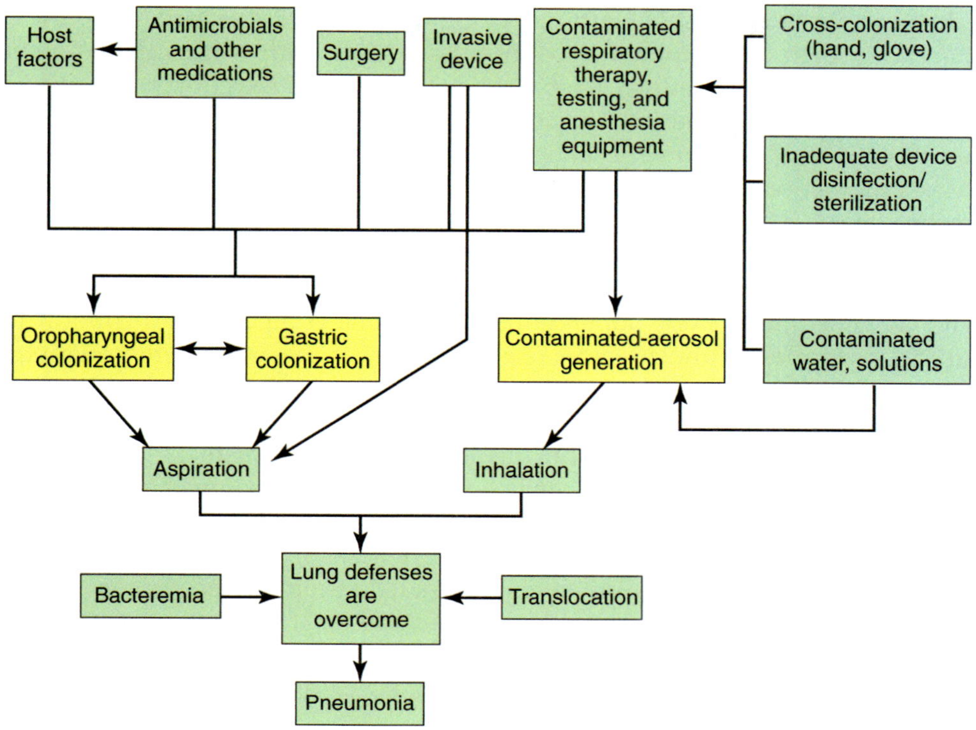

Recent epidemiologic studies have identified other subsets of patients who are at high risk for acquiring health-care-associated bacterial pneumonia. Such patients include persons older than 70 years; persons who have endotracheal intubation and/or mechanically assisted ventilation, a depressed level of consciousness (particularly those with closed-head injury), or underlying chronic lung disease; and persons who have previously had an episode of a large-volume aspiration. Other risk factors include 24-hour ventilator circuit changes, hospitalization during the fall or winter, stress-bleeding prophylaxis with cimetidine (either with or without antacid), administration of antimicrobials, presence of a nasogastric tube, severe trauma, and recent bronchoscopy.

HCAP, HAP, or VAP has been associated with mortality rates of 20% to 50%. Patients receiving mechanically assisted ventilation have higher mortality rates than patients not receiving ventilation support; however other factors (e.g., the patient's underlying disease and organ failure) are stronger predictors of death in patients who have pneumonia. Ventilator-associated pneumonia (VAP) is difficult to diagnose, but seems to correlate with the duration of mechanical ventilation.

The high incidence of gram-negative bacillary pneumonia in hospitalized patients might result from factors that promote colonization of the pharynx by gram-negative bacilli and the subsequent entry of these organisms into the lower respiratory tract. Although aerobic gram-negative bacilli are recovered infrequently or are found in low numbers in pharyngeal cultures of healthy persons, the likelihood of colonization increases substantially in comatose patients, in patients treated with antimicrobial agents, and in patients who have hypotension, acidosis, azotemia, alcoholism, diabetes mellitus, leukocytosis, leukopenia, pulmonary disease, or nasogastric or endotracheal tubes in place.

Bacteria also can enter the lower respiratory tract of hospitalized patients through inhalation of aerosols generated primarily by contaminated respiratory therapy or anesthesia-breathing equipment. Outbreaks related to the use of respiratory therapy equipment have been associated with contaminated nebulizers. When the fluid in the reservoir of a nebulizer becomes contaminated with bacteria, the aerosol produced may contain high concentrations of bacteria that can be deposited deep in the patient's lower respiratory tract. Contaminated aerosol inhalation is particularly hazardous for intubated patients, because endotracheal and tracheal tubes provide direct access to the lower respiratory tract.

Several large studies have examined the potential risk factors for bacterial pneumonias acquired in a health-care setting. Although specific risk factors have differed among study populations, they can be grouped into the following general categories: (1) host factors (e.g., extremes of age and severe underlying conditions, including immunosuppression); (2) factors that enhance colonization of the oropharynx and/or stomach by microorganisms (e.g., administration of antimicrobials, acid-suppression medications, admission to an ICU, underlying chronic lung disease, or coma); (3) conditions that favor aspiration or reflux (e.g., endotracheal intubation, insertion of a nasogastric tube, or supine position); (4) conditions that require prolonged use of mechanical ventilatory support with potential exposure to contaminated respiratory equipment and/or contact with contaminated or colonized hands of health-care workers (HCWs); and (5) factors that impede adequate pulmonary toilet (e.g., undergoing surgical procedures that involve the head, neck, thorax, or upper abdomen, or being immobilized as a result of trauma or illness).

By sorting out these risk categories, the clinician can better define the likely pathogens and then choose the most appropriate empiric antibiotic therapy. Each patient is different, and individual analyses must be made. Table 14-7 showed some of the likely pathogens causing pneumonia in a health-care setting and the general antibiotic choices. Most of these antibiotics can be considered the "big guns" of the antibiotic world. They are costly, require parenteral therapy, have significant toxicities, and require close monitoring. In general selection of antibiotics for a patient with HCAP, VAP, or HAP requires an antibiotic to cover gram-negative pathogens as well as the more common pneumonia pathogens. Most patients require more than one antibiotic to cover the entire spectrum of likely organisms. If a culture is obtained and the pathogenic organisms are isolated, the antibiotic regimen may be simplified or narrowed to specifically cover the isolated organisms.

Antibiotic Therapy Recommendations for the Treatment of Pneumonia Acquired in a Health-Care Setting (HCAP, VAP, HAP) Patients with pneumonia acquired in a health-care setting require many supportive and symptomatic therapies. They may be mechanically ventilated, they may be in an ICU, and they may be very sick. It is not possible to go over all of their potential therapies in detail; you will need to use your clinical knowledge of respiratory illness to help the prescriber know what symptomatic therapies will be needed. We will focus on the antibiotic therapies at this point.

Antibiotic resistance in hospitals is variable, and specific institutions have their own guidelines. The newer antibiotics for resistant cases tend to be expensive and restricted in use. The 2005 joint American Thoracic Society/Infectious Diseases Society of America guideline recommends that empiric therapy should cover MRSA, *Pseudomonas aeruginosa,* gram-negative bacilli, and *Legionella.* Empiric therapy decisions can be modified based on local data indicating the most frequent bacterial pathogens isolated and their respective susceptibility patterns. Moderately ill patients with pneumonia may receive intravenous ceftriaxone, levofloxacin, or ertapenem. Alternatively, in patients who have been hospitalized for more than 5 days and have been receiving antibiotics previously, intravenous cefepime or ceftazidime, meropenem or doripenem, or piperacillin-tazobactam plus either gentamicin or tobramycin should be considered along with a drug that has activity against MRSA such as vancomycin or linezolid. If a pathogen is identified, the initial broad-spectrum, empiric regimen should be de-escalated by discontinuing drugs that are not necessary.

Aspiration Pneumonia

Aspiration pneumonia can be either chemical (exposure to stomach acid) or bacterial. Bacteria can invade the lower respiratory tract by aspiration of oropharyngeal organisms, inhalation of aerosols containing bacteria, or, less frequently, hematogenous spread from a distant body site. In addition bacterial translocation from the gastrointestinal tract has been hypothesized recently as a mechanism for infection. Of these routes, aspiration is believed to be the most important for both health-care-associated and community-acquired pneumonia.

Aspiration pneumonia brings a different set of possible pathogens. If the pneumonia is due to the acid exposure, antibiotics won't help. Only symptomatic therapy can be used as the lungs heal. Empiric antibiotic therapy generally consists of agents with anaerobic and gram-negative coverage in their spectrums of activity.

Patients who develop aspiration pneumonia in the community setting should be treated with an antibiotic that is effective against gram-positive anaerobes. Such antibiotics include clindamycin or penicillins. If the patient aspirated while hospitalized or is significantly debilitated by coexisting disease, broader-spectrum therapy should be used to expand the coverage to gram-negative pathogens. Generally clindamycin or a penicillin combined with a β-lactamase inhibitor (such as piperacillin-tazobactam) plus an aminoglycoside (tobramycin, gentamicin, or amikacin) should be considered.

Clinical pearl

In radioisotope tracer studies, 45% of healthy adults were found to aspirate during sleep. Persons who swallow abnormally (e.g., those who have depressed consciousness, respiratory tract instrumentation and/or mechanically assisted ventilation, or GI tract instrumentation or diseases) or who have just undergone surgery are particularly likely to aspirate.

time for review

Why are gram-negative pathogenic bacteria more common in aspiration?

Pneumocystis Jiroveci *Pneumonia*

Pneumocystis jiroveci pneumonia (PJP), formerly known as *Pneumocystis carinii,* is a complication of HIV infection. It should be noted that it can also occur in non-HIV-infected patients. Like tuberculosis, *Pneumocystis* can be asymptomatic and latent.

Diagnosis and Treatment Symptoms, when present, may include fever, cough, tachypnea, and dyspnea. Treatment is divided into acute and chronic. Arterial blood gases are one of the key factors in therapy decisions. The disease can be classified as mild, moderate, or severe on the basis of oxygenation.

Clinical pearl

Patients often have worse hypoxemia during the first 3 to 5 days after treatment is started. Although this might appear to be a poor prognostic indicator, many patients do well despite needing mechanical ventilation.

Factors to consider when starting drug therapy for PJP are whether it is a first episode, arterial blood gases, history of drug reaction, and route of therapy. Drugs used for acute treatment are intravenous trimethoprim–sulfamethoxazole (TMP–SMX), dapsone, parenteral clindamycin, primaquin, atovaquone, or IV pentamidine. These drugs are toxic. For example more than 50% of patients who receive trimethoprim–sulfomethoxazole may develop rash, fever, leukopenia, hepatitis, or thrombocytopenia. Pentamidine can cause azotemia, pancreatitis, hypocalcemia, or leukopenia, to name a few complications. Corticosteroids have a role in patients with acute, moderate to severe PJP, and calculation of PaO_2 gradient can guide their use.

Cystic Fibrosis and Pneumonia

Cystic fibrosis is a genetic disease of exocrine gland secretions. Recurrent respiratory infections play a big role in this chronic pulmonary disease. At different times during the course of the disease, different pathogens are found. It's common to have multiple bacterial isolates that have different antibiotic sensitivities. Systemic antibiotics may be used to treat pulmonary infections in cystic fibrosis, frequently in combination therapy. Agents used may be an aminoglycoside combined with an extended-spectrum penicillin or third-generation cephalosporin. Antibiotic use is controversial, and goals differ in individual patients because of resistance, changes in host defense, and bacterial growth patterns. Intuitively one would expect that suppressive antibiotic therapy would prolong the time between disease exacerbations and slow progression of lung disease.

Because antibiotics penetrate poorly in lung tissue, aerosolized antibiotics have been utilized with some success. One of the limiting factors in aerosol antibiotic administration is the bronchospasm that can result from aerosolized antibiotics. However aerosolized preservative-free tobramycin should be considered in cystic fibrosis patients 6 years of age and older with moderate to severe lung disease to reduce exacerbations and to improve lung function.

Clinical pearl

Giving a bronchodilator before administering aerosolized antibiotics is recommended to prevent or lessen the possibility of bronchospasm.

Therapeutic Guidelines

Because care of patients with pneumonia is quite common, therapeutic guidelines for the care of pneumonia patients are published and updated frequently. Individual institutions may have guidelines as well. It is important to stay updated with the current recommendations. The American Thoracic Society, the British Thoracic Society, the Canadian Infectious Diseases Society, and the Infectious Diseases Society of America all publish sets of guidelines, and each of those societies updates them regularly.

PATIENT & FAMILY EDUCATION

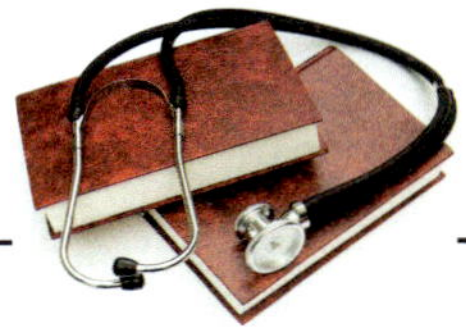

Counseling patients and their families on the proper use of aerosolized antibiotics is important. Education should include specific instructions on what to do before using the aerosol, complete directions for use, safety considerations for aerosol antibiotic therapy, and monitoring.

Prevention of Pneumonia

Prevention of pneumonia may be possible with use of pneumonia and influenza vaccines. Influenza virus vaccine is formulated each year to contain antigens of expected prevalent strains. Immunization is promoted for those who might experience serious complications from influenza, such as patients with underlying heart disease, lung disease, chronic renal disease, and the elderly.

14.4c Tuberculosis

No chapter on respiratory infectious diseases would be complete without a short discussion of **tuberculosis** (TB). Tuberculosis is a chronic disease caused by *Mycobacterium tuberculosis*. Although it can affect any part of the body, it most commonly affects the lungs. There has been a gradual decline in the number of active cases over the years, but there are still millions of people with TB infection that has progressed to active TB. TB is spread by microscopic droplets and is an airborne disease. It can be spread when an infected person coughs or sneezes. Once the droplet is inhaled, it becomes encapsulated, and the infection is latent.

Diagnosis and Treatment

When the infection droplets, called bacilli, escape, the disease becomes active. Symptoms of active TB can range from none to weight loss, fever, night sweats, or bloody sputum. Diagnosis is made with a skin test, blood test, sputum sample, and chest X-ray. See Figure 14-5 for an illustration of the Mantoux skin test or purified protein derivative (PPD) test to diagnose TB. Drug therapy for TB is aimed at preventive therapy for latent infection or treatment of active TB disease.

Pharmacologic Treatment

Preventive therapy is usually with isoniazid for 6 to 12 months, which decreases the risk that the infection will progress to disease. Research is always in progress to determine the easiest yet most effective method of prophylaxis. Certain people are at a higher risk for developing TB; this group includes people who are in close contact with others with TB, people with a chest X-ray suggesting previous TB that was not treated, persons with HIV, and people who are substance abusers, for example. Patients on corticosteroids also may be at increased risk of disease progression.

FIGURE 14-5 The Mantoux or PPD Testing Procedure to Diagnose TB

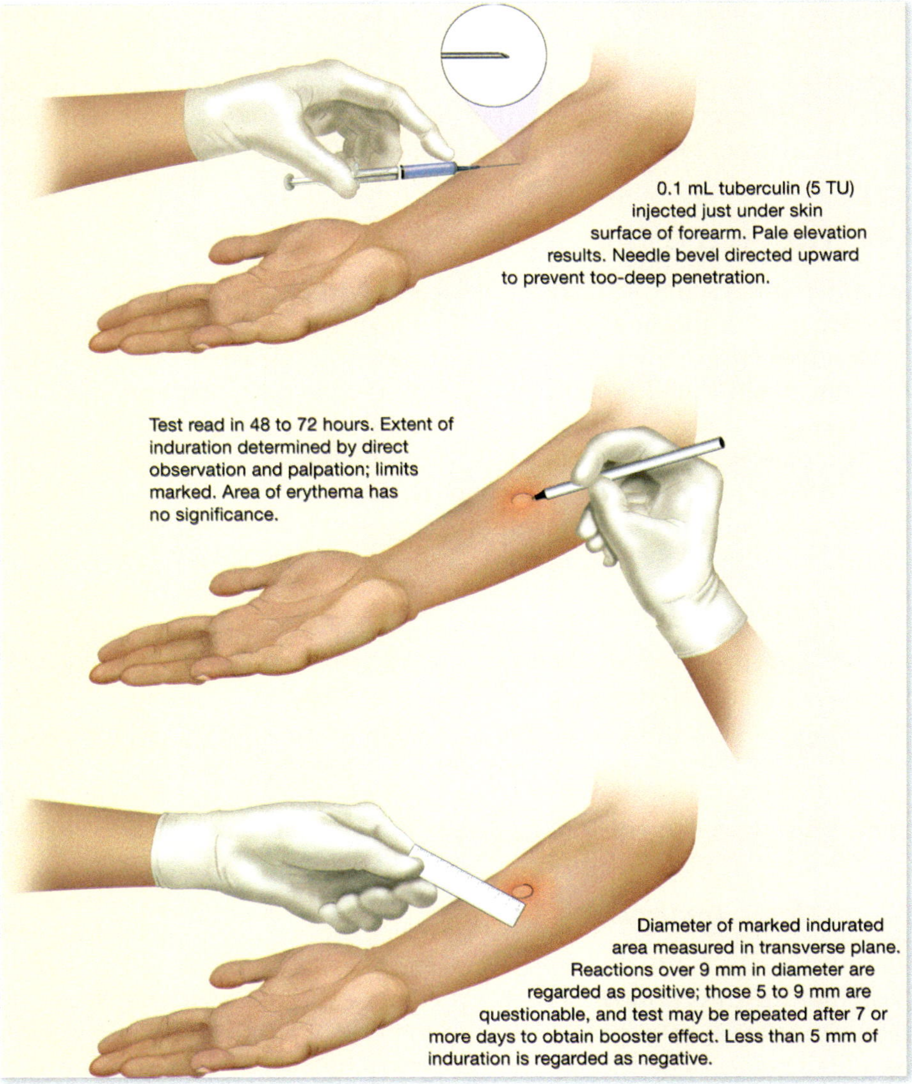

Clinical pearl

One way to try to reduce TB treatment failures is to use DOT, or directly observed treatment, to make sure a patient is medication-compliant. This is now considered a standard component of therapy.

Treatment of TB takes 6 to 24 months. The current recommendations for TB treatment include a combination of case management and directly observed therapy to ensure completion of therapy and minimize drug resistance. Drug treatment must be in combination, because resistance is a problem. Drugs used are isoniazid, rifampin, pyrazinamide, ethambutol, and streptomycin. Bedaquiline (Sirturo™) was recently approved by the U.S. FDA for multidrug-resistant TB to be used in combination with at least three drugs that are also active against the patient's TB isolate. Because of resistance, adherence to the drug regimen is the key point for TB.

14.4d Avian Influenza

Avian influenza (bird flu) is a type of influenza virus carried in the intestines of wild birds. Although the wild birds themselves may not get sick, they transmit the virus to domestic birds. Poultry industry conditions may make it possible for humans to be exposed and a humanized strain to evolve. Because the human immune system has not been previously exposed, it does not have any antibodies, making for a potentially devastating outbreak. Some of the clinical features that may present after an incubation period of 2 to 5 days are high fever, cough, rhinorrhea, diarrhea, vomiting, abdominal pain, shortness of breath, myalgia, and headache. Some patients may have lymphopenia, thrombocytopenia, or pulmonary infiltrates. Symptoms appear like a viral pneumonia, with progression to acute respiratory distress syndrome a possibility. There is a lack of treatment for avian influenza, making prophylaxis and supportive treatment the reality.

CONTROVERSY

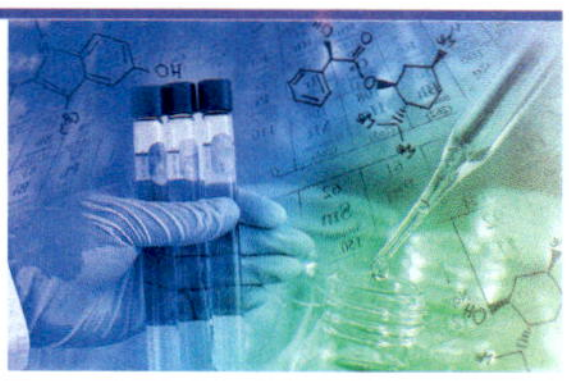

The lack of a vaccine and proven treatment makes the public and medical community nervous about a bird flu pandemic. What do you think of "hoarding" antiviral medications?

14.5 CHEMICAL TERRORISM

Chemical terrorism agents include nerve agents such as cholinesterase inhibitors, pulmonary irritants, and chemical asphyxiants—making them a very pertinent topic. Because antibiotics have a role in treatment and/or prophylaxis, the topic needs to be mentioned in this chapter.

Pulmonary irritants such as chlorine and phosgene have been used since World War I. Through biochemical reactions, these irritants can cause laryngospasm and pulmonary edema. Cyanide warfare was used as far back as Napoleon III with bayonets and more recently in Tylenol® tampering in 1982. Cyanide binds to cytochrome oxidase to interfere with aerobic cell metabolism, given a cutaneous or inhalational exposure.

Anthrax acts as a biologic weapon through cutaneous or inhalational exposure. Spore inhalation by host is transported lymphatically until spores germinate and toxins are produced. Anthrax is best treated prophylactically with antibiotics such as ciprofloxacin.

Plague is a potential bioweapon because it is contagious with close contact and aerosol transmission is possible. Systemic illness warrants parenteral antibiotic therapy with agents such as streptomycin or gentamicin. Postexposure prophylaxis is usually oral treatment with doxycycline and ciprofloxacin. Vaccination was discontinued in 1999.

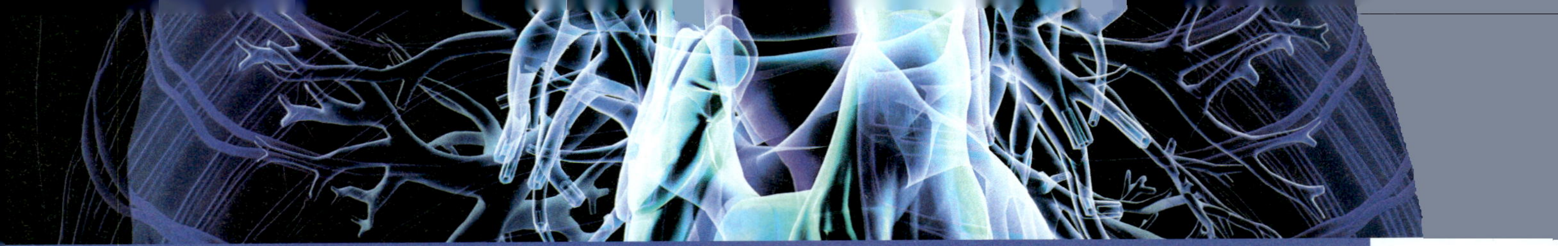

Summary

Respiratory infections are the major cause of morbidity and mortality from acute illness in the United States. The majority of these infections follow colonization of the upper respiratory tract with potential pathogens. Less commonly the pathogen may gain access to the lungs via the blood or by inhalation of infected aerosol particles. The patient's own immune status will have much to do with his or her susceptibility to a respiratory tract infection.

Appropriate therapy for respiratory tract infections is a multifaceted decision. The clinician must consider patient's history, physical examination, chest X-ray, culture results, and local pathogen incidence and resistance patterns. The most common pathogen in respiratory illness is *Streptococcus pneumoniae,* but this is changing. Other pathogens are becoming more virulent and deadly, and *S. pneumoniae* has changed significantly in its resistance to antimicrobial therapy.

REVIEW QUESTIONS

1. A usual first-line antibiotic agent for children with acute otitis media is
   (a) tetracycline (Achromycin®)
   (b) metronidazole (Flagyl®)
   (c) amoxicillin (Amoxil®)
   (d) cefaclor (Ceclor®)
   (e) any of the above
2. Most cases of acute sinusitis develop from what causative organism?
   (a) anaerobic bacteria
   (b) *Streptococcus pneumoniae*
   (c) *Escherichia coli*
   (d) influenza virus
3. The treatment of choice for pharyngitis is
   (a) penicillin
   (b) tetracycline
   (c) cephalexin
   (d) erythromycin
4. A patient presents with a high white blood cell count, fever, bronchial breathing, and rhonchi on auscultation. What type of infectious process do you suspect?
   (a) otitis media
   (b) sinusitis
   (c) croup
   (d) pneumonia

5. Gram-negative bacteria are frequently colonized in
   (a) healthy persons
   (b) hypertensive patients
   (c) patients with nasogastric tubes
   (d) patients with community-acquired pneumonia
   (e) all of the above
6. What is empiric therapy? What are some of the questions that need to be answered when treating infections?
7. Give an example of an indication when an antibiotic may not be appropriate.
8. Why does an ear or sinus infection have respiratory implications?
9. What is community-acquired pneumonia, and what are some problems with its treatment?
10. A 62-year-old man presents to the walk-in clinic with a chief complaint of headache, sore throat, and cough. A sputum sample isolates *Streptococcus* and *Haemophilus*. The physician is debating whether to treat the patient with an antibiotic. What would you recommend?
11. A child is brought to the emergency department in respiratory distress, and the mother states that the child has difficulty swallowing and has been drooling for the last 3 hours. What infection would you suspect, and what antibiotic therapy would be indicated? What respiratory intervention might be needed?

CASE STUDY 1

A 60-year-old man

A 60-year-old man is admitted to the hospital from work with fever, cough, tachypnea, and increased sputum production. His past medical history is significant for smoking two packs per day and prn 2-week amoxicillin antibiotic courses for sputum color changes. His blood pressure is 140/85 mmHg and RR 30 breaths/minute. He has an elevated WBC count and crackles in the lower base of the right lung. A Gram stain shows predominant gram-negative rods.

What findings are consistent with pneumonia in this man? What more information would you need to confirm this? What empiric treatment might you consider? How would you decide if inpatient treatment is necessary?

Chapter 15

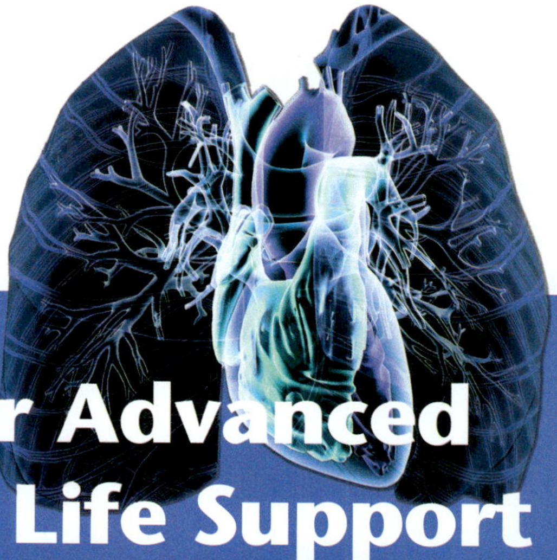

Medications for Advanced Cardiovascular Life Support

OBJECTIVES

Upon completion of this chapter you will be able to

- Define key terms related to advanced cardiac life support.
- Identify the conduction pathway for a normal heartbeat.
- Describe the pharmacologic effects of the drugs commonly used in the treatment of acute myocardial infarction, cardiac arrest, cardiogenic shock, bradycardia, tachycardia, and pulseless arrest.
- Review algorithms for treatment of bradycardia, tachycardia, and pulseless arrest.

KEY TERMS

acute myocardial infarction
arrhythmia
asystole
automaticity
bolus
cardiac arrest
defibrillate
infusion
ischemia
stroke

ABBREVIATIONS

ACLS Advanced Cardiac Life Support
AMI acute myocardial infarction
AV atrioventricular
BLS basic life support
CPR cardiopulmonary resuscitation
ECC emergency cardiovascular care
HF heart failure
IO intraosseous
mEq milliequivalent
mV millivolt
PEA pulseless electrical activity
PSVT paroxysmal supraventricular tachycardia
SA sinoatrial
VF ventricular fibrillation
VT ventricular tachycardia

A variety of health-care practitioners participate in the emergency treatment of patients who have suffered **acute myocardial infarctions**, cardiogenic shock, **cardiac arrest**, and **stroke**. The American Heart Association offers courses in Advanced Cardiac Life Support (ACLS) to help health-care practitioners recognize important signs and symptoms and treat patients accordingly. These courses emphasize the skills and knowledge necessary to ensure that members of the resuscitation team will be prepared to act quickly and efficiently to treat and resuscitate a victim of cardiac arrest. Some of these practitioners may have the primary responsibility for administering medications, while others may be more concerned with airway management and support of circulation. Regardless of the specific role, to be truly prepared for emergencies, members of the resuscitation team need to be knowledgeable about the entire process and be prepared to act.

In this chapter we discuss some of the drugs and treatment algorithms used for serious, life-threatening **arrhythmias** and acute myocardial infarction. You will no doubt recognize many of these drugs from previous chapters, but in this chapter we will be looking at their specific roles in the context of the emergency setting. This chapter is not intended to be a substitute for the 2010 American Heart Association's Guidelines for cardiopulmonary resuscitation (CPR) and emergency cardiovascular care (ECC), but rather a brief overview of its basic components. The potential effects of any drugs or ACLS therapy on outcome are less than the potential effects of immediate, high-quality CPR and early defibrillation.

In order for any discussion of the pharmacologic agents used in ACLS to be meaningful, the reader should have a general understanding of rhythm disturbances. We begin with an overview of some common arrhythmias, and you may also want to refer to the cardiac section of Chapter 9. Then we discuss pharmacologic treatments for serious arrhythmias and cardiac arrest. Current guidelines place much less emphasis on drug therapy during cardiac arrest and more emphasis on CPR. Finally we review several examples of treatment algorithms to show how the pharmacology fits into the complete management of the patient. Remember that an *algorithm* provides practitioners with a systematic approach to treat the victim of a cardiac emergency. It is intended to help guide and standardize treatment. Algorithms should not limit the physician from implementing alternative therapy based on assessment of each individual patient or situation.

Clinical pearl

The American Heart Association website provides updates and a visual depiction of the color version of the algorithms; see http://circ.ahajournals.org/content/122/18_suppl_3/S729.figures-only

Information in this chapter is based on the 2010 American Heart Association guidelines for cardiopulmonary resuscitation and emergency cardiovascular care. These guidelines are based on an extensive evidence review of resuscitation literature. They have been streamlined from the 2000 guidelines to reduce the information needed to learn and to clarify the most important skills. If you are familiar with the 2005 guidelines, it may serve you well to look at the website to review some of the most significant new recommendations in the 2010 guidelines. Advanced Cardiac Life Support begins with high-quality basic life support (BLS). Changes in ACLS treatment of cardiac arrest have been designed to minimize interruptions in chest compressions.

Patient & Family Education

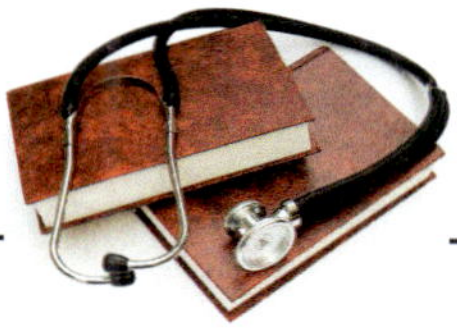

The use of cardiopulmonary resuscitation (CPR) dates back to 1740, even though today most Americans don't know how to perform it. CPR can save lives if given immediately and properly to sudden cardiac arrest victims. Health-care professionals should encourage patients and their families to learn CPR.

15.1 NORMAL CONDUCTION AND ARRHYTHMIAS

15.1a Electrophysiology

The heart's conduction network coordinates organized muscle contraction. The conduction cells transmit impulses by depolarization. In its resting or polarized state, the cell has about –90 mV of stored energy. This charge is maintained by differences in concentrations of sodium (Na) and potassium ions. An electrical, chemical, or mechanical stimulation causes this stored energy to be released by opening cell membrane channels and allowing a rapid influx of Na^+ ions into the cell, reversing the polarity to about +20 mV. This is called *depolarization* and causes muscle contraction. Calcium also begins to enter the cell to aid in muscle contraction.

The depolarized cell now needs to *repolarize* before it can conduct another impulse. During repolarization the sodium channels close and potassium channels open, thereby restoring the membrane potential to the resting level of –90 mV. In the last phase of repolarization, sodium ions are actively extruded from the cell, while potassium reenters (see Figure 15-1).

FIGURE 15-1 Depolarization of a Myocardial Conduction Cell

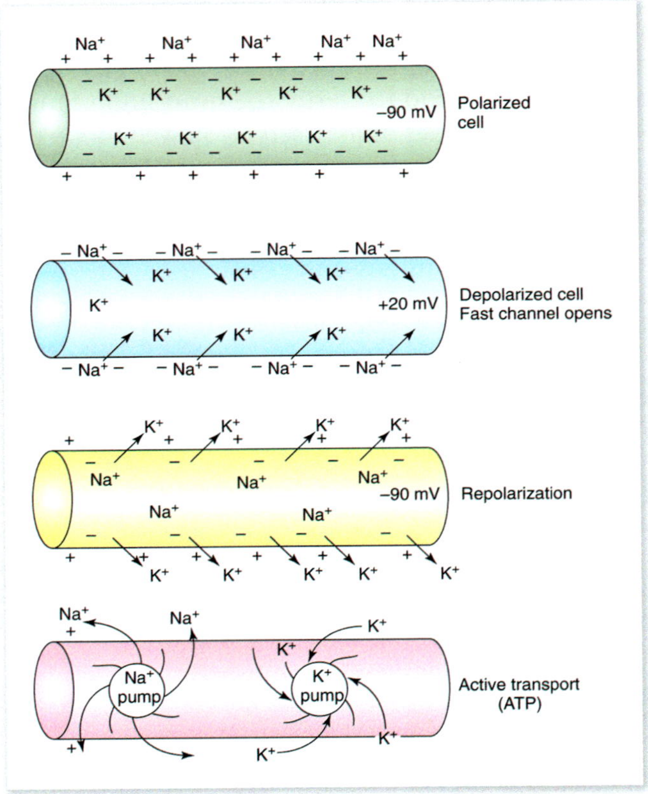

15.1b Normal Conduction

Normally the electrical impulses begin in the sinoatrial (SA) node. The wave of depolarization spreads through the atria, then to the atrioventricular (AV) node, where there is a brief pause (0.1 second). The pause allows time for the atria to contract and the blood from the atria to flow into the ventricles. Now that the ventricles are fully loaded, the impulse travels to the AV bundle, or bundle of His, to the right and left bundle branches. The bundle branches terminate in Purkinje fibers. The numerous fibers of the Purkinje system serve to rapidly transmit the impulse to the contractile ventricles, so that they depolarize and contract in unison (see Figure 15-2).

FIGURE 15-2 Normal Conduction System and Normal ECG

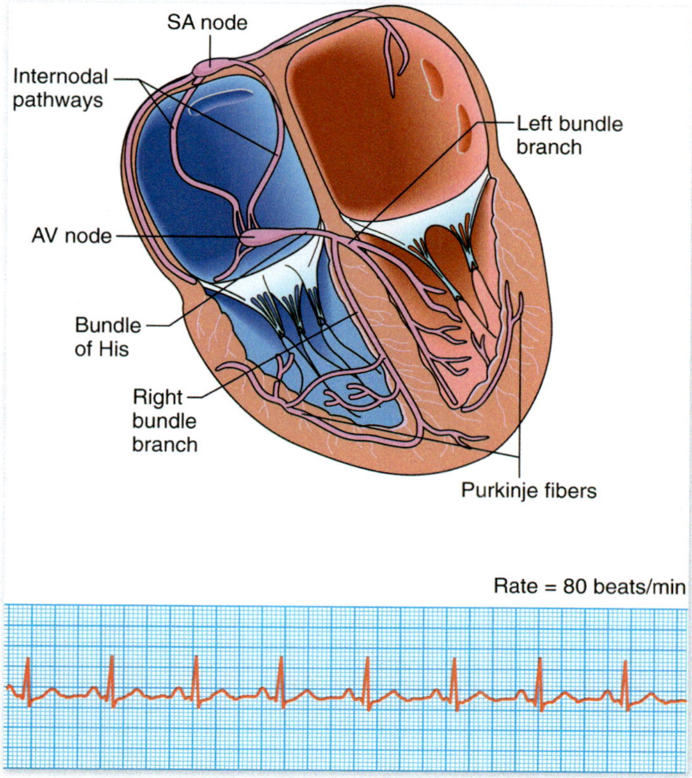

15.1c Acute Myocardial Infarction

The heart contracts with amazing regularity. It also manages to compensate for a variety of pathologic conditions. In spite of this ability, however, coronary heart disease remains the leading cause of death in the United States. Approximately 50% of deaths from acute myocardial infarction (AMI) occur outside the hospital, usually within 4 hours of symptoms. High-fat/high-calorie diets, a sedentary lifestyle, cigarette smoking, and high blood pressure are just a few of the contributing factors in heart disease. High levels of cholesterol in the bloodstream build up, narrowing the walls of the arteries. Smoking causes constriction of the arteries, which can further reduce oxygen delivery to the heart. High blood pressure and narrowed arteries make the heart work harder and consume more oxygen as it pumps blood and oxygen to the rest of the body. When the heart is no longer getting the full supply of oxygen it needs, the myocardial cells become more irritable. The patient may begin to experience chest pain, which is referred to as angina. Symptoms of AMI usually last more than 15 minutes. If the interruption in the supply of oxygen continues, tissue damage occurs, and the damaged myocardium becomes electrically unstable. The ability of the myocardial cells to depolarize and repolarize normally may be affected, and abnormal beats can then develop. If the oxygen supply is not reestablished quickly, myocardial cells will die. Death of myocardial cells is irreversible, and this is what is known as myocardial infarction.

Learning Hint

Beats that begin anywhere outside the normal conduction system are called *ectopic beats.* Ectopic beats can be further defined as premature if they come earlier than a normal beat would or as escape beats if they come later.

15.1d Bradycardia

Clinical pearl

Although bradycardia is defined clinically as a heart rate of less than 60 beats per minute, it may not always need to be treated. For example conditioned athletes typically have resting bradycardia because of a highly efficient and conditioned heart muscle.

Bradycardia simply means a slow heart rate. The SA node is the "pacemaker" of the heart, and it normally fires 60 to 100 times per minute. Various conditions such as increased parasympathetic tone, profound hypoxia, and damage to the conduction system of the heart (heart block) may result in a rate that is too slow for the patient (normally, less than 60). When the heart rate becomes too slow, the cardiac output decreases and the patient's blood pressure drops. Oxygen delivery to the tissues may also be compromised. This can cause serious signs and symptoms, such as chest pain, hypotension, altered acute mental status, and loss of consciousness.

time for review

How might damage to the heart's conduction system affect cardiac output and tissue perfusion?

15.1e Tachycardia

Tachycardia (fast heart) is when the heart rate increases to more than 100 beats per minute. The increased heart rate increases the cardiac output and blood pressure. In sinus tachycardia, the heart rate ranges between 100 and less than 180. This is usually an appropriate physiologic response to stress, fever, exercise, hypovolemia, or hypoxemia. Heart rates faster than 150 are usually due to some type of pathologic arrhythmia, such as another pacemaker or pacemakers that override the SA node, an electrical short-circuit called reentry, or increased irritability in the myocardial cells.

Fast heart rates may actually compromise the heart's function. The heart may not get enough oxygen or the ventricles may not have enough time to fill, and the cardiac output and blood pressure begin to drop. Arrhythmias that are extremely fast (greater than 150) may be so compromising (e.g., cause hemodynamic instability, which is a fancy term for a drop in blood pressure) that they may require direct-current countershock.

When the tachycardia originates in the atria or AV node, the QRS complexes are usually narrow, as on the normal electrocardiogram (ECG). These are often called supraventricular tachycardias, because they originate "above" the ventricles, but a more appropriate term based on the mechanism of this type of arrhythmia is AV nodal reentrant tachycardia. There are actually several different supraventricular tachycardias with narrow complexes (atrial tachycardia, atrial fibrillation, and atrial flutter, to name a few), but it is not critical to differentiate them immediately in the emergency setting.

When the impulses originate *in* the ventricles, the QRS complexes take on a wide, tall, and bizarre appearance. When we see these very unusual QRS complexes on an ECG, we can *usually* assume that they are originating from the ventricles. There are some important exceptions to this rule, but we will not get into that now. Ventricular tachycardia is a very serious rhythm, because some patients with it do not have a pulse. It is important to assess the patient's pulse quickly and treat the patient accordingly.

Patients with either tachycardia should be quickly evaluated to determine whether they are stable or having serious signs and symptoms, and whether it is a ventricular or supraventricular rhythm. If the patient is stable, then he or she can be treated pharmacologically. Unstable patients need synchronized cardioversion. Figures 15-3a and 15-3b show the atrial and ventricular tachycardia, respectively.

FIGURE 15-3A Multifocal Atrial Tachycardia (Supraventricular)

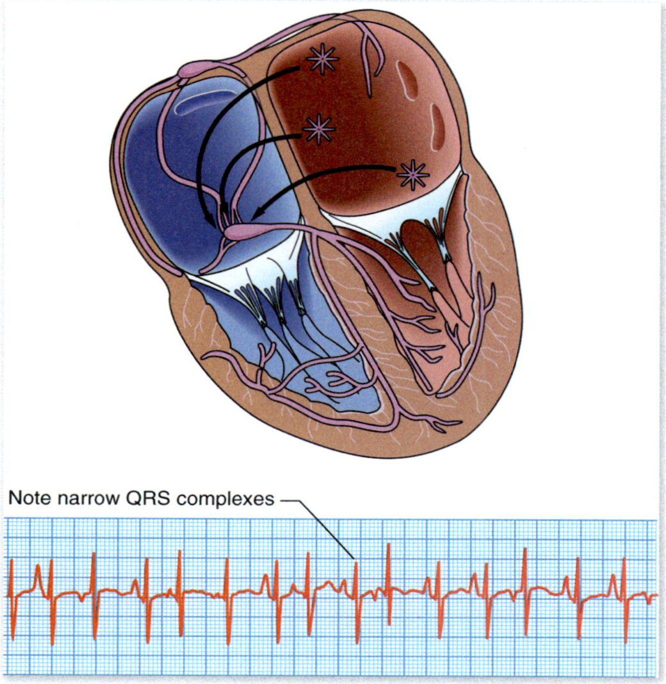

FIGURE 15-3B Ventricular Tachycardia

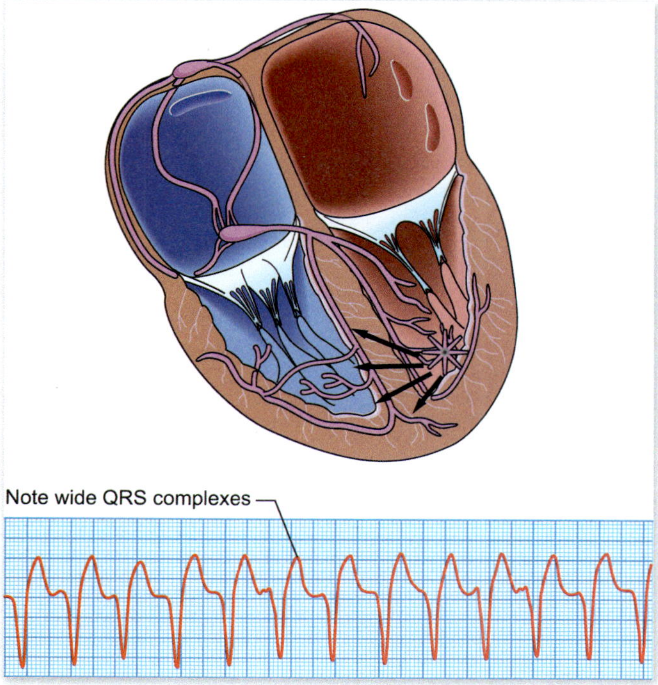

time for review

How can you tell where a tachycardia is originating?

Learning Hint

The prefix "de-" means to take away from. If the heart is fibrillating, the proper treatment is to remove the ineffective fibrillation, or to **defibrillate**.

15.1f Ventricular Fibrillation

Ventricular fibrillation occurs when multiple rapid ventricular pacemakers are firing. The patient's heart is not contracting. Instead, the ventricles quiver, or fibrillate. This is a very serious rhythm, in which the patient never has a pulse. The treatments for pulseless ventricular tachycardia and ventricular fibrillation are exactly the same. CPR must be initiated while defibrillation and appropriate drug therapy are provided. Please see Figure 15-4, which illustrates ventricular fibrillation.

15.1g Asystole

Asystole means without rhythm. The heart is electrically silent. Of course the patient is pulseless, and CPR needs to be initiated immediately. Epinephrine and vasopressin are drugs used in the treatment of asystole.

FIGURE 15-4 Ventricular Fibrillation

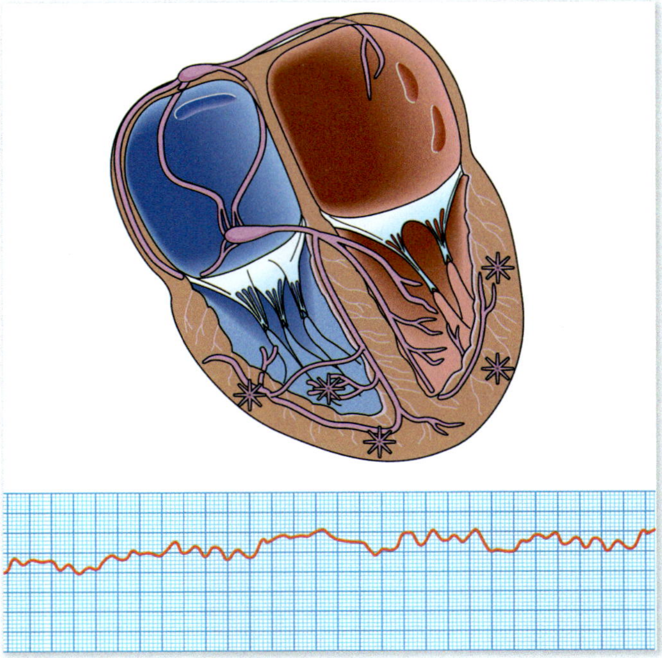

time for review

What is the relationship between a fibrillating heart and cardiac output?
What is the main treatment for fibrillation?

15.1h Pulseless Electrical Activity

Pulseless electrical activity (PEA) is the presence of some type of electrical activity (other than ventricular tachycardia or ventricular fibrillation) even though the patient has no pulse. Because the patient has no pulse, treatment of this condition and asystole are identical. They both require rapid assessment to determine the cause of the pulselessness. The patient must be supported immediately with excellent CPR, and epinephrine and vasopressin can be given, as in asystole. Ultimately, successful resuscitation will depend on correcting the underlying problem. Causes include severe hypovolemia, tension pneumothorax, cardiac tamponade, hypoxia, hypothermia, massive pulmonary embolism, some types of drug overdose, hyperkalemia, acidosis, and massive acute myocardial infarction.

Learning Hint

Always search for and treat reversible causes of cardiac arrest and failure to respond to resuscitation. Comorbidity factors can be remembered as the "H"s (hypovolemia, hypoxia, hydrogen ion, hypokalemia, hyperkalemia, hypoglycemia, hypothermia) and "T"s (toxins, tamponade, tension pneumothorax, thrombosis, trauma).

Life Span Considerations

Cardiopulmonary arrests in children are most often due to a primary respiratory problem, while in adults the most common cause is a primary cardiac problem.

time for review

In both asystole and PEA, patients do not have a pulse. What are the similarities in recognizing and treating these two conditions?

15.2 PHARMACOLOGIC AGENTS FOR ADVANCED LIFE SUPPORT

Resuscitation guidelines are evidence-based recommendations. This means that international resuscitation experts have met to evaluate published research and have drawn conclusions in the form of recommendations. When drug administration is indicated, the drugs should be given during CPR, as soon as possible after the rhythm is checked. Drug delivery should not interrupt CPR.

15.2a Medication Access

Clinical pearl

The optimal dose for endotracheal delivery is not known, but the dose is usually increased to 2 to 2.5 times the IV dose, which is then injected down the endotracheal tube.

Few drugs used in cardiac arrest are supported by strong research evidence. When drugs are used, they typically require 1 to 2 minutes to reach the central circulation when given by peripheral access. Resuscitation drugs are usually administered by **bolus** injection, followed by a 20-ml bolus of IV fluid and elevation of the extremity. The intraosseous (IO) route may be used if IV access is not available, with endotracheal administration being another alternative. Endotracheal administration results in lower blood concentrations than the same dose given intravascularly.

15.2b Categories of ACLS Drugs

The drugs used in Advanced Cardiac Life Support can be divided into two categories: medications used for cardiovascular support and medications used for arrest rhythms. Drugs for cardiovascular support are used to alter cardiac output, cardiac rate, and peripheral vascular resistance. These are sometimes referred to as Pharmacology I category drugs (see Table 15-1). These medications alter vasomotor tone and cardiovascular contractility. They stabilize hemodynamics, avert cardiovascular collapse, restore perfusing rhythm, and improve cardiac output and organ perfusion. Adrenergic and noradrenergic vasopressors increase diastolic pressure.

TABLE 15-1 **Medications for Cardiovascular Support (Pharmacology I Category Drugs)**

Medication	Effect
epinephrine	Inotrope/vasopressor
vasopressin	Nonadrenergic peripheral vasoconstrictor
norepinephrine	Inotrope/vasopressor
dobutamine	Inotrope
dopamine	Adrenergic agonist/dopamine agonist
digoxin	Inotrope/ventricular rate control
milrinone	Inotrope/vasodilator
nitroglycerin	Vasodilator
sodium nitroprusside	Peripheral vasodilator

The drugs used for arrest rhythms include agents to control rate and rhythm, as listed in Table 15-2. Pulseless cardiac arrest is produced by four rhythms: ventricular fibrillation, rapid ventricular tachycardia, pulseless electrical activity, and asystole. For patients with acute coronary ischemia, the greatest risk for arrhythmias is in the first 4 hours after the onset of symptoms. Treatment decisions are based on rhythm interpretation and clinical evaluation. Electrical and drug treatment options are important for unstable or immediately life-threatening rhythms.

TABLE 15-2 **Agents to Control Rate and Rhythm**

Agent	Indication
procainamide	Stable monomorphic VT, atrial fibrillation or flutter, SVT
lidocaine	Stable monomorphic VT
atenolol	Narrow-complex tachycardias associated with either reentry or ectopic foci, rate control in atrial fibrillation or flutter
esmolol	Same as atenolol
labetalol	Same as atenolol (used infrequently as a rate control agent due to alpha-blockade properties that may cause or worsen hypotension)
metoprolol	Same as atenolol
propranolol	Same as labetalol
amiodarone	Narrow complex tachycardias, hemodynamically stable VTs
ibutilide	Pharmacologic cardioversion of atrial fibrillation or flutter
sotalol	Rhythm control of atrial fibrillation or flutter, monomorphic VT
verapamil	Stable narrow-complex tachycardias (SVT), rate control in atrial fibrillation or flutter
diltiazem	Same as verapamil *and* is used more often clinically than verapamil for these indications
adenosine	Stable, narrow-complex tachycardias
atropine	Symptomatic bradycardia
magnesium	Torsades de pointes VT
dopamine	Bradycardia unresponsive to atropine

VF, ventricular fibrillation; VT, ventricular tachycardia; SVT, supraventricular tachycardia; AV, atrioventricular.

15.3 MEDICATIONS FOR CARDIOVASCULAR SUPPORT

15.3a Oxygen

Oxygen is a key component in resuscitation and emergency cardiac care, yet it is frequently taken for granted or overlooked as a drug. The atmosphere that we breathe contains 21% oxygen. This is enough to maintain a partial pressure in the blood (PaO_2) of 80–100 mmHg. In healthy individuals, this keeps the red blood cells saturated with oxygen. During mouth-to-mouth or mouth-to-mask ventilation, the breath exhaled by the rescuer to the victim contains only 16% to 17% oxygen. In addition the cardiac output of the victim during CPR is only about 25% to 30% of normal. Low perfusion makes it necessary for the body to extract much more oxygen than usual from the blood. In turn the venous blood will be extremely depleted of oxygen, and 21% oxygen may not be enough to resaturate the blood of the cardiac arrest victim. Administering 100% oxygen as quickly as possible is critical in preventing organ damage in the cardiac arrest victim.

Indications

Oxygen is indicated in any suspected cardiopulmonary emergency, especially (but not limited to) complaints of shortness of breath and suspected ischemic chest pain.

Dosage

Oxygen delivery devices for spontaneously breathing patients are described in Chapter 12. Patients who are not breathing on their own must have their breathing assisted with positive-pressure ventilation or with a manual resuscitator bag and 100% oxygen.

Precautions

Problems associated with the overuse of oxygen depend on the concentration and the duration of exposure. This should never be a concern during short-term exposure to oxygen during resuscitation. Although occurrence is rare, observe closely for hypoventilation when using oxygen with chronic obstructive pulmonary disease patients. Pulse oximetry can be inaccurate in low-cardiac-output states or with vasoconstriction.

15.3b Epinephrine

Epinephrine is a natural catecholamine with both α and β effects. It plays a critical role in cardiac arrest. In fact, if you look at the algorithms for cardiac arrest, you will see that it is the first drug (after oxygen) administered in all of them. The reason is that the primary beneficial effect is to produce peripheral vasoconstriction, which leads to improved myocardial and cerebral perfusion. This is important because, as we said before, cardiac output is low during CPR.

Epinephrine appears to improve cerebral blood flow more than other adrenergic agents. It also makes the heart more susceptible to direct countershock, improving the likelihood of converting ventricular fibrillation and ventricular tachycardia to rhythms with spontaneous circulation. Epinephrine increases the rate and force of myocardial contraction through β-adrenergic effects. This tends to increase the oxygen consumption of the heart, which could increase **ischemia** of the myocardial tissue. During cardiac arrest, it is felt that the beneficial effects of epinephrine outweigh any potential risk of cardiac ischemia. If IV/IO access is not available, epinephrine may be given by the endotracheal route at a dose of 2 to 2.5 mg. Higher doses may be needed for specific overdoses, such as with β-blockers or calcium-channel blockers.

Learning Hint

Sometimes it is difficult to comprehend that epinephrine, which increases blood flow to the tissues, can cause ischemia. It all has to do with supply and demand. Epinephrine makes the heart work harder to increase its rate and force of contraction. This requires more oxygen, but the myocardial muscle is perfused with oxygen-rich blood during diastole (the resting phase of the cardiac cycle). So, as the rate increases, there is less time for diastole and therefore for coronary artery perfusion, and myocardial ischemia can become worse.

Indications

Indications include cardiac arrest of any kind (ventricular fibrillation, pulseless ventricular tachycardia, pulseless electrical activity, and asystole). It can also be considered for treatment of profoundly symptomatic bradycardia, severe hypotension, or severe allergic anaphylactic reactions.

Dosage

The standard dose of epinephrine is 1 mg (not based on body weight) given IV/IO every 3 to 5 minutes. One dose of vasopressin may be given instead of either the first or second dose of epinephrine.

Precautions

Epinephrine should not be mixed in alkaline solutions (including sodium bicarbonate). Its positive inotropic and chronotropic effects can increase myocardial oxygen demand. Large doses in patients who are not in cardiac arrest can cause hypertension. It can also cause ventricular ectopy, especially in patients receiving digoxin. High doses do not improve survival or neurologic outcome and may contribute to postresuscitation myocardial dysfunction.

time for review

Based on what you know about general principles of pharmacodynamics, are higher doses always better?

15.3c Vasopressin

Vasopressin is a naturally occurring antidiuretic hormone. In high doses it acts as a noradrenergic peripheral, coronary, and renal vasoconstrictor. Its half-life is 10–20 minutes. Advantages over epinephrine include lack of blunted vasoconstriction in acidosis and lack of β-receptor stimulation, which could increase myocardial demand and complicate the postresuscitative phase of CPR.

Indications

Given the similarly equivocal evidence of efficacy for epinephrine, vasopressin could be considered as an alternative to either the first or second dose of epinephrine in treatment of pulseless arrest. It may be effective in patients with asystole or pulseless electrical activity and in patients who remain in cardiac arrest after treatment with epinephrine. It is sometimes used for hemodynamic support in vasodilatory shock.

Dosage

Vasopressin is given one time only as 40 units IV/IO.

Precautions

The current evidence for the use of vasopressin in cardiac arrest is promising, but its use has not improved rates of intact survival to hospital discharge.

15.3d Norepinephrine

Norepinephrine is a potent α-vasoconstrictor and β_1-inotrope. Low doses result primarily in inotropic effects, with higher doses producing mixed effects.

Indications

Norepinephrine is used primarily for severe hemodynamically significant hypotension and low total peripheral vascular resistance that is refractory to other sympathomimetics.

Dosage

Norepinephrine is mixed and infused through a central venous catheter to minimize risk of extravasation. The usual starting dose is 0.5–1 mcg/min titrated to achieve a systolic blood pressure of at least 90 mmHg. The average adult dose is 2–12 mcg/min.

Precautions

Evidence does not currently support benefits with norepinephrine, with some trends toward worse neurologic outcome.

15.3e Sodium Bicarbonate

Sodium bicarbonate is a buffer (base) that combines with acid (in effect, neutralizing the acid). In the process, carbon dioxide and water are produced, and of course the carbon dioxide is excreted by the lungs. Sodium bicarbonate is indicated in situations where there has been a bicarbonate-responsive metabolic acidosis prior to arrest, hyperkalemia, or some drug overdoses.

During CPR, cardiac compressions produce only about 25% to 30% of the normal cardiac output. This low perfusion may mean that insufficient amounts of oxygen are delivered to the tissues. This results in anaerobic metabolism and production of lactic acid. The decreased blood flow to the lungs also decreases carbon dioxide excretion by the lungs, further contributing to the acidosis. Because administration of sodium bicarbonate increases the amount of CO_2 in the blood, and CO_2 removal is compromised, bicarbonate must be used very judiciously during cardiac arrest. Increased amounts of carbon dioxide in the blood also lower the pH of the blood, and this leads to a respiratory acidosis.

Indications

Sodium bicarbonate is indicated when there is severe hyperkalemia or tricyclic antidepressant overdose. It may be used upon return of spontaneous circulation after a long arrest interval. It is not effective in hypercarbic acidosis (cardiac arrest and CPR without intubation).

Dosage

An IV bolus of 1 mEq/kg can be given as an initial dose, followed by half of this dose every 10 minutes. Administration of bicarbonate should be guided by arterial blood gas analysis to monitor the patient's acid–base status. Inducing alkalosis should always be avoided.

Precautions

Sodium bicarbonate rapidly combines with acid to produce carbon dioxide, so good ventilation is essential to eliminate the carbon dioxide, or the patient will remain acidotic because of the excess carbon dioxide. Administration of bicarbonate can cause alkalosis, increased serum sodium, and hyperosmolality. It also compromises oxygen release at the tissues, which further endangers survival. It is not recommended for routine use in cardiac arrest patients.

15.4 POSITIVE INOTROPIC DRUGS

Positive inotropic drugs increase the force of contraction of the heart. This in turn increases cardiac output, blood pressure, and tissue perfusion. These drugs depress the sodium pump, which increases intracellular sodium and calcium. Calcium increases the force of the heart's contraction. There is also an increase in heart rate and increased conduction through the AV node. Digoxin, on the other hand—due to its enhancement of parasympathetic tone—decreases heart rate and AV conduction. The decrease in heart rate and the slower conduction are beneficial because they allow for more ventricular filling time coupled with a more efficient ventricular contraction.

15.4a Digoxin

Indications

Digoxin is used in advanced cardiac life support to slow ventricular response in atrial fibrillation or atrial flutter. It is also an alternative drug for paroxysmal supraventricular tachycardia (PSVT).

Dosage

Loading IV **infusion** doses of 10–15 mcg/kg lean body weight provide therapeutic effect with minimum risk of toxic effects. Maintenance dose is determined by body size and renal function.

Precautions

Digoxin toxicity is frequently associated with serious arrhythmias. Electrical cardioversion is usually avoided if the patient is receiving digoxin, unless the condition is life-threatening. Lower settings can be used.

15.4b Milrinone

Milrinone is a phosphodiesterase inhibitor (also called inodilators). It has a positive inotropic effect and a vasodilating effect, which decreases afterload. Together these effects result in an increased cardiac output. These agents inhibit intracellular phosphodiesterase, leading to an increase in the concentration of cAMP.

Indications

Milrinone is used in the treatment of heart failure (HF) that is refractory to diuretics, vasodilators, and conventional inotropic agents.

Dosage

Intravenous loading doses of 50 mcg/kg are used, followed by an infusion of 0.375–0.75 mcg/kg per minute titrated to clinical effect. Hemodynamic monitoring optimizes use.

Precautions

Milrinone may cause tachyarrhythmias, hypotension, or thrombocytopenia. It can cause myocardial ischemia and should not be mixed with other drugs. Loading doses are generally not recommended but if used should be administered over at least 10 minutes.

15.4c Dopamine

Dopamine is a chemical precursor of norepinephrine.

Indications

Dopamine is a second-line drug after atropine for symptomatic bradycardia. It is used for hypotension (systolic blood pressure < 90 mmHg) with signs and symptoms of shock.

Dosage

Effects are dose-dependent. Low doses (1–2 mcg/kg/min) stimulate the dopaminergic receptors to produce cerebral, renal, and mesenteric vasodilation, but overall venous tone is increased because of concurrent α-adrenergic effect.

When administered at 2–10 mcg/kg/min, dopamine stimulates the β_1- and α-receptors. The main effect is to increase cardiac output. At doses of greater than 10 mcg/kg/min, dopamine's α-adrenergic effect predominates. There is marked vasoconstriction (arterial and venous), which increases preload, afterload, and blood pressure. This effect may be useful when there is hypotension or shock without hypovolemia. If the dose of dopamine exceeds 20 mcg/kg/min, it produces a potent α-adrenergic effect and increases systemic vascular resistance, similar to norepinephrine.

Precautions

Dopamine may be used in patients with hypovolemia after volume replacement. It can be used cautiously in cardiogenic shock with accompanying HF. It may cause tachyarrhythmias and excessive vasoconstriction. Dopamine should not be mixed with sodium bicarbonate.

15.4d Dobutamine (Dobutrex®)

Dobutamine is a synthetic catecholamine (analog of dopamine) that stimulates β_1-receptors. It has a strong positive inotropic effect, with less chronotropic effect than dopamine. It does not increase peripheral vascular resistance and renal vasoconstriction, as dopamine does.

Indications

Dobutamine is used for heart failure or pulmonary congestion with systolic blood pressure of 70–100 mmHg and no signs of shock.

Dosage

The usual infusion rate for dobutamine is 2–20 mcg/kg/min. It should be titrated so the heart rate does not increase more than 10% of baseline.

Precautions

Dobutamine should be avoided with systolic blood pressure less than 100 mmHg and signs of shock. It may cause tachyarrhythmias, fluctuations in blood pressure, headache, and nausea. It is contraindicated in suspected or known poison- or drug-induced shock.

15.5 ANTIARRHYTHMIC DRUGS

15.5a Atropine

Atropine sulfate is a parasympatholytic drug. Patients with advanced heart disease frequently have increased parasympathetic tone. As you may recall, one of the effects of the parasympathetic nervous system is to slow the heart rate, and the result can be bradycardia or even asystole. Atropine increases the heart rate by increasing the automaticity of the sinus node and conduction through the AV node.

Indications

Atropine is indicated for treatment of symptomatic bradycardia (Class I). Symptomatic bradycardia is a slow heart rate accompanied by serious signs and symptoms such as chest pain, shortness of breath, decreased level of consciousness, very low blood pressure, and acute heart failure. Atropine may be beneficial in the presence of AV block at the nodal level (Class IIa). Relative bradycardia is the term used for a heart rate in the "normal range" of 60–100 when a tachycardia would be more appropriate for the patient's condition. For example tachycardia is a normal physiologic response to hypotension. A patient with a blood pressure of 80/40 and a heart rate of 70 is not "normal"; the heart rate needs to be faster to maintain adequate circulation.

Dosage

For patients who have symptomatic bradycardia but still have a pulse, 0.5–1 mg of atropine is administered IV. The dose can be repeated at 3- to 5-minute intervals until the patient's heart rate is up to 60 beats/min or more, or until the signs and symptoms subside. The total dose should not exceed 2–3 mg (0.03–0.04 mg/kg). If the bradycardia is recurrent, an electrical pacemaker may be used to keep the heart rate up.

Precautions

Particularly in the setting of severe symptomatic bradycardia, hazards may seem to be of little consequence, but there are still a few things to keep in mind when administering atropine. Tachycardia may occur, and this tends to increase myocardial oxygen consumption, increasing incidence of ischemia and risk of myocardial infarction. Ventricular tachycardia and fibrillation have also occurred. Excessive doses of atropine can cause an anticholinergic syndrome that may include delirium, tachycardia, coma, flushed hot skin, ataxia, and blurred vision. Finally doses of less than 0.5 mg can produce paradoxical worsening of bradycardia. Atropine should be avoided in hypothermic bradycardia. It is not effective for intranodal AV block and new third-degree block with wide QRS complexes.

15.5b Amiodarone (Cordarone®)

Amiodarone is an antiarrhythmic that is useful in treating both atrial and ventricular tachycardias and for ventricular fibrillation. Its actions are complex. It affects sodium, potassium, and calcium channels. It also has α- and β-adrenergic-blocking properties. Its ability to block the AV node makes it useful in the treatment of supraventricular tachycardias.

Indications

Amiodarone is indicated for supraventricular tachycardia, ventricular tachycardia, ventricular tachycardia without a pulse, and ventricular fibrillation. It is not indicated for torsades de pointes (a specific subtype of ventricular tachycardia that is treated with magnesium sulfate). For cardiac arrest, amiodarone may be administered for ventricular fibrillation or pulseless ventricular tachycardia unresponsive to shock delivery, CPR, and a vasopressor (Class IIb).

Dosage

150 mg of amiodarone is given over 10 minutes, followed by a 1 mg/min infusion for 6 hours and then 0.5 mg/min. Supplementary infusions at the higher dose can be repeated if necessary for recurrence of the arrhythmia, but the maximum recommended daily dose is 2.2 g over 24 hours. If VF or pulseless VT continues or recurs after the fourth shock, amiodarone (300 mg IV/IO push) is used, with administration of a second dose of 150 mg IV/IO considered.

Precautions

Major adverse effects are hypotension and bradycardia, which can be prevented by slowing the rate of drug infusion and giving fluid, vasopressor, or chronotropic agents.

15.5c Lidocaine

Lidocaine is said to decrease automaticity, increase the fibrillation threshold, and decrease the defibrillation threshold. This means that it makes the heart more resistant to fibrillation and more responsive to defibrillation. Lidocaine does not usually affect myocardial contractility, blood pressure, or atrial arrhythmias.

time for review

If lidocaine metabolism depends on hepatic blood flow, will clearance decrease or increase with the decrease in cardiac output that occurs in cardiac arrest?

Indications

Lidocaine has long been considered the "gold standard" antiarrhythmic, but although it is still considered to be clinically useful, it is no longer the first-line antiarrhythmic drug used to treat ventricular tachycardia and ventricular fibrillation. Wide-complex PSVT may also be treated with lidocaine. It has no proven short-term or long-term efficacy in cardiac arrest. Lidocaine is considered an alternative treatment to amiodarone.

Clinical pearl

The main reason for using antiarrhythmic agents post–cardiac arrest is to raise the threshold for fibrillation.

Dosage

For ventricular fibrillation and pulseless ventricular tachycardia that has not responded to epinephrine and defibrillation, and if amiodarone is not available, the initial lidocaine dose is 1.0 to 1.5 mg/kg IV. If ventricular fibrillation (VF) or pulseless ventricular tachycardia (VT) persists, a 0.5 to 0.75 mg/kg IV push may be given. It may be repeated in 5 to 10 minutes for a maximum total dose of 3 mg/kg. On occasion a maintenance infusion of 1–4 mg/min (30–50 mcg/kg/min) may be used. Tracheal administration is 2–4 mg/kg. Lidocaine is only recommended if amiodarone is not available.

Precautions

Lidocaine is a long-standing drug that is familiar to many. In general it has fewer immediate side effects than other antiarrhythmics. Excessive doses and prolonged administration of lidocaine can result in toxicity. The dosage may need to be reduced in patients over age 70, those with hepatic dysfunction, and those with low cardiac output states. Signs of toxicity include slurred speech, drowsiness, disorientation, decreased hearing ability, paresthesia, and muscle twitching. Severe toxicity can occur, resulting in generalized seizures.

15.5d Procainamide (Pronestyl®)

Procainamide decreases **automaticity** in the ventricular muscle and Purkinje fibers and slows intraventricular conduction. It can be effective even when lidocaine has failed to suppress ventricular ectopic rhythms. It has also been shown to be useful in some types of supraventricular rhythms. Its limitation in cardiac arrest is the need for prolonged administration time.

Indications

- Procainamide may be used for treatment of PSVT uncontrolled by adenosine and vagal maneuvers if blood pressure is stable.
- Procainamide can be used to treat stable, wide-complex supraventricular tachycardias of unknown origins (though not as a first-line drug).

Dosage

For hemodynamically stable VT, the dose is 20–50 mg/min by infusion, until any one of the following occurs:

- The rhythm is suppressed.
- Hypotension develops.
- The QRS complex widens by 50% of its original width.
- A total dose of 17 mg/kg has been administered.

The maintenance dose is an IV infusion of 1–4 mg/min.

Precautions

The most common problem with procainamide is that it can cause hypotension, especially if it is given too rapidly, if blood levels get too high, or if the patient has impaired left ventricular function. When the QRS complex widens by more than 50%, it can cause heart block or even cardiac arrest. The patient needs to be carefully monitored, and blood levels of the drug should be monitored in patients receiving continuous infusions and those with cardiac or renal failure. Procainamide may be proarrhythmic in the setting of AMI, hypokalemia, or hypomagnesemia. It should be used cautiously with other drugs that prolong the QT interval (e.g., amiodarone, sotalol).

15.5e Magnesium Sulfate

Magnesium plays a role in several important enzymatic reactions, such as the sodium–potassium ATPase pump, and it is a physiologic calcium-channel blocker. Low magnesium increases the incidence of cardiac arrhythmias and sudden cardiac death.

Indications

Magnesium is recommended for use in cardiac arrest only if torsades de pointes with a pulse or hypomagnesemia is present. Prophylactic administration in hospitalized patients with AMI is not recommended.

Dosage

In cardiac arrest (for hypomagnesemia or torsades de pointes), the dose is 1–2 g of magnesium sulfate (2–4 ml) of 50% solution, diluted in 10 ml of 5% dextrose solution given IV/IO push, typically over 5 to 20 minutes. In non–cardiac arrest, torsades de pointes is treated with a loading dose of 1–2 g mixed in 50–100 ml for D_5W over 5 to 60 minutes IV. This is followed by 0.5–1.0 g/hr IV.

Precautions

When magnesium is given too fast to a patient who has a pulse, hypotension and even asystole can occur. Caution should be used if renal failure is present.

15.5f Ibutilide (Corvert®)

Ibutilide (Corvert®) prolongs the action potential duration and increases the refractory period of cardiac tissue.

Indications

Ibutilide is used for acute pharmacologic conversion of atrial fibrillation or flutter in patients with normal cardiac function and arrhythmia duration $\leq$ 48 hours (Class IIb). It is also used to control rate when calcium-channel blockers or β-blockers are ineffective.

Dosage

For adults weighing ≥ 60 kg, ibutilide is administered intravenously 1 mg over 10 minutes. If needed, a second dose can be given at the same rate 10 minutes after the first.

Precautions

Ibutilide minimally affects blood pressure and heart rate, but can cause ventricular arrhythmias. It must be monitored for at least 4 to 6 hours after administration with baseline electrolyte check before use. It is contraindicated in QT prolongation.

15.6 CALCIUM-CHANNEL BLOCKERS

Calcium-channel blockers are drugs that inhibit the slow-channel activity of the cardiac and vascular smooth muscle. The slow channels, as you may recall, allow for the influx of calcium and sodium ions. This results in several effects that can be clinically useful, and as you will see, the effects of the following two calcium-channel blockers are somewhat different from each other. Diltiazem has fewer hemodynamic effects than verapamil, but both dilate coronary arteries and slow conduction through the AV node, which makes them useful in terminating supraventricular tachycardias that are due to reentry pathways at the AV node. They also slow the ventricular response rate in atrial fibrillation.

15.6a Verapamil (Calan®, Isoptin®)

Verapamil has potent negative chronotropic and negative inotropic effects. It is highly effective for the treatment and prevention of supraventricular tachycardias. Slowing the flux of calcium and sodium ions by way of the slow channels decreases the rate and force of contraction. This results in reduced myocardial oxygen consumption and less ischemia. The drug's negative inotropic effect tends to reduce the patient's stroke volume and cardiac output, but it is counterbalanced by a concurrent reduction in systemic vascular resistance secondary to vasodilation.

Indications

Verapamil is an alternative drug (after adenosine) to terminate paroxysmal supraventricular tachycardia with narrow QRS complex and adequate blood pressure and preserved left ventricular function. It may control ventricular response in patients with atrial fibrillation and atrial flutter or multifocal atrial tachycardia.

Dosage

The does for verapamil is 2.5 to 5.0 mg IV bolus, given over 1 to 2 minutes. The peak effect is achieved within 15 minutes of the bolus injection. If this dose is not adequate, repeat doses of 5 to 10 mg can be given every 15 to 30 minutes to a total dose of 20 mg. Alternatively a 5-mg bolus can be given every 15 minutes until the desired response is achieved or a total dose of 30 mg.

Precautions

A transient decrease in blood pressure due to vasodilation may occur. Verapamil should be avoided or used with great caution in patients with severe left ventricular dysfunction, or tachycardia that is due to Wolff-Parkinson-White syndrome, as the heart rate may actually speed up and cause ventricular fibrillation. Verapamil is not effective for most types of wide-QRS ventricular tachycardia, and it may induce severe hypotension and ventricular fibrillation. Avoid using it in patients with sick sinus syndrome or second- or third-degree AV block without a pacemaker.

15.6b Diltiazem (Cardizem®)

Diltiazem has potent negative chronotropic effects, with only mild negative inotropic action. It produces less myocardial depression than verapamil, particularly in patients with left ventricular dysfunction.

Indications

Diltiazem is used to control the ventricular response rate in patients with atrial fibrillation and atrial flutter. It may terminate reentrant arrhythmias that require AV nodal conduction for their continuation.

Dosage

The initial bolus dose is 0.25 mg/kg (about 20 mg for the average-sized patient), followed by a second dose of 0.35 mg/kg, which can be followed with an IV infusion that is titrated to achieve the desired rate.

Precautions

Although it is less likely to occur with diltiazem than with verapamil, hypotension can still occur. The use of IV β-blockers with IV calcium-channel blockers (verapamil or diltiazem) is relatively contraindicated, because their hemodynamic effects may be synergistic. Even if the β-blockers are given orally, calcium-channel blockers should be used only with great caution. Circumstances when diltiazem should not be used are the same as for verapamil.

15.6c Adenosine (Adenocard®)

Adenosine is an endogenous purine nucleoside that slows conduction through the AV node and interrupts reentry pathways at the AV node. It can convert PSVT (including that associated with Wolff-Parkinson-White syndrome) to a normal sinus rhythm. Adenosine will not terminate atrial fibrillation, atrial flutter, or ventricular tachycardia, because they are caused by the rapid firing of atrial ectopic foci rather than a reentry mechanism. There are also some atrial tachycardias that are not due to reentry, so adenosine will not convert them but may produce a transient AV block. However adenosine is still indicated, because the response to adenosine may help to clarify the diagnosis. Adenosine has a very short duration of action, owing to rapid uptake by the red blood cells. It has a half-life of only 10 seconds.

Indications

Adenosine is the first drug used for treating narrow-complex paroxysmal supraventricular tachycardia.

Dosage

The initial dose is usually a 6 mg bolus given rapidly over 1 to 3 seconds. It is common for a long pause to occur (up to 15 seconds) in the heart rhythm after administration of adenosine. Be careful—this can be very scary and your own heart may want to skip a beat, too! A second dose of 12 mg can be given if there has been no response within 1 to 2 minutes after the first dose.

Precautions

Patients should be placed in mild reverse Trendelenburg position before administration of the drug. Side effects of adenosine are quite common, but they usually last only 1 or 2 minutes. They include flushing, dyspnea, and chest pain. Sinus bradycardia and ventricular ectopy are also common. Also, it should be noted that therapeutic levels of methylxanthines block the action of adenosine by blocking its receptors. Adenosine has a precise injection technique that must be followed for appropriate administration.

15.6d β-Adrenergic Blockers

When a patient has an acute myocardial infarction, his or her body responds to the stress by releasing a lot of endogenous catecholamines. You should recall that this increases the patient's heart rate and force of contraction, which increases blood pressure and increases the heart's demand for oxygen. The result can be more ischemia and injury to the heart muscle. The β-blockers inhibit the action of circulating catecholamines by blocking the adrenergic receptor sites. This results in decreased heart rate and decreased contractility, decreased blood pressure, and reduced myocardial oxygen consumption. It may also prevent recurrent episodes of ventricular tachycardia and fibrillation when these arrhythmias are caused by myocardial ischemia. In emergency situations, rapid action is critical, so once again using the IV preparations of these drugs is indicated. This includes atenolol (Tenormin®), metoprolol (Lopressor®), propranolol (Inderal®), esmolol (Brevibloc®), and labetalol (Normodyne®).

The effects of these agents vary slightly depending on their degree of β_1- and β_2-specificity. Propranolol is nonspecific; it blocks both β_1- and β_2-receptors, which results in decreased heart rate, decreased force of contraction, and bronchoconstriction. Metoprolol, atenolol, and esmolol are β_1-specific at low doses but may still cause bronchoconstriction when used at higher doses.

Propanolol and metoprolol sustain their effects for 6 to 8 hours following IV administration. Esmolol is β_1-selective and has a short duration (15 to 20 minutes), which may make it safer.

Indications

Because β-blockers are effective antianginal agents and can reduce the incidence of ventricular fibrillation, they are administered to almost all patients with suspected myocardial infarction and unstable angina in the absence of complications. β-Blockers are useful as adjunctive agents with fibrinolytic therapy and may reduce nonfatal reinfarction and recurrent ischemia. β-Blockers can be used to convert to normal sinus rhythm or to slow ventricular response, or both, in supraventricular tachyarrhythmias.

Dosage

Each of the drugs mentioned in this category has its own specific initial IV dose, interval for repeat dose, and IV drip rate. There are many good references for these specifics, including the ACLS manual.

Precautions

It is important to note that any of these agents can precipitate hypotension, heart failure, and/or bronchoconstriction. Administering β-blockers is particularly hazardous when cardiac function is already depressed. The β-blockers are contraindicated or should be used with caution in patients with cocaine-induced acute coronary syndrome, second-degree or third-degree heart block, hypotension, severe congestive heart failure, HR < 60 beats/min, or lung disease associated with bronchospasm. When it does occur, HF can be managed with diuretics and vasodilators, and of course bronchospasm requires treatment with bronchodilators. As was mentioned before, adverse effects increase when β-blockers are combined with calcium-channel blockers, antihypertensive agents, and antiarrhythmic agents.

Learning Hint

Remember from the Learning Hint in Chapter 5: You have one heart and two lungs, corresponding to β_1 effects in the heart and β_2 effects in the lungs. A nonselective β-blocking agent may also block the β_2-receptors in the lungs, causing bronchoconstriction in susceptible individuals.

15.6e Sotalol (Betapace®)

Like amiodarone, sotalol prolongs action potential duration and increases cardiac tissue refractoriness. It also acts as a nonselective β-blocker.

Indications

Sotalol is used to control rhythm in atrial fibrillation or atrial flutter with preexcitation (Wolff-Parkinson-White syndrome) in patients with preserved left ventricular function when the duration of the arrhythmia is ≤ 48 hours.

Dosage

Oral sotalol is given at an initial dose of 80 mg twice daily and may be increased every three days by 80 mg per day to a maximum dosage of 320 mg per day if necessary.

Precautions

Side effects may include bradycardia, hypotension, and arrhythmia.

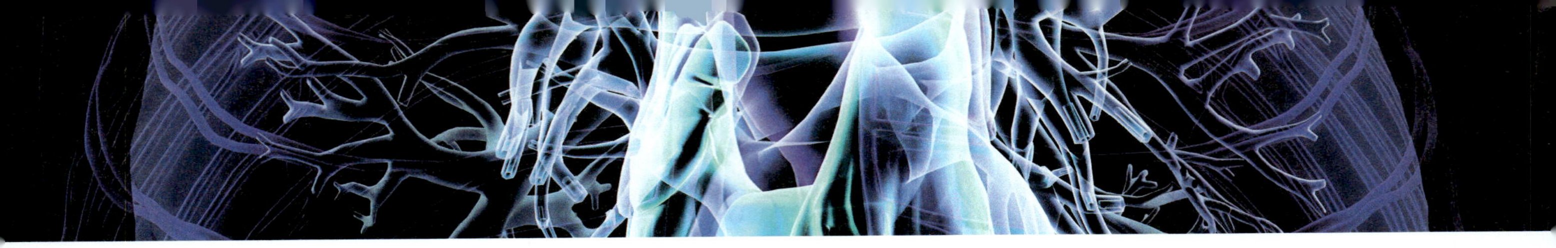

REVIEW QUESTIONS

1. Which of the following is indicated for any patient who is in cardiac arrest?
   (a) atropine
   (b) dopamine
   (c) amrinone
   (d) epinephrine

2. A patient is experiencing chest pain that radiates down his left arm. Which of the following would you do first?
   (a) Administer oxygen by nasal cannula.
   (b) Give a bolus of lidocaine.
   (c) Start an infusion of lidocaine.
   (d) Defibrillate.

3. In which of the following heart rhythms is the patient most likely to have a pulse?
   (a) ventricular fibrillation
   (b) ventricular tachycardia
   (c) atrial fibrillation
   (d) asystole

4. Which of the following are precautions associated with amiodarone?
   (a) hypotension and bradycardia
   (b) nausea and vomiting
   (c) vasoconstriction
   (d) AV node block

5. Magnesium sulfate is best used to treat
   (a) torsades de pointes VT
   (b) atrial tachycardia
   (c) ventricular fibrillation
   (d) non-torsades pulseless arrest

6. What percentage of oxygen should be administered to a victim in cardiac arrest?
   (a) 16% to 17%
   (b) 21%
   (c) 5% to 30%
   (d) 100%

7. Which of the following is indicated for a patient in ventricular tachycardia who is seriously hypotensive and having chest pain?
   (a) sodium bicarbonate
   (b) amiodarone
   (c) epinephrine
   (d) defibrillation

8. Describe how medications can be given to a cardiac arrest victim when no IV can be established.
9. List three antiarrhythmic drugs that can be used to treat a patient in ventricular tachycardia.
10. Explain why it may be hazardous to administer epinephrine to a bradycardic patient who is having an acute myocardial infarction. What drug would you suggest?

CASE STUDY 1

A 67-year-old woman

A 67-year-old woman is brought to the emergency department by her husband. She is complaining of chest pain that radiates to her left arm and jaw, and she is short of breath. She is being placed on a heart monitor and a nurse is getting set up to start her on IV. What else needs to be done immediately?

Ten minutes later the patient becomes bradycardic. Her heart rate is 35 and her blood pressure is 40/0. What drug should be administered? What dose?

An hour later, her heart rate is 78 and her blood pressure is 120/80, but she is exhibiting frequent premature ventricular contractions. What would you recommend now?

Glossary

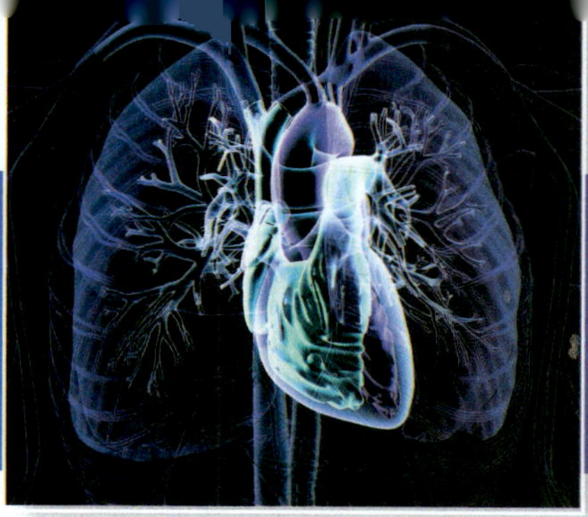

absorptive atelectasis a hazard of breathing high concentrations of oxygen, which can wash out the inert nitrogen in the lungs and lead to collapse of lung tissue when the oxygen is absorbed into the bloodstream.

acetylcholine (ACh) the chemical neurotransmitter of skeletal muscles, the preganglionic sites of both the parasympathetic and the sympathetic nervous system, and the postganglionic sites of the parasympathetic nervous system.

acetylcholinesterase (AChE) also known as cholinesterase; the enzyme that deactivates acetylcholine.

action potential change in membrane voltage when the membrane is excited.

acute myocardial infarction (AMI) new or recent onset of a cardiac event that leads to the death of myocardial tissue; this process is irreversible.

additive describing two drugs whose sum effect when given together is equal to the effect from each given separately but at the same time.

adrenergic agents that stimulate the sympathetic nervous system.

adrenergic receptors receptors of the sympathetic nervous system that include alpha- and beta-receptors.

adverse drug reaction (ADR) a harmful or unpleasant reaction resulting from the use of a drug.

aerobic refers to bacteria that need oxygen to survive.

aerosol suspension of liquid or solid particles in a gas.

aerosol therapy delivery of aerosol particles into the respiratory system for therapeutic purposes.

afferent nerves nerves that carry impulses to the brain and spinal cord. Also known as sensory nerves.

afterload force against which the heart must pump, including tension that develops in the ventricular wall during systole.

agonist drug that activates its receptor upon binding.

aliquot equally divided portions of a total amount of solution.

alpha-receptors receptors found in the sympathetic nervous system that generally cause vasoconstriction.

anaerobic refers to bacteria that do not need oxygen to survive.

analeptic a drug that stimulates the central nervous system.

analgesic an agent that relieves pain.

anemic hypoxia hypoxia due to low levels of hemoglobin or dysfunctional hemoglobin.

angina a severe pain, often described as a heavy pressure, caused by reduced blood supply to the heart.

antagonist drug that binds to its receptor without activating it.

antiadrenergic agents that block the effects of the sympathetic nervous system.

antibiogram hospital compilation of microbial culture results from the laboratory.

antibiotic substance that destroys or inhibits the growth of other microorganisms.

anticholinergic agents that block the effects of the parasympathetic nervous system.

anticoagulant drug used to prevent formation of fibrin clot.

antigen foreign material that stimulates the immune and inflammatory response.

antiplatelet drug used to inhibit the release and aggregation of platelets.

anxiolytic a drug that reduces anxiety.

arrhythmia technically an absence of rhythm, but the term is also used to refer to an abnormal rhythm or any deviation from the normal electrocardiogram tracing.

asthma inflammatory process characterized by reversible airway narrowing and airway hyperreactivity.

asthma COPD overlap syndrome the coexistence of increased variability of airflow in a patient with incompletely reversible airway obstruction.

asthma paradox the phenomenon of increasing incidence of, and mortality from, asthma in recent years despite a better understanding of the pathophysiology and improved drugs for treatment of asthma. The reasons for the asthma paradox are still open to debate.

asystole without rhythm.

automaticity characteristic of cardiac cells that allows them to spontaneously depolarize without innervation from the central nervous system.

autonomic nervous system (ANS) the nervous system that controls the involuntary responses; divided into the parasympathetic and sympathetic branches.

bactericidal refers to drugs that kill bacteria.

bacteriostatic inhibiting of bacterial growth.

baroreceptor homeostatic mechanism the body uses to maintain blood pressure.

base the number being multiplied in an exponential expression.

beta-agonist (β-agonist) a drug that combines with a β-receptor and stimulates the activity of that receptor.

beta-receptors (β-receptors) receptors found in the sympathetic nervous system that are divided into $beta_1$ and $beta_2$ subcategories. $Beta_1$-receptors are found primarily in the heart; when stimulated, they cause an increase in rate and force of contraction. $Beta_2$-receptors are found primarily in the lungs; when stimulated, they cause bronchodilation.

bioavailability fraction of drug dose that reaches the systemic circulation.

bland aerosol therapy nonmedicated aerosol therapy.

bolus a large dose of medication that is usually pushed manually into an IV for rapid effect.

breath-actuated nebulizer (BAN) a newer type of nebulizer device that creates aerosol only when a patient is inhaling.

broad-spectrum antibiotic classification system based on bacteria types against which the drug is effective.

bronchial gland mucus-producing exocrine glands found in the submucosa. They are stimulated by parasympathetic nerves and secrete a relatively watery fluid.

bronchial hyperresponsiveness (BHR) a state characterized by easily triggered bronchospasm.

bronchiolitis inflammatory condition of the small airways, usually associated with respiratory infection.

bronchitis inflammatory condition of the large airways, usually associated with respiratory infection.

bronchoconstriction narrowing of the bronchioles due to swelling, mucus obstruction, or spasm of the smooth muscle of the airway.

bronchorrhea excessive discharge of respiratory tract secretions.

bronchospasm narrowing of the bronchioles due to contraction of the smooth muscle surrounding the airways.

cancelling units method of changing starting units to desired units.

cardiac arrest absence of pulse.

central nervous system (CNS) the nervous system comprised of the brain and spinal cord.

chemical mediators initiators of the inflammatory process that are released in response to a stimulus.

chemotherapy prevention or treatment of disease by administration of chemical substances.

chlorofluorocarbons (CFCs) older propellant for metered dose inhalants; because they damage the ozone layer and are reactive in some patients, they are currently banned.

cholinergic referring to the parasympathetic nervous system, where acetylcholine is the neurotransmitter substance at all ganglionic sites.

chronic bronchitis respiratory condition characterized by productive cough, mucous gland enlargement, and hypertrophy of airway smooth muscle.

chronic obstructive pulmonary disease (COPD) global term used to describe abnormal pulmonary conditions associated with cough, sputum production, dyspnea, airflow obstruction, and impaired gas exchange.

chronotropic affecting the time or rate of cardiac contractions.

community-acquired pneumonia (CAP) infection of lung tissue that is contracted outside the institutional setting.

compliance flexibility of the blood vessels responding to pressure.

conduction transmission of electrical impulses through fibers in the heart, causing heart muscle contraction.

corticosteroid any steroid hormone produced by the adrenal cortex.

cross-allergenicity drug allergy reaction with one antibiotic class that crosses over and presents with another antibiotic class as well.

croup infection of the respiratory tract that can cause airway obstruction; usually affects young children.

culture laboratory testing process that involves growing microorganisms to determine which drugs might fight the infection.

cyanosis bluish discoloration of the skin.

cyclic adenine monophosphate (cAMP) enzyme produced when β_2-receptors are stimulated; it affects the activities of a variety of cells, including the relaxation of bronchial muscle.

cyclic guanosine monophosphate (cGMP) enzyme that has the opposite effect of cAMP; it causes bronchoconstriction.

defibrillate to apply direct countershock to the heart in order to depolarize the myocardial cells simultaneously.

demand hypoxia hypoxia as a result of a hypermetabolic state.

dependence drug use that may result in withdrawal symptoms upon discontinuation; symptoms can be psychologic or physiologic.

depolarizing agent an agent that causes skeletal muscle paralysis by persistent depolarization of the neuromuscular endplate.

deposition aerosol particles falling out or "raining out" of suspension.

desensitization loss of tissue responsiveness that can occur with drug exposure.

disease management all-inclusive management of a patient's disease that includes pharmacotherapy.

dopamine receptors adrenergic receptors found in renal tissue that, when stimulated, relax the renal arteries and therefore increase renal perfusion.

downregulation the long-term process of decreasing the sensitivity of β-receptors to β-agonists because of a reduction in the number of receptors.

dromotropic a drug that alters the rhythm or electrical conduction of the heart.

dry-powder inhaler (DPI) medicated aerosol delivery device that delivers a powdered (solid) aerosol to the respiratory system.

dyspnea labored or difficult breathing.

efferent nerves nerves that carry impulses away from the brain and spinal cord. Also known as motor nerves.

efficacy the capacity for a therapeutic effect of a given intervention.

emetics agents that induce vomiting.

emphysema respiratory condition characterized by permanent, abnormal enlargement of airway spaces and destruction of alveolar walls.

empiric therapy antimicrobial therapy begun before a specific pathogen has been identified with laboratory tests.

endogenous surfactant complex mixture of phospholipids and proteins produced in the lung by the type II pneumocytes. It plays a crucial role in reducing alveolar surface tension and preventing alveolar collapse.

English system of measurement the common system of measurement using miles, feet, ounces, pounds, etc.

enteral route the route comprising oral, sublingual, nasogastric, or rectal routes of drug absorption.

epiglottitis infection usually caused by *Haemophilus influenzae* type B that causes airway obstruction in children.

epinephrine also called adrenaline; a hormone produced by the adrenal medulla. It acts as the circulating neurotransmitter for the sympathetic nervous system, stimulating both α- and β-receptors; it is also a potent catecholamine administered for its effects on the sympathetic nervous system.

essential hypertension high blood pressure with no identifiable cause.

exercise-induced bronchospasm (EIB) bronchospasm triggered by vigorous physical activity.

exogenous surfactant surfactant drugs that are produced outside of the patient's own body. They may be obtained from humans or animals or synthesized in the laboratory.

expectorant substance that improves expectoration of respiratory secretions by increasing the output from the bronchial glands.

exponent the number of times the base is multiplied in an exponential expression.

factor-label method or fraction method method for changing units or converting between the English and metric systems.

fibrinolytic drug used to dissolve the fibrin of an existing clot.

first-pass effect elimination of drug that happens after administration but before it reaches the systemic circulation.

flora normally harmless microbial organisms in the body.

forced expiratory volume in 1 second (FEV_1) pulmonary function test that measures the volume of air forcefully exhaled in one second.

formulary list of drugs stocked by the pharmacy.

free radicals charged particles or oxidants that are formed with excess oxygen; they can disrupt tissue function.

ganglion nerve cell body outside of the brain and spinal cord.

general anesthesia state of deep sleep with no response to stimulation.

glucocorticoid one of two main groups of corticosteroids needed for stress response and utilization of carbohydrates, fat, and protein by the body.

goblet cell found in the mucosal epithelium, these secretory cells produce gelatinous mucus. Topical irritation and exposure to irritants increase their size and number.

gram (g) a basic unit of mass in the metric system.

Gram stain method of staining bacterial cells, used to identify the type.

half-life ($T_{1/2}$) time it takes for the drug concentration to fall to 50% in the body.

heated humidified high-flow therapy (HHHF) a type of respiratory therapy that delivers a high flow of heated, humidified gas to a patient through an interface intended to provide total ventilatory support.

heliox mixture of oxygen and helium gas.

hemoglobin molecule that transports oxygen by binding with it in a reversible manner.

high-flow oxygen systems oxygen delivery devices that provide the patient's total ventilatory requirement.

high-flow therapy (HFT) a type of respiratory therapy that delivers a high flow of medical gas to a patient through an interface intended to provide total ventilatory support.

histamine vasodilator that mediates inflammation and allergic reactions.

histotoxic hypoxia hypoxia as a result of the tissue's inability to utilize oxygen for metabolism.

hydrofluoroalkanes (HFAs) replacing chlorofluorocarbons (CFCs) as metered-dose inhalant (MDI) propellants, because HFAs do not damage the ozone layer and are not as reactive in patients.

hydrophilic molecule or substance that is attracted to water.

hypertension high blood pressure.

hypertonic a solution containing a greater concentration of salt than is normally found in the body.

hypnotic a drug that induces sleep.

hypotonic a solution containing a lower concentration of salt than is normally found in the body.

hypoxemia an abnormally low concentration of oxygen in the blood.

hypoxemic hypoxia hypoxia caused by impairment of oxygen delivery to the alveoli.

hypoxia low levels of oxygen at the tissues.

hypoxic drive the ventilatory drive when it is stimulated by the peripheral chemoreceptors' response to low levels of oxygen in the blood.

inertial impaction the impacting of aerosol particles on airway walls because of inertial energy.

infusion medication or fluid that is given gradually and continuously into an IV by an infusion pump, often used to maintain the effect achieved by bolus administration of the drug.

inhaled nitric oxide (INO) colorless, odorless gas that is inhaled to treat pulmonary hypertension due to its selective pulmonary vasodilation.

inotropic affecting the force or energy of cardiac contraction.

ischemia a decrease in perfusion to an organ or body part that may result in pain and organ dysfunction.

isotonic a solution containing the same concentration of salt as that found in the body.

jet mixing mask (air entrainment mask) a high-flow oxygen mask that utilizes the Bernoulli principle to mix oxygen and room air to deliver a precise fraction of inspired oxygen (FIO_2).

large-volume nebulizers nebulizers that can deliver oxygen and aerosol particles.

leukotriene group of biologically active compounds that regulate allergic and inflammatory reactions.

liter (l) a basic unit of liquid measure in the metric system.

loading dose starting dose that is administered to achieve a therapeutic concentration rapidly.

local anesthesia condition that results when sensory transmission from a local area of the body to the central nervous system is blocked.

long-term control type of asthma medication used to achieve and maintain control of persistent asthma.

low-flow oxygen systems oxygen delivery devices that provide only a portion of the patient's ventilatory requirement.

maintenance dose dose given to keep a drug at a therapeutic level in the blood.

maintenance therapy medications that provide long-term control of symptoms, such as shortness of breath and wheezing; usually taken daily.

malignant hyperthermia increase in temperature to 42°C or higher; this can be a lethal complication of anesthetics.

medicated aerosol medicine that has been made into an aerosol to be delivered into the respiratory system.

meter (m) a basic unit of length in the metric system.

metered-dose inhaler (MDI) a medicated aerosol delivery device that delivers measured doses (metered puffs) of aerosol from a small gas propellant-powered canister.

metric system of measurement a system of measurement based on powers of 10.

micron one-millionth of a meter; the order of magnitude of how small therapeutic aerosol particles are.

mineralocorticoid one of two main groups of corticosteroids necessary for regulation of salt and water balance.

muscarinic receptors receptors found at the postganglionic site of the parasympathetic nervous system.

narrow-spectrum antibiotic classification system based on bacteria types against which the drug is effective.

nasal cannula a common low-flow oxygen device inserted into the nostrils.

nicotinic receptors receptors found at the skeletal muscles in the somatic system and at all preganglionic sites in the parasympathetic and sympathetic nervous systems.

nondepolarizing agent an agent that causes skeletal muscle paralysis by blockade of the nicotinic endplate.

nonrebreathing mask an oxygen mask with a reservoir and valves to increase the amount of delivered oxygen or fraction of inspired oxygen (FIO_2).

norepinephrine (NE) the chemical neurotransmitter substance found at the postganglionic junction of the sympathetic nervous system.

opioid a class of drugs that mimic actions of opiates, which are drugs derived from opium.

otitis media middle ear inflammation that is common in children.

oxygen therapy the delivery of oxygen for therapeutic value.

oxygen toxicity serious condition that can occur if excess oxygen is delivered.

parasympathetic branch of the peripheral nervous system that maintains normal body functions and homeostasis.

parasympatholytic agent that blocks or antagonizes the effects of the parasympathetic system.

parasympathomimetic agent that stimulates the parasympathetic system.

parenteral route drug administration routes that bypass the alimentary tract; injectable routes.

pathogen disease-producing microorganism.

peak expiratory flow rate (PEFR) measurement of maximum flow rate generated during a forced exhalation. Used to indicate the degree of airflow obstruction.

penetration how deep the aerosol particles travel into the respiratory system.

percentage of solution strength of solution as parts of solute per 100 ml of solution.

peripheral chemoreceptors receptors in the carotid and aortic bodies that respond to low levels of oxygen.

peripheral nervous system (PNS) part of the nervous system comprised of all nerves outside the brain and spinal cord; includes the somatic and autonomic nervous systems.

pharmacodynamics actions of a drug on the body.

pharmacogenomics science that examines how genes affect the action of drugs within the body.

pharmacokinetics actions of the body on a drug.

pharmacology study of drugs and their action on the body.

pharmacotherapy application of drug therapy to disease treatment.

pharyngitis inflammation of the pharynx and surrounding tissue; may be bacterial or viral.

pneumonia inflammation of lung tissue in the alveoli and interstitial tissue.

polycythemia higher-than-normal levels of hemoglobin.

potentiation the effect of two drugs given together when one drug has no effect but increases the response of the other drug, which normally has a lesser effect.

preload filling pressure of the heart during diastole.

premature ventricular contraction (PVC) potentially serious abnormal heartbeats that originate in the ventricles.

proarrhythmia arrhythmia induced by antiarrhythmic drugs.

proportion a statement that compares two ratios.

prostaglandin (PG) one of many hormone-like substances present throughout the body.

protein binding refers to sites such as albumin where the drug is connected or bound and inactive; influences drug distribution.

quick-relief medications type of asthma medications used to provide rapid relief in treating asthma symptoms and exacerbations.

racemic refers to drugs that contain two chemical components that may have different activities.

ratio solution a method of expressing the strength of solution as a ratio that represents parts of solute related to parts of solution.

receptor target for drugs to act on.

refractory period period of time before a new action potential can be initiated.

rescue therapy rapid-acting medications used to provide prompt relief of symptoms such as shortness of breath and wheezing in asthma.

resistance degree to which a disease-causing organism remains unaffected by antibiotics.

respiration process of gas exchange of oxygen and carbon dioxide.

reuptake process wherein norepinephrine is deactivated at the sympathetic postganglionic sites.

rhinorrhea excessive secretion from the nose.

scientific notation a means of representing very large or very small numbers.

sedative a drug that produces sedation.

selectivity extent to which a drug acts on one specific site or receptor.

simple mask a low-flow oxygen mask.

sinusitis inflammation of the mucosal lining of the paranasal sinuses.

small-volume nebulizer (SVN) a medicated aerosol delivery device that uses a pneumatic-powered source to form and deliver the aerosol continuously over a period of usually 8–12 minutes.

solute a liquid or solid that is dissolved in a liquid to form a solution.

solution a physically homogeneous mixture of two or more substances.

solvent the liquid that dissolves the solute.

somatic nervous system the part of the nervous system that controls skeletal muscles and therefore voluntary movement.

spacer reservoir device used with aerosol delivery devices such as MDIs to optimize aerosol drug delivery.

stability tendency of an aerosol to remain in suspension.

stagnant hypoxia hypoxia due to an impairment in the circulatory system's ability to transport oxygen.

steady state state reached when input of the drug is equal to output of the drug over the dosing interval.

stomatitis inflammation of the mucous lining in the mouth.

stroke a sudden loss of neurologic function due to a vascular injury or blockage to blood flow within the brain.

sublingual refers to drug absorption under the tongue.

surface tension force of contraction at the surface of a liquid that pulls the molecules at the surface inward and down.

surfactant complex mixture of phospholipids and proteins produced in the lung by the type II pneumocytes. It plays a crucial role in reducing alveolar surface tension and preventing alveolar collapse.

susceptibility test a laboratory microbiology test that establishes the drug sensitivity of a bacterium.

sympathetic the branch of the peripheral nervous system that prepares the body for stress and emergencies (also called the "fight-or-flight" system).

sympatholytic agent that blocks or antagonizes the effects of the sympathetic system.

sympathomimetic agent that stimulates the sympathetic system.

synergism the result when two drugs are given together and their effect is greater than the sum of the effects from each given separately.

teratogenic having an effect on prenatal development that results in abnormal structure or function.

therapeutic range range of drug concentration in the body in which the drug produces the desired response.

therapeutics study of drugs used to cure, treat, or prevent disease.

thromboembolism (TE) a traveling thrombus that leads to obstruction and blood flow occlusion.

tolerance decrease in susceptibility to a drug's effect from continued use.

toxicology study of drugs as they relate to poisonings and environmental toxins.

train-of-four (TOF) a type of monitoring used to determine the depth of muscle paralysis during neuromuscular blockade drug administration. It involves the application of four electrical stimuli, each separated by 1/12 of a second, to a nerve that innervates a muscle while observing the muscle twitch during the stimuli.

transdermal delivered through the skin.

tuberculosis (TB) chronic disease caused by *Mycobacterium tuberculosis*.

ultrasonic nebulizer (USN) aerosol delivery device that provides increased speed and capacity while minimizing noise.

volume/volume (v/v) solution a solution represented by the volume of the liquid solute in the volume of solution.

vasodilator a drug that selectively dilates blood vessels.

ventilation the movement of gas into and out of the respiratory system.

ventilatory drive the strength of the stimulus to breathe, controlled by the CNS; influences the rate and depth of breathing.

ventilatory stimulant a drug that acts on the respiratory center in the medulla to increase the rate and depth of ventilation.

viscoelastic having the ability to change from thick to thin and back.

weight/volume (w/v) solution a solution in which the solute being dissolved is a solid.

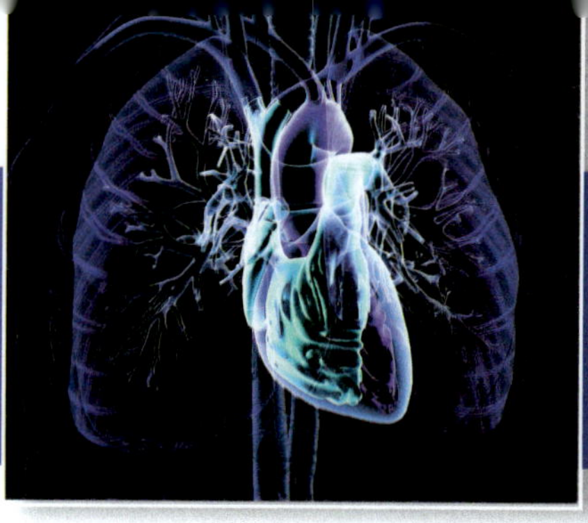

Index

A

D

E

F

G

H

I

Q

R